# ABC OF
# NUTRITION

## Fourth Edition

WITHDRAWN

2 1 JUN 2018

Dublin Dental University
Hospital Library

RES

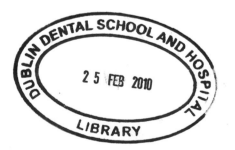

Acc No: B2010009

Class No: 612.3 TRU

Price/Inv. ...........................

Dublin Dental School
& Hospital
Library & Information
Service
Ph: 6127205  Fax: 6127251

DUBLIN DENTAL SCHOOL AND HOSPITAL
2 5 FEB 2010
LIBRARY

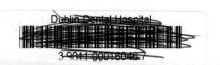

Dublin Dental Hospital

3 9011 000180457

WITHDRAWN

2 1 JUN 2018

Dublin Dental University
Hospital Library

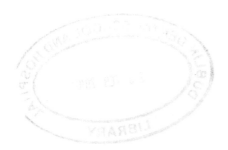

# ABC OF NUTRITION

## Fourth Edition

**A STEWART TRUSWELL**

*Emeritus Professor of Human Nutrition,*
*University of Sydney, Australia*

*with contributions from*
PATRICK G WALL
CIARA E O'REILLY
*the late* CHRISTOPHER R PENNINGTON
NIGEL REYNOLDS

© BMJ Publishing Group 1986, 1992, 1999, 2003

All rights reserved. No part of this publication may be reproduced, stored in a retrieval
system, or transmitted, in any form or by any means, electronic, mechanical, photocopying,
recording and/or otherwise, without the prior written permission of the publishers.

First published in 1986
by BMJ Books, BMA House, Tavistock Square,
London WC1H 9JR
www.bmjbooks.com

First edition 1986
Second edition 1992
Third edition 1999
Fourth edition 2003

4  2008

**British Library Cataloguing in Publication Data**
A catalogue record for this book is available from the British Library

ISBN 978 0 7279 1664 8

Typeset by Newgen Imaging Systems (P) Ltd., Chennai, India
Printed and bound in Singapore by Fabulous Printers Pte Ltd

Cover shows halved apple, with permission
from Gusto productions/Science Photo Library

# Contents

# Contributors

**Ciara E O'Reilly PhD**
Technical Executive, Food Safety Authority of Ireland, Dublin, Ireland

**Christopher R Pennington MD, FRCPEd**
Late Professor of Gastroenterology,
Ninewells Hospital and Medical School, Dundee, Scotland

**Nigel Reynolds MB, ChB, MRCP**
Medicine and Cardiovascular Group, Department of
Digestive Diseases and Clinical Nutrition, Ninewells Hospital
and Medical School, Dundee, Scotland

**A Stewart Truswell AO, MD, DSc, FRCP, FRACP**
Emeritus Professor of Human Nutrition, University of Sydney,
Australia

**Patrick G Wall MB, BCh, BAO, MRCVS, MFPMM**
Chief Executive, Food Safety Authority of Ireland, Dublin,
Ireland

# Preface

**Preface to 3rd edition**

Nutrition is one of those subjects which comes up every day in general practice—or should do—yet in most undergraduate medical schools it is crowded out by the big clinical specialities and high technology procedures. It is for subjects like nutrition that the British Medical Journal's ABC series is extremely useful.

This book was started when Dr Stephen Lock, previous editor of the BMJ asked me to write a series of weekly articles for an imagined general practitioner, in an unfashionable provincial town who had been taught almost no nutrition at medical school. They now felt the need to use nutrition in the practice, but could spare only 15 to 20 minutes a week to read about it.

The brief was that the writing must be practical and relevant; about half the page was to be for tables, figures, photographs or boxes (that is, not text) and these have to tell part of the story. The writing was to "come down off the fence", to make up its mind on the balance of evidence and state it plainly. The first edition had no references but some reviewers asked for them and now in the era of evidence-based medicine some well chosen references seem indispensable when writing about nutrition.

Nutritional concepts, of course, are not as tightly evidence-based as information about drugs because randomised controlled trials, so routine for drug therapy, are rare for nutrition.

This book does not deal with all aspects of human nutrition, only those that are useful in everyday medical practice. The latest fads and controversies are not here either. This is the ABC of Nutrition, not the XYZ.

A Stewart Truswell
1999

**Preface to 4th edition**

When the first edition of this ABC was written in 1985 there was no "evidence-based medicine", no human genome, no BSE or nvCJD, no epidemic of obesity and associated type II diabetes; there were no statins to lower plasma cholesterol and no genetically modified foods. *Helicobacter pylori* had just been discovered. The role of folate in neural tube defects had not been established, or raised plasma homocysteine as a risk factor for heart disease. The Barker hypothesis had not been propounded. These recent discoveries and ideas affect nutritional practice and they appear or influence what is in this new edition.

A Stewart Truswell
2003

# 1   Reducing the risk of coronary heart disease

For some doctors in affluent countries the first question about prevention of coronary heart disease (CHD) nowadays is whether to write a prescription for one of the statins (simvastatin, pravastatin, fluvastatin, atorvastatin, etc) which inhibit an early step of cholesterol biosynthesis in the body (see p 7). Tables are available to show whether the 5- or 10-year risk justifies the cost of long term statin medication, but the relation of diet and CHD is still of primary importance for the majority of people. **What we eat is bound up with the aetiology of CHD**. Many people do not know their current plasma cholesterol, many coronary deaths occur before medical help and most countries cannot afford these expensive drugs.

Coronary heart disease is the largest single cause of death in Britain and the disease that causes most premature deaths, but it is only one-seventh as common in industrial Japan and rare in the masses in most developing countries. Its incidence must be environmentally determined because **immigrant groups** soon take on the incidence rate of their new country and there have been large changes in mortality over time. Coronary heart disease was uncommon everywhere before 1925 and then increased steadily in Western countries until the 1970s, except for a dip during the Second World War. Age-standardised mortality rates from coronary heart disease in the United States of America and Australia **started to decline** from 1966 and have reduced by more than 70%. In Britain rates are higher in Scotland and Ireland than in England, and higher in the north of England than the south. They have been declining since 1979 and have fallen by about 25%. Most EU countries have shown similar recent modest reductions of coronary mortality, but in the countries of eastern Europe coronary mortalities have risen. They have, however, recently fallen in Poland and the Czech Republic.

Coronary heart disease is a **multifactorial disease**, but diet is probably the fundamental environmental factor. The pathological basis is **atherosclerosis**, which takes years to develop. **Thrombosis** superimposed on an atherosclerotic plaque, which takes hours, usually precipitates a clinical event. Then whether the patient dies suddenly, has a classic **myocardial infarct**, develops **angina**, or has asymptomatic electrocardiographic changes depends on the state of the myocardium. Each of these three processes is affected by somewhat different components in the diet.

The characteristic material that accumulates in atherosclerosis is **cholesterol ester**. This and other lipids in the plaque, such as yellow carotenoid pigments, come from the blood where they are carried on low density lipoprotein (LDL). In animals, including primates, atheroma can be produced by raising plasma cholesterol concentrations with high animal fat diets. Much of this cholesterol is present in modified macrophages that have the histological appearance of foam cells. Experimental pathology studies indicate that these cells only take up large amounts of LDL if *it has been oxidised*.[2] This oxidation probably occurs within the artery wall.

People with genetically raised LDL-cholesterol (*familial hypercholesterolaemia*) tend to have premature coronary heart disease. This is accelerated even more in homozygotes who have plasma cholesterols four times normal and all develop clinical coronary heart disease before they are 20.

Thousands of papers have been written on diet and CHD. Since early in the century scientists have suggested links

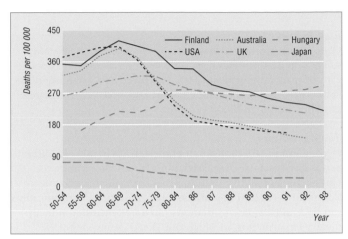

Coronary heart disease death rates in six countries, for men aged 25-74, 1950-83. (Adapted from *Heart and Stroke Facts* published by the National Heart Foundation of Australia, from WHO data.) CHD mortality in USA and Australia started to fall 10 years before any decline in UK coronary deaths and fell more profoundly. Smoking rates and medical treatments cannot explain these phenomena. They may have been due to dietary changes (increased polyunsaturated and decreased saturated fatty acids)[1]

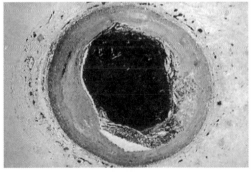

Photomicrograph of coronary artery with atherosclerosis

## Evidence linking diet and CHD

This comes from:
- animal experiments
- pathology studies
- genetic polymorphisms
- epidemiology: ecological and cohort/prospective studies
- randomised controlled trials with dietary changes.

The strongest body of evidence comes from cohort studies which demonstrate environmental factors that are either associated with increased subsequent risk of CHD events (risk factors) or decreased subsequent risk (protective factors).

between a series of dietary components and CHD. Some of these were subsequently found to be unconnected or of little importance, for example sucrose, soft water, milk. The latest component to be associated is in the news, but this does not mean that the older components have been disproved—just that well-established facts are not newsworthy.

## Risk factors

Over 50 prospective (cohort) studies in more than 600 000 subjects in 21 countries have reported on risk factors associated with or protective against CHD. The three best established risk factors are: raised plasma total and LDL-cholesterol, cigarette smoking, and high blood pressure.[3]

### Two step reasoning

High plasma LDL- (and total) cholesterol is firmly established as a major risk factor for CHD, both from cohort study epidemiology and from randomised controlled trials with statins. In turn, how diet affects LDL-cholesterol concentration can be—and has been—demonstrated in controlled human dietary experiments, in which one dietary component is changed in the experimental period, with control periods on either side or in parallel.

## Plasma total and low density lipoprotein cholesterol (LDL-cholesterol)

About three quarters of plasma total cholesterol is normally in LDL-cholesterol and the higher the total cholesterol the higher the percentage of LDL-cholesterol because HDL-cholesterol rarely exceeds 2 mmol/l (and never exceeds 3). The **mean** plasma total cholesterol of healthy adults ranges widely in different communities, from 2.6 mmol/l (Papua New Guinea highlanders) to 7.2 mmol/l (in east Finland some years ago). Only in countries whose average total cholesterol exceeds 5.2 mmol/l (200 mg/dl)—as in Britain—is coronary heart disease common.

## Dietary components that affect plasma LDL-cholesterol: type of fat

The major influence is the type of fat. Fats in the diet are mostly in the form of triglycerides (triacylglycerols): three fatty acids joined to glycerol. The most abundant fatty acid(s) determine(s) the effect. *Saturated fatty acids* raise LDL-cholesterol; these are mostly 12:0 (lauric), 14:0 (myristic), and 16:0 (palmitic). Palmitic may be less potent but is the most abundant of these saturated fatty acids in foods. 18:0 (stearic) has little or no cholesterol-raising effect.

*Monounsaturated fatty acids*—the main one is 18:1 (oleic)—in the natural *cis* configuration have an intermediate effect on LDL-cholesterol: lower than on saturated fatty acids, not as low as on linoleic.

*Polyunsaturated fatty acids* (PUFA), (with two or more double bonds) lower LDL-cholesterol. The most abundant of these in foods is 18:2 (linoleic) which belongs to the ω-6 (omega-6 or n minus 6, n−6) family of polyunsaturated fatty acids (first double bond, numbering from the non-carboxylic acid end is at 6th carbon). The omega-3 (ω-3) series of PUFAs are less abundant in most foods 18:3, ω-3, α-linolenic occurs in plants and some vegetable oils. 20:5, ω-3, eicosapentaenoic acid (EPA) and 22:6, ω-3, docosahexaenoic acid (DHA) are mostly obtained from fatty fish and fish oils. The cholesterol-lowering effect of ω-3 PUFAs is less important than their other properties (p 6).

In unsaturated fatty acids the double bond is normally in the *cis* configuration and the carbon chain bends at the double

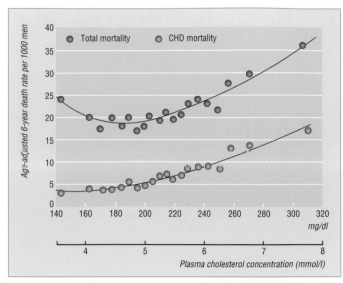

Within-population relation between plasma cholesterol and CHD and total mortality based on 6-year follow up of 350 000 US men. (Adapted from Martin *et al.*[4]) The increased total mortality at (only) the lowest cholesterol concentration is thought to reflect acute and chronic illnesses (which often lower plasma cholesterol)

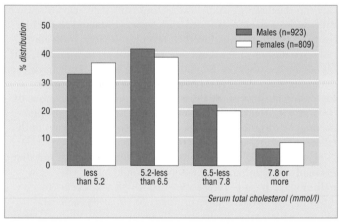

Percentage distribution of serum total cholesterol in British adults by sex (Adapted from Gregory *et al.*[5])

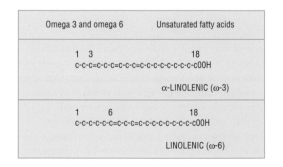

bond. If the configuration is *trans*, straight at the double bond, the fatty acid behaves biologically like a saturated fatty acid. The usual *trans* fatty acid is 18:1 *trans* (elaidic) acid, found in foods produced by hydrogenation in making older-type hard margarines.

*Dietary cholesterol and phytosterols*
Cholesterol is only found in animal foods. Dietary cholesterol has less plasma cholesterol-raising effect than saturated fats. This is because about half the plasma cholesterol comes from the diet and half is biosynthesised in the liver from acetate. When more cholesterol is absorbed it tends to switch off this endogenous synthesis.

Plant oils also contain sterols, but these are **phytosterols**, for example, β-sitosterol, campesterol, brassicasterol. These typically have one or two more extra carbons on the side chain of the cholesterol molecule. They interfere competitively with cholesterol absorption and are poorly absorbed themselves. Phytosterols in vegetable oils (200-500 mg/100 g) add a little to their cholesterol-lowering effect. They are also present in nuts and seeds. Some premium PUFA margarines (introduced 1999) are enriched with concentrated natural phytosterols (or-stanols) to enhance cholesterol lowering.

*Overweight and obesity*
Overweight people tend to have raised plasma triglycerides and to a lesser extent total and LDL-cholesterol. Weight reduction by diet and/or exercise will usually reduce their cholesterol. Overweight, especially abdominal visceral adiposity, is itself a direct risk factor for CHD.

*Dietary fibre*
The effect of dietary fibre depends on the type. Wheat fibre (bran or wholemeal breads) does not lower plasma cholesterol but viscous ("soluble") types, pectin and guar and oat fibre, in large intakes, produce moderate cholesterol reductions. Although wheat fibre does not lower plasma cholesterol cohort studies consistently show less subsequent CHD in people who eat more wheat fibre and whole grain foods.[7]

*Vegetable protein*
Most vegetable foods are low in protein. Soya is an exception. When soya protein replaces animal protein in the diet there has usually been a reduction of plasma total and LDL-cholesterol. Although many human trials have been carried out, the mechanism has been elusive.

*Coffee*[9]
Coffee contains small amounts of diterpenes (lipids), cafestol and kahweol—not caffeine—that raise plasma total and LDL-cholesterol. Several cups a day of boiled, plunger or espresso coffee can raise the cholesterol but filtered or instant coffee does not—the diterpenes have been removed from the beverage.

**Mechanisms for LDL-cholesterol lowering**
Many complex experiments have been done to elucidate how different fatty acids affect LDL-cholesterol. The main mechanism appears to be by effect on the number and activity of the LDL-receptors in cell membranes. Saturated fatty acids downregulate these receptors, so less cholesterol is taken up from the plasma; unsaturated fatty acids have the opposite effect. In overweight people there is increased secretion of very low density lipoprotein (VLDL) from the liver.

**Effect of dietary fatty acids on plasma LDL-cholesterol**

| | |
|---|---|
| • Up to 10:0 (MCTs) | 0 |
| • 12:0 (lauric) | ↑ |
| • 14:0 (myristic) | ↑↑ |
| • 16:0 (palmitic) | ↑ |
| • 18:0 (stearic) | (↑) |
| • 18:1 *cis* (oleic) | (↓) |
| • 18:1 *trans* | ↑↑ |
| • 18:2 6-*cis* (linoleic) | ↓ |
| • Other polyunsaturates | (↓) |

MCTs = medium chain triglycerides

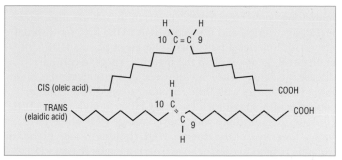

*Cis* unsaturated fatty acids are bent at the double bond(s), *trans* fatty acids are not

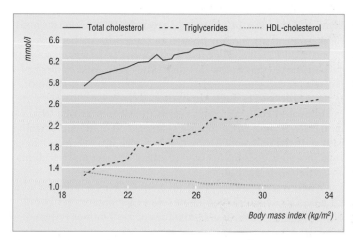

The relation between body mass index (weight/height²) and total cholesterol, HDL-cholesterol and triglycerides (all in mmol/l). (Adapted from Thelle *et al.*[6])

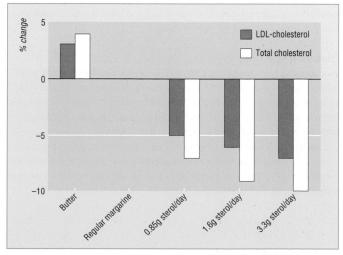

Plasma LDL and total cholesterol change over 3.5 weeks (double-blind, controlled trial) in 100 healthy human subjects who took in turn (randomised) butter, standard PUFA margarine or this enriched with different amounts of phytosterols. 20 g/day of the commercial product provides 1.6 g phytosterols[8]

Large amounts of viscous (soluble) dietary fibre increase viscosity in the lower small intestine and reduce reabsorption of bile acids, so producing negative sterol balance, hence increased cholesterol → bile acids (cholestyramine effect). The mechanism for the potent plasma cholesterol-raising effect of coffee lipids has not yet been worked out (plasma aminotransferase goes up too); no animal model has been found.

## Plasma high density lipoprotein cholesterol (HDL-cholesterol)

HDL-cholesterol is a potent protective factor in communities with high LDL- and total cholesterols.[2] It appears to act by mobilising cholesterol from deposits in peripheral tissues, including arteries, and transporting it to the liver for disposal ("reverse cholesterol transport"). Levels of plasma HDL-cholesterol do not explain the big differences of coronary disease incidence between countries; its concentration is often lower in countries with little coronary heart disease. But in countries with a high incidence of CHD and high plasma-LDL-cholesterol, individuals with above average HDL-cholesterol have a lower risk of the disease. HDL-cholesterols are higher in women (related to oestrogen activity), a major reason why coronary disease usually affects women at older ages than men.

Low HDL-cholesterols are often associated with raised plasma triglycerides and the latter metabolic dysfunction may compound the risk of coronary disease. HDL-cholesterols tend to be lower in overweight people, in those with diabetes, and in those who smoke. They may be reduced by a high carbohydrate (that is, low fat) diet. They are raised by alcohol consumption, by moderate or heavy exercise, by reduction of body weight, and by high fat diets.

Increased HDL concentration is the clearest reason why moderate alcohol consumption is associated epidemiologically with reduced risk of CHD. Note that above two drinks per day, total mortality goes up because of other diseases and accidents associated with alcohol.

When someone changes from a typical Western diet to a low fat (therefore high carbohydrate) diet LDL-cholesterol goes down, (good!) because percentage saturated fat was reduced, but HDL-cholesterol goes down as well (may not be so good). If instead the fat intake is maintained but saturated fat is replaced by polyunsaturated and monounsaturated fats, LDL also goes down but with little or no reduction of HDL-cholesterol. Changing fat type like this should give a lower risk of coronary disease but reducing total fat intake is better for the management of overweight.

## Plasma triglycerides

If a patient has raised plasma triglycerides the first question is whether they had been fasting when the blood was taken. The next question is whether the hypertriglyceridaemia is a pointer to other risk factors that tend to be associated with it: high plasma cholesterol, overweight, lack of exercise, glucose intolerance, low-HDL-cholesterol or other metabolic disease (renal disease, hypothyroidism). A common cause of increased plasma triglycerides is excessive alcohol indulgence the evening before blood was taken.

---

### Risk factors for coronary heart disease

- High plasma total cholesterol
- High plasma LDL-cholesterol
- Low plasma HDL-cholesterol
- High plasma triglycerides
- High blood pressure
- (Cigarette smoking)
- Obesity; high intra-abdominal fat
- Diabetes mellitus
- (Lack of exercise)
- Increased plasma coagulation factors
- Increased platelet adhesiveness
- High plasma homocysteine
- Increased Lp(a)
- (Apo E4 genotype)

Factors in parentheses are not influenced by diet.

---

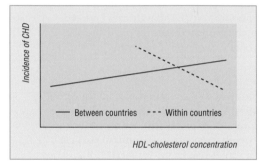

Relation of HDL-cholesterol to incidence of CHD. (Adapted from Knuiman and West[10])

---

### Alcohol intake, coronary heart disease (CHD), and total mortality*

| | Mortality-relative risk | | |
| Stated alcohol consumption | From CHD | From accidents | Total |
| --- | --- | --- | --- |
| Non-drinkers | 1.00 | 1.00 | 1.00 |
| 1/day | 0.79 | 0.98 | 0.84 |
| 2/day | 0.80 | 0.95 | 0.93 |
| 3/day | 0.83 | 1.32 | 1.02 |
| 4/day | 0.74 | 1.22 | 1.08 |
| 5/day | 0.85 | 1.22 | 1.22 |
| 6+/day | 0.92 | 1.73 | 1.38 |

* 12-year follow up of cohort of 276 802 US men by stated alcohol habits at entry. Reduced risk of CHD brought down total mortality at 1 and 2 drinks/day but not above
Reproduced from Boffeta and Garfinkel[11]

The management of hypertriglyceridaemia consists of looking for and dealing with any of the common associations. The non-pharmacological treatment is more exercise, fewer calories (weight reduction), and less alcohol. Reduced carbohydrate is not advised; it implies an increased fat intake which can only increase lipaemia during the day. People with exaggerated postprandial lipaemia appear to have an increased risk of coronary heart disease. Fish oil (for example, Maxepa) is a nutritional supplement with a powerful plasma triglyceride-lowering effect and regular consumption of fatty fish also lowers plasma triglycerides.

## Other risk factors
**High blood pressure** is discussed in chapter 2; **overweight and inactivity** in chapter 11.

Increased levels of two of the **coagulation factors**, Factor VII and fibrinogen, have been clear in some prospective studies (they were not assayed in most studies).[13] **Factor VII** activity is increased during alimentary lipaemia after a fatty meal and is persistent in people with hypertriglyceridaemia. Plasma **fibrinogen** is raised in people who smoke and in obesity; it is reduced by alcohol consumption.

## Antioxidants
The LDL oxidation hypothesis of atherogenesis predicts that if LDL carries more lipid-soluble antioxidants they should provide some protection against CHD. The principal antioxidant in LDL is $\alpha$-tocopherol, vitamin E (average 7 tocopherol molecules per LDL particle). Its concentration can be raised by intake of vitamin E supplements. *In vitro* (outside the body) extra vitamin E delays the oxidation of LDL (by copper). In two large prospective studies, one in US nurses, the other in health professionals, those with high intakes of vitamin E experienced less subsequent CHD. But these high intakes of vitamin E were achieved by taking supplements, and people who regularly take vitamin supplements are likely to have more health conscious lifestyles than the average citizen.

Five large randomised controlled prevention trials, in Western populations, with acronyms ATBC,[14] GISSI,[15] HOPE, PPP, and CHAOS involving 56 000 subjects have now been reported. There was no reduction of cardiovascular disease or mortality. LDL contains smaller amounts of carotenoids, which are also lipid-soluble antioxidants. But supplements of $\beta$-carotene have also not prevented CHD in large randomised controlled trials.[14]

Polyunsaturated fatty acids, 18:2, 20:5 and 22:6 are more susceptible to peroxidation *in vitro* than saturated or monounsaturated acids but in the whole body there is a lot of evidence that PUFA intake is **negatively** associated with CHD.[16]

## Plasma homocysteine
In the inborn error of metabolism homocystinuria, plasma homocysteine is so high that it spills into the urine and vascular diseases are among the complications. Then during the 1990s evidence accumulated (many case-control studies and several prospective studies) that lesser degrees of elevated plasma homocysteine (above 16 $\mu$mol/l total homocysteine, tHcy) are a largely independent risk factor for CHD. They also increase the risk of cerebral and peripheral arterial diseases and even venous thrombosis.[18] Raised plasma homocysteine appears to both damage the endothelium and increase liability to thrombosis.

Homocysteine is an intermediary metabolite of the essential amino acid, methionine (it is methionine minus its terminal methyl group). Folic acid is co-factor for the enzyme in a pathway that re-methylates homocysteine back to methionine.

## Plasma triglycerides

- Triglycerides in the blood after overnight fast are mainly in VLDL (very low density lipoprotein), synthesised in the liver, hence endogenous. Triglycerides in casual blood samples taken during the day may be mainly in chylomicrons, after a fatty meal, and hence exogenous.
- In prospective studies, raised fasting triglycerides have often shown up as a risk factor for coronary heart disease in single-factor analysis. But hypertriglyceridaemia is likely to be associated with raised plasma cholesterol, or overweight/obesity, or glucose intolerance, or lack of exercise or low HDL-cholesterol. When these are controlled, increased triglycerides is certainly not as strong a risk factor as hypercholesterolaemia but it has emerged in some studies as an independent coronary risk factor, more often in women.[12]

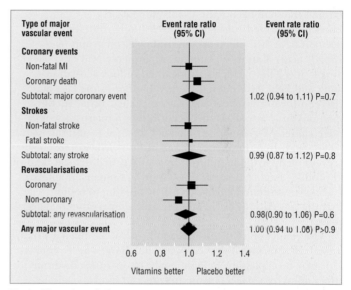

No significant benefit from vitamins C and E and $\beta$-carotene in MRC/BHF secondary prevention trial in over 20 000 subjects[17]

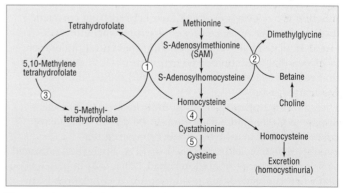

Homocysteine metabolism in humans. Enzymes [vitamins involved]:
1. N-5-methyltetrahydrofolate:homocysteine methyltransferase (methionine synthase) [folate, vitamin B-12]; 2. betaine:homocysteine methyltransferase; 3. methylene-tetrahydrofolate reductase (MTHFR) [folate]; 4. cystathione beta-synthase [vitamin B-6]; 5. gamma-cystathionase [vitamin B-6]

In apparently well-nourished people folic acid lowers elevated homocysteine by about a quarter.[19] A dose of 0.5 mg or even 200 $\mu$g folic acid is effective. Plasma homocysteine is also increased in mild vitamin B-12 deficiency. Folic acid may be a safe, inexpensive way of reducing vascular disease. Randomised controlled trials are under way.

### Dangerous arrhythmias

Dangerous arrhythmia is one of the two major causes of death in CHD. Over half the deaths occur before the arrival of paramedical or medical help. Then in the ambulance or coronary care unit the treatment of ventricular fibrillation saves lives. Developments in nutrition research are showing, with animal experiments, that electrical instability of ischaemic myocardium is influenced by the fatty acid pattern of the diet and hence of myocardial membranes. In rats or marmoset monkeys fed polyunsaturated oils, fewer animals had sustained ventricular arrhythmia when a coronary artery was tied, than in animals that had been fed on saturated fat or (monounsaturated) olive oil.[20] The fish oil group were more resistant to arrhythmia than the sunflower oil group ($\omega$-6 linoleic acid). Canola oil containing linolenic acid (18:3, $\omega$-3), the plant $\omega$-3 fatty acid, also appears to reduce arrhythmias. Kang and Leaf have studied the mechanism of the fatty acid effect with cultured, neonatal, rat ventricular myocytes whose spontaneous contractions are recorded by a microscope and video camera. Eicosapentaenoic acid (20:5, $\omega$-3) and the plant oil $\omega$-3 acid, 18:3 (linolenic) as well as linoleic acid (18:2, $\omega$-6) prevent tachyrhythmia induced by a variety of chemicals known to produce fatal ventricular fibrillation in humans. It appears that polyunsaturated fatty acids act by binding to sodium channel proteins in the membrane and altering their electrical charge.[21]

The reduction of deaths outside hospital has been a striking feature in countries where coronary death rates have reduced. This may be explained, at least partly, by an anti-arrhythmic effect of increased $\omega$-6 polyunsaturated fat intake (national fish intakes have not increased).

### Platelet function and thrombosis

In patients with symptomatic CHD tests of platelet function have usually indicated activation. Available tests of platelet function are not on lists of risk factors predicting coronary disease; they are *in vitro* tests and are inevitably indirect. However platelet activation is of course a central phenomenon in myocardial infarction or recurrent angina, so that any diet that reduces platelet aggregation should reduce the risk of coronary disease.

Following up an observation that the rarity of coronary disease in Greenland Eskimos might be due to their heavy consumption of marine fat, it was discovered that eicosapentaenoic acid (20:5, $\omega$-3) or EPA, a principal fatty acid of fish oil, displaces arachidonic acid (20:4, $\omega$-6) in platelets, so that when stimulated they produce an inactive thromboxane TXA$_3$ instead of the active TXA$_2$ derived from arachidonic acid. EPA is only present in traces in the body fat of land animals and is absent from vegetable oils. In human experiments fish oil also reduced the levels of PAI-I, plasminogen activator inhibitor-1. Fish oil is therefore a pharmaceutical alternative (for example Maxepa) to aspirin to reduce the tendency to thrombosis. Results have been mixed in trials with fish oils to see if they delay restenosis after coronary angioplasty.

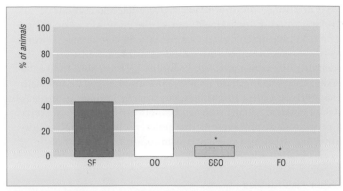

Total mortality from irreversible ventricular fibrillation during ischaemia or reperfusion in rats fed a saturated fat (SF), olive oil (OO), sunflower seed oil (SSO), or fish oil (FO) diet for 12 weeks from 18 weeks of age. *Significantly different from SF, $P < 0.05$. (Adapted from McLennan *et al.*[20])

### Coronary deaths per 100 000 in men in three Australasian cities using standardised MONICA criteria

|  | 1984 | 1993 | Change |
| --- | --- | --- | --- |
| Coronary deaths before patient in hospital |  |  |  |
|    Auckland (NZ) | 188 | 141 | 47 |
|    Newcastle (NSW) | 186 | 102 | 84 |
|    Perth (WA) | 128 | 78 | 50 |
| Coronary deaths after patient in hospital |  |  |  |
|    Auckland (NZ) | 57 | 24 | 33 |
|    Newcastle (NSW) | 78 | 28 | 50 |
|    Perth (WA) | 41 | 30 | 11 |

Reproduced from Beaglehole R *et al.*[22] with permission from Oxford University Press

### Effects of fish oil

↑ EPA and DHA in plasma and red cells
↓ Arrhythmias in ischaemic myocardium
↓ Platelet aggregation
↓ PA1-1, ↓ fibrinogen, ↓ TPA
↓ Fibrinolysis
↑ Bleeding time
↓ Fasting plasma VLDL and triglycerides
↓ Postprandial lipaemia

DHA = docosahexaenoic acid (22:6, $\omega$-3), TPA = tissue plasminogen activator

### More on diets and platelet function

- Several prospective studies (in countries with intermediate fish intake) and a secondary prevention trial in Cardiff [23] suggest that a modest intake of fatty fish (for example sardines, herring, mackerel, or salmon) two or three times a week may help to prevent coronary heart disease. The EPA in this amount of fish is less than that needed (at least 2 g of EPA per day) to inhibit platelet aggregation.
- $\omega$-6 polyunsaturated oils also appear to have an inhibiting effect on platelet function. They are less active but people eat more plant seed oils than fish oil.
- Heavy alcohol ingestion exerts an inhibitory effect on platelet function, which is reversible on abstinence.

## Dietary components associated directly with coronary disease in cohort epidemiological studies

Most of the many prospective studies involving coronary heart disease have not measured diet. It is much more complex and expensive to estimate all the different foods, and thence to compute all the nutrients, than to measure blood pressure or plasma lipids. Of all the parts of a total diet there have been most reports of **alcohol** intake. It is simpler to include in a questionnaire than to tackle the intricacies of type of fat intake.

In the minority of prospective studies that did report on foods or food components, most have used food frequency questionnaires (chapter 12), which are easier to handle than open-ended dietary records. Another method, occasionally used, is to measure objective biomarkers of food intake such as plasma fatty acid pattern. Interpretation of associations in the table must allow for uncertainties in assessing usual food intake, and confounding between different food components and with lifestyle. Vitamin E findings have not been confirmed in randomised controlled trials.

### Adding a statin to the diet

Treatment with statins lowers raised plasma cholesterol by average 20% and LDL-cholesterol 25%, without lowering HDL-cholesterol, and reduces subsequent CHD events significantly. Statin treatment has also been shown to reduce CHD events by about 24% in people who had survived a myocardial infarction and had average plasma cholesterols of around 5.4 mmol/l.[26]

Note that a statin is prescribed (as the manufacturers state) as an **adjunct to diet** and normally after a proper trial of a cholesterol lowering diet. The dietary principles described in this chapter lower plasma cholesterol by different mechanisms from the HMG COA reductase inhibition by statins. Parts of diets used to protect against CHD do not act by lowering LDL-cholesterol, for example, only by diet and exercise can overweight be treated.

Statins are very expensive at present, either for the patient or the health service, and we do not yet know if there might be long-term complications. Put very simply the indications for adding a statin to diet are for patients with:

- existing clinical CHD
- two or more coronary risk factors and high plasma cholesterol
- no or one coronary risk factor and very high plasma cholesterol.

In assessing the plasma cholesterol, LDL-cholesterol should be used or total cholesterol/HDL-cholesterol (after repeat measurements in a good laboratory). Risk factors are diabetes, hypertension, smoking, strong family history.

### The dietary prescription (consistent with NCEP[27] and DOH[28]

*Total fat*
Reduction is not essential for improving plasma lipids but should reduce coagulation factors and daytime plasma triglycerides and contribute to weight reduction.

*Saturated fatty acids*
Principally 14:0, 16:0 and 12:0 should be substantially reduced from around 15% of dietary energy in many Western diets to 8-10%.

*Polyunsaturated fatty acids*
Mainly linoleic acid (18:2, $\omega$-6): they should be about 7% of dietary energy (present British level), up to 10%. Omega-3

### Dietary components directly related to CHD

| Component | No. of studies |
|---|---|
| Alcohol ↓ | 29/38 |
| Fruits and vegetables ↓ | many |
| Cereal fibre ↓ | several |
| Saturated fatty acids ↑ | 4/4 |
| $\omega$-6 PUFA ↓ | 6/12 |
| *Trans* fatty acids ↑ | 2/3 |
| $\alpha$-linolenic ($\omega$-3) ↓ | 2/3 |
| Fish ↓ | 5/11 |
| Coffee ↑ or 0 | 14 |
| Nuts ↓ | 3/3 |
| Vitamin E ↓ | 3/3 |
| Folate ↓ | 3/3 |
| And 0 for eggs (2/2) and iron intake (7/9) | |
| ↑ Increased risk | ↓ Protective |

### Randomised controlled trials (RCTs) with diet or nutrients

- **Reduced saturated, increased $\omega$-6 PUFA diets**
8 RCTs in UK, USA, Finland and Norway, published 1965-1992. Total 17 529 subjects. In intervention groups plasma cholesterol fell. Combined result CHD events 81% of control ($P < 0.05$) and total mortality 95%.[24]

- **Lyon "Mediterranean" diet**[25]
Intervention group used a canola margarine, rich in linolenic acid (18:3, $\omega$-3): they ate more bread, fruit, legumes, fish, less meat and butter but showed no fall in plasma cholesterol. CHD events were significantly reduced but the mechanism and dietary components responsible are not clear.

- **Fish and fish oil**
One secondary prevention RCT with fish (DART)[22] and another with fish oil (GISSI)[15] reduced CHD events significantly.

- **Vitamin E and $\beta$-carotene** have both been ineffective in several RCTs.

polyunsaturated fatty acids should be increased, both 20:5 and 22:6 from seafoods and 18:3 from canola (rapeseed) oil, etc.

### Monounsaturated fatty acids
Ideal intake if total fat 30%, saturated 10% and polyunsaturated 8% would be 12% of total dietary energy.

### Trans fatty acids
With the help of margarine manufacturers these have been reduced. The Department of Health recommends no more than 2% of dietary energy. Avoid older hard margarines.

### Dietary cholesterol
This boils down to the question of egg yolks. Eggs are a nutritious, inexpensive and convenient food. The Department of Health recommends for the general population no rise in cholesterol intake.

### Salt (NaCl)
Restriction to under 6 g/day is advised for the general population (100 mmol Na). It is more important for coronary patients.

### Fish
The Department of Health recommends at least twice a week, preferably fatty fish. It should not be fried in saturated fat.

### Fibre
Eat plenty of high fibre and whole grain cereal foods, including oatmeal.

### Vegetables and fruit
These are low in fat, and contain pectin and other fibres, flavonoids and other antioxidants, and they contain folate. Expert Committees in Britain and the USA recommend five servings of different vegetables and fruit per day (400 g/day average weight).[28]

### Soy products
(Not salty soy sauce) recommended.

## Fatty acid patterns of fats, oils, and some meats (as % total fat in the food)

| | Saturated | | | | | |
|---|---|---|---|---|---|---|
| | C4-12 | C14-18 (myristic, palmitic, stearic) | Mono-unsaturated | Linoleic | Other poly-unsaturated | P:S* |
| Butter, cream, milk | 13 | 48 | 30 | 2 | 1 | 0.05 |
| Cocoa butter | — | 61 | 36 | 3 | — | 0.05 |
| Beef | — | 48 | 48 | 2 | 1 | 0.06 |
| Coconut oil | 58 | 31 | 8 | 2 | | 0.1 |
| Bacon and pork | — | 42 | 50 | 7 | 1 | 0.2 |
| Palm oil (used in ice cream) | — | 45 | 45 | 9 | — | 0.2 |
| Margarine (old style, hard) | 3 | 37 | 33** | 12 | 1 | 0.3 |
| Chicken | — | 34 | 45 | 18 | 2 | 0.6 |
| Olive oil | — | 14 | 73 | 11 | 1 | 0.9 |
| Groundnut oil | — | 15 | 53 | 30 | 1 | 2.1 |
| Fish oil | — | 23 | 27 | 7 | 43† | 2.2 |
| Margarine, polyunsaturated | 2 | 21 | 22 | 52 | 1 | 2.3 |
| Corn (maize) oil | — | 14 | 24 | 53 | 2 | 3.9 |
| Soya bean oil | — | 14 | 24 | 53 | 7 | 4.3 |
| Canola oil | — | 7 | 63 | 20 | 10‡ | 4.3 |
| Sunflower seed oil | — | 12 | 33 | 58 | — | 4.8 |
| Flaxseed oil | — | 9 | 18 | 16 | 57‡ | 8.0 |
| Safflower oil | — | 9 | 14 | 77 | — | 8.5 |

* These are in ascending order of ratio of polyunsaturated to saturated fats, but this is not the only consideration in choosing dietary fats and oils
† Includes varying amounts of 20:5 ω-3 and 22:6 ω-3 (depending on species).
‡ α Linolenic acid
** Includes variable amounts of trans 18:1

### Alcohol
In moderation, one or two drinks per day is beneficial for middle-aged people at risk of CHD but cannot be recommended for the general population because of the greater danger of accidents in younger people and of all the medical complications of excessive intake.

### Coffee
Should be instant or filtered.

## References

1 Truswell AS. Cholesterol controversy. *BMJ* 1992; **304**: 912-13.
2 Steinberg D, Parthasarathy S, Carew TE, Khoo JC, Witztum JL. Beyond cholesterol: modifications of low-density lipoprotein that increase its atherogenicity. *N Engl J Med* 1989; **320**: 915-24.
3 Keys A, Aravanis C, Blackburn H *et al. Seven countries: a multivariate analysis of death and coronary heart disease.* Cambridge, Massachusetts: Harvard University Press, 1980.
4 Martin MJ, Hulley SB, Browner WS, Kuller LH, Wentworth D. Serum cholesterol, blood pressure and mortality implications from a cohort of 361 662 men. *Lancet* 1986; **ii**: 933-6.
5 Gregory J, Foster K, Tyler H, Wiseman M. *The dietary and nutritional survey of British adults.* London: HMSO 1990: 266.
6 Thelle DS, Shaper AG, Whitehead TP, Bullock DG, Ashby D, Patel J. Blood lipids in middle-aged British men. *Br Heart J* 1983; **49**: 205-13.
7 Truswell AS. Cereal grains and coronary heart disease. *Eur J Clin Nutr* 2002; **56**: 1-14.
8 Hendricks HFJ, Westrate JA, Van Vliet T, Meijer GW. Spreads enriched with three different levels of vegetable oil sterols and the degree of cholesterol lowering in normocholesterolaemic and mildly hypercholesterolaemic subjects. *Eur J Clin Nutr* 1999; **53**: 319-27.

9 Urgert R, Meybom S, Kuilman M *et al.* Comparison of effect of cafetiere and filtered coffee on serum concentrations of liver aminotransferases and lipids: six month randomised controlled trial. *BMJ* 1996; **314**: 1362-6.
10 Knuiman JT, West CA. Differences in HDL cholesterol between populations: no paradox? *Lancet* 1983; **i**: 296.
11 Boffeta P, Garfinkel L. Alcohol drinking and mortality among men enrolled in an American Cancer Society prospective study. *Epidemiology* 1990; **1**: 342-8.
12 Tunstall-Pedoe H, Woodward M, Tavendale R, Brook RA, McClusky MK. Comparison of the prediction by 27 different factors of coronary heart disease and death in men and women of the Scottish heart health study: cohort study. *BMJ* 1997; **315**: 722-9.
13 Miller GJ. Postprandial lipid metabolism and thrombosis. *Proc Nutr Soc* 1997; **56**: 739-44.
14 Rapola JM, Virtamo J, Ripatti S *et al.* Randomised trial of α-tocopherol and β-carotene supplements on incidence of major coronary events in men with previous myocardial infarction. *Lancet* 1997; **349**: 1715-20.
15 GISSI-Prevenzione Investigators. Dietary supplement with n-3 polyunsaturated fatty acids and vitamin E after myocardial infarction: results of the GISSI-Prevenzione trial. *Lancet* 1999; **354**: 447-55.

16 Hu FB, Stampfer MJ, Manson J *et al.* Dietary fat intake and the risk of coronary heart disease in women. *N Engl J Med* 1997; **337**: 1491-9.

17 Heart Protection Study Group. MRC/BHF Heart Protection Study of antioxidant vitamins supplementation in 20,536 high-risk individuals: a randomised placebo-controlled trial. *Lancet* 2002; **360**: 23-33.

18 Bouskey CJ, Beresford SAA, Omenn GS, Motulsky AG. A quantitative assessment of plasma homocysteine as a risk factor for vascular disease. Probable benefits of increasing folic acid intake. *JAMA* 1995; **274**: 1049-57.

19 Homocysteine Lowering Trialists' Collaboration. Lowering blood homocysteine with folic acid based supplements: meta-analysis of randomised trials. *BMJ* 1998; **316**: 894-8.

20 McLennan PL. Relative effects of dietary saturated, monounsaturated and polyunsaturated fatty acids on cardiac arrhythmias in rats. *Am J Clin Nutr* 1993; **57**: 207-12.

21 Kang JX, Leaf A. Antiarrhythmic effect of polyunsaturated fatty acids. Recent studies. *Circulation* 1996; **94**: 1774-80.

22 Beaglehole R, Stewart AW, Jackson R. Declining rates of coronary disease in New Zealand and Australia. *Am J Epidemiol* 1997; **145**: 707-13.

23 Burr ML, Fehily AM, Gilbert JF *et al.* Effects of changes in fat, fish and fibre intakes on death and myocardial reinfarction: Diet and Reinfarction Trial (DART). *Lancet* 1989; **ii**: 757-61.

24 Truswell AS. Review of dietary intervention studies: effect on coronary events and on total mortality. *Aust NZ J Med* 1994; **24**: 98-106.

25 de Lorgeril M, Renaud, Mamalle N *et al.* Mediterranean alpha-linolenic acid-rich diet in secondary prevention of coronary heart disease. *Lancet* 1994; **343**: 1454-9.

26 Sacks FM, Pfeffer MA, Moye LA *et al.* The effect of pravastatin on coronary events after myocardial infarction in patients with average cholesterol levels. *N Engl J Med* 1996; **335**: 1001-9.

27 Expert Panel on Detection, Evaluation and Treatment of High Blood Cholesterol in Adults. Executive summary of the third report of the National Cholesterol Education Program (NCEP) Expert Panel of Detection, Evaluation and Treatment of High Blood Cholesterol in Adults (Adult Treatment Panel III). *JAMA* 2001; **285**: 2486-97.

28 Department of Health. Nutritional Aspects of Cardiovascular Disease. *Report on the Cardiovascular Review Group, Committee on Medical Aspects of Food Policy.* London: HMSO, 1994.

29 National Heart Forum. *At least five a day. Strategies to increase vegetable and fruit consumption.* London: The Stationery Office, 1997.

# 2  Diet and blood pressure

Essential hypertension is a multifactorial disease. It is common in older people not only in urban and industrialised areas but also in a quiet Hebridean island, in tropical Africa, where Albert Schweizer used to work, and in an isolated Solomon Islands' tribe minimally influenced by Western ways, which cooks in sea water.[1]

## Salt (sodium)

*To what extent is essential hypertension related to an unnecessarily high intake of salt?*
Hypertension is not an inevitable accompaniment of ageing. Evidence showed that hypertension did not occur in a few isolated communities, such as Yanomamo Indians (in the Amazon), Kalahari Bushmen (Botswana),[2] and remote Pacific islanders. These people typically had no access to salt and their urinary sodiums (reflecting salt intake) were under 30 mmol/day.

---

**Salt and blood pressure history**

Salt is the best known of the dietary factors affecting blood pressure. It has been hypothesised for the longest time, first by Ambard and Beaujard in 1904. Then in 1922 Allen first documented reduction of blood pressure by sodium restriction.

---

In the Intersalt study,[3] 10 000 people were examined by standardised methods in 52 different communities in 30 countries around the world. The rise in blood pressure with age was significantly related to 24-hour urinary sodium.

Within communities correlation between individuals' blood pressure and sodium intake (or excretion) is difficult to see. This is partly because of large day-to-day swings in people's sodium intake,[4] partly because people should only be compared in the same age group, and also because not all individuals are sensitive to salt—this can be demonstrated by a week of 12 g NaCl, followed by a very low salt diet.[5] However, in the dietary and nutritional survey of British adults blood pressure was found to correlate with 24-hour urinary sodium, reflecting salt intake.[6] A cohort study in 2436 Finnish men and women found that those who started with high 24-hour urine sodiums had more cardiovascular and total mortality over the following 8 years.[7]

The requirement for sodium in health is usually under 25 mmol Na/day (equivalent to 1.5 g NaCl).[9] Normal kidneys can shut down sodium excretion almost to zero and sweat loss is reduced in people on low salt intakes or adapted to hot climates. Human milk contains only 7 mmol Na/litre, so young infants' sodium intake per megajoule is only about one-sixth that of their parents'!

Salt intakes in Britain are around 9 g NaCl (150 mmol Na) per day and in parts of Asia considerably higher, over 250 mmol Na/day. To prove that our unnecessarily high intakes of salt contribute to the development of essential hypertension, blood pressures of a group of adults eating only their sodium requirement (25 mmol Na/day) would have to be compared over many years with another group, similar in all respects, eating the usual 150 mmol sodium/day. Such a human trial is probably impossible, so a trial in chimpanzees, who have 98% the same DNA as humans and half our life span, is important.

**Causal factors in essential hypertension**
- **Genetic**—several mechanisms
- **Tension from anxiety**—via increased sympathetic tone or circulating catecholamines
- **Dietary—positive correlation—negative correlation**
  Overweight and obesity   Potassium
  Sodium (salt) intake       ?Calcium
  Alcohol

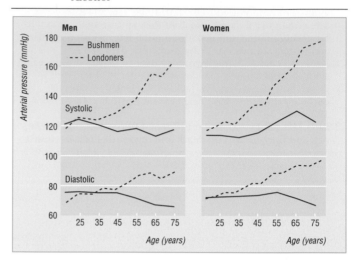

Blood pressure with age of 152 Bushmen, hunter gatherers (aged 15-83 years) in NW Botswana (continuous lines) compared with standard figures from London measured in 1954. (Adapted from Truswell *et al.*[2])

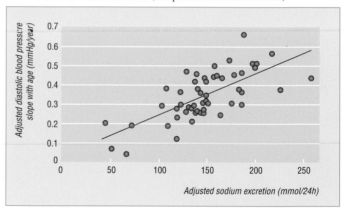

Cross-centre plots of diastolic blood pressure slope with age and median sodium excretion; $P < 0.001$. (Adapted from Intersalt study[3]). For an additional 100 mmol Na/day, the increase of BP over 30 years (25 to 55) was 10 systolic/6 diastolic mmHg greater[8]

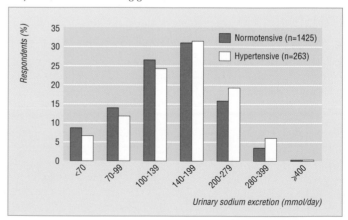

Distribution of normotensive and hypertensive respondents by urinary sodium excretion rate in the Dietary and Nutritional Survey of British Adults, 1986-87. (Adapted from Beard *et al.*[6])

Chimpanzees, living on a natural (low sodium) vegetarian and fruit diet in Gabon (West Africa) were given a liquid infant formula with or without salt up to 15 g/day for 1.5 years.[10] Blood pressures rose progressively in eight of the 10 animals given typical human salt intakes and in none of the controls.

Salt has been used since Neolithic times by most cultures as an important food preservative. Most of mankind has become used to the taste of more salt than we need now that canning, freezing, refrigeration, etc, are widely used to preserve our food.

For the general adult population, mainly as a measure to help prevent hypertension, Australia (from 1982), the USA (from 1989), WHO (1990) and the UK Department of Health (1994)[11] all recommend a target intake of 100 mmol sodium per day equivalent to 6.0 g NaCl or 2.3 g Na *or less*.

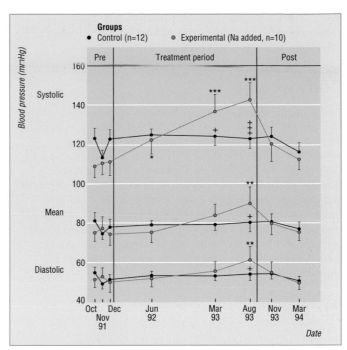

Mean systolic and diastolic blood pressures of 10 salt-added (experimental) and 12 control chimpanzees over 2.5 years. Blood pressure rose in most of the experimental chimpanzees. It returned to normal when the salt was discontinued (post treatment). (Adapted from Denton *et al.*[10])

## Sodium accumulation and arterioles

The mechanism of action of sodium is undoubtedly complex and involves kidney tubules and several hormones. One aspect is that if sodium tends to accumulate in cells it interferes with calcium transport, and elevated free calcium in the cytosol of arteriolar smooth muscle cells increases their tone and consequently the arterial blood pressure.

*In people with hypertension, how much reduction of blood pressure can be achieved with a low salt diet and how difficult is this to organise (and persist with)?*

Elevated blood pressure can usually be lowered by salt restriction.[12] Diuretic drugs work by increasing urinary sodium excretion. Alternatively a sufficient reduction of dietary sodium can achieve the same degree of negative sodium balance. In mild to moderate hypertension, a reduction of sodium intake (which can be monitored with 24-hour urinary sodium) by 50 mmol/day will usually give a useful reduction of blood pressure, so that the patient may be able to come off the hypotensive drugs (or not start them) or reduce the dose (and with this the probability of side effects). Salt restriction increases sensitivity to all hypertensive drugs except slow channel calcium blockers, like nifedipine. Some people are more responsive than others. Older people may be more responsive to salt reduction and they are particularly susceptible to the side effects of drugs.

When people change to a lower salt diet their taste adjusts after a few weeks. Other flavours are perceived and appreciated more. The major obstacle to eating low salt is that most of the salt in food is put in during processing and is outside the individual's control.

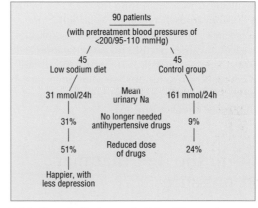

Trial of low-salt diet in people with mild to moderate hypertension[13]

## Sodium in foods

Most of the salt that we eat is not that added at the table or in cooking water (much of which goes down the sink). It is salt added in food processing, particularly of staple foods. Wheat flour contains 3 or 4 mg sodium/100 g but average breads have 520-550 mg/100 g. Oils like sunflower or olive oil contain only traces of sodium but butter averages 750 mg/100 g and margarines 800 mg/100 g. Many cereal products—biscuits, cakes and breakfast cereals (though not all)—are very high in sodium, which consumers cannot taste (being masked by the sugar content). Salted peanuts contain less sodium than breads; consumers can taste the salt because it is all on the surface. Anyone wanting to reduce salt intake must find low-salt breads and breakfast cereals and cheeses as well as cutting out the more obvious bacon and olives in brine which people eat less

### Average percentages of sodium from different sources[14]

| | |
|---|---|
| • **Discretionary** | |
| Added at table | 9.0 |
| Used in cooking | 6.0 |
| • **Food** | |
| Naturally occurring | 18.5 |
| Added salt in processing | 58.7 |
| Non-salt additives | 7.2 |
| • **Salt in water supply** (average) | 0.6 |
| | 100.0 |

often. Other sodium compounds in food, bicarbonate and glutamate, have less effect on blood pressure than sodium chloride.

## Body weight

Obese people are likely to have a higher blood pressure than lean people. In a cohort of over 5000 people born in Britain in the same week, blood pressures at the age of 36 were progressively higher in those with a body mass index (weight (kg)/height (m$^2$)) above 26. Typically a 3 mmHg higher diastolic pressure may be expected for every 10 kg increase in body weight.[3] In a large Swedish study of 60-year-old men, a quarter of the fattest fifth were taking antihypertensive drugs compared with only 4% of the thinnest fifth.[16] Raised blood pressure and hyperlipidaemia are both major risk factors for cardiovascular disease, and effective weight reduction will improve both.

## Alcohol

Alcohol intake is emerging as one of the important environmental factors associated with raised blood pressure. Heavy drinkers have higher blood pressure than light drinkers and abstainers. The effect starts above about three (stated) drinks a day. Systolic pressure is more affected than diastolic.

The pressor effect of alcohol can be demonstrated directly. It was seen, for example, in men with essential hypertension who were moderate to heavy drinkers. They continued their habitual intake of beer and antihypertensive drugs; when low alcohol beer (0.9% alcohol) was substituted for the same intake of regular beer (5% alcohol), their blood pressure fell 5/3 mmHg.[18] The mechanism(s) have not yet been established. Acute ingestion of alcohol causes peripheral vasodilatation, but there are features of a hyperadrenergic state in the withdrawal syndrome. Plasma cortisol concentrations are sometimes raised in alcoholics. Increased red cell volume, and hence increased blood viscosity, is a possible mechanism.

## Components in the diet that may lower blood pressure

### Potassium
In a placebo-controlled, crossover trial in mild to moderate hypertension, blood pressure fell by (average) 7/4 mmHg with a supplement of eight Slow-K tablets (64 mmol potassium) a day. But the same (London) clinic found little or no effect in similar hypertensive patients who had managed to reduce their sodium intake (and urinary sodium) to around 70 mmol a day—potassium acts as a sodium antagonist and has little effect when sodium intake has been halved.[19]

### Calcium
Analyses of a diet and health study in the USA suggested that people with low calcium intakes had more hypertension, and in Britain less cardiovascular disease is reported in areas with hard water (which contains more calcium). Over 30 controlled trials with calcium supplements have been summarised in three meta-analyses,[21] which showed that 1000 mg per day or more of calcium has only a trivial effect on systolic (not diastolic) blood pressure. Increased calcium, by diet or supplements, might be useful in a very small number of hypertensive patients who have a low calcium intake or increased plasma parathyroid levels.

---

### Reduced food energy and falling blood pressure
- People who do not eat enough food energy and lose weight usually have a fall of (normal) blood pressure.
- If hypertensive obese patients reduce their weight they show falls of blood pressure like 10 mmHg systolic/5 mmHg diastolic for a 5-kg weight loss.
- Less food means less sodium eaten. Some weight loss occurs even if sodium intake is maintained, but the combination of weight loss and a low sodium intake is more effective.
- In a randomised placebo-controlled trial of first-line treatment of mild hypertension in overweight patients, the weight reduction group (mean loss 7.4 kg) had a 13 mmHg fall of systolic blood pressure while those treated with metoprolol *(200 mg/day) had a 10 mmHg fall. Plasma lipids improved in the weight reduction group, but changed adversely in those on drug therapy.*[15]

---

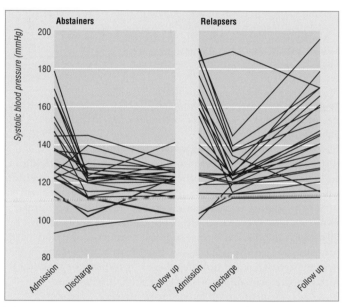

When alcoholic patients were admitted to hospital for detoxification their systolic blood pressure fell by about 20 mmHg; it stayed down if they continued to abstain, but rose again if drinking was resumed. The same pattern was seen with diastolic pressure[17]

---

### Potassium in foods
- **Moderate to high (mmol per usual serving):**
  Potatoes (12-26), pulses (19), dried fruits (5-12), fresh meat and fish (8-10), All Bran (8), fresh fruit (2-10), vegetables (2-10), orange juice (6), oatmeal (5), cows' milk (5), nuts (2-6), wine (3-4), beer (3), coffee (2).
- **Low (1-3 mmol per usual serving):**
  Rice, chocolate, egg, biscuits, bread, cheese, flour, cornflakes.
- **Very low or absent:**
  Sugar, jam, honey, butter, margarine, cream, oils, spirits.

Potassium is the major intracellular cation; the more concentrated the cells in a food, the higher the potassium is likely to be.

In Britain potassium intakes are around 70 mmol/day in men and 60 mmol/day in women: 17% from potatoes (10% from fried potatoes), 14% from cereals, 14% from milk products, 13% from meat and products, 11% from other vegetables, 5% from fruit and 16% from beverages (coffee 6%, tea 4%, beer 3%, fruit 2%).[20]

## Magnesium

Magnesium can sometimes lower blood pressure. In patients who had received long term diuretics (mostly for hypertension) and potassium supplements, half were also given magnesium aspartate hydrochloride for six months. Their blood pressure fell significantly. The diuretics had presumably led to subclinical magnesium depletion.

## Vegetarianism

Healthy (normotensive) hospital staff in Perth, Western Australia, were provided with all their meals as one of two diets—mixed omnivore or (lacto-ovo) vegetarian. Sodium intakes were kept the same. After six weeks the subjects were changed to the other diet. Blood pressures were significantly lower by about 6/3.5 mmHg while on the vegetarian diet.[23] The responsible ingredient(s) have not been clearly demonstrated.

## DASH 1 and 2

*D*ietary *A*pproaches to *S*top *H*ypertension was a multicentre randomised controlled dietary trial in over 400 middle aged US adults with BP in the normal or mildly elevated range. In DASH 1 three diets were compared for eight weeks.[24] Blood pressures were lower with extra fruits and vegetables than on control diet and lower still with a combination of low fat dairy food and low saturated fat with the extra fruits and vegetables (cf control diet): $-7.2/-2.8$ on extra fruits plus vegetables and $-11.4/-5.5$ mmHg on the combination diet. Sodium and alcohol intakes and body mass index were held the same between groups.

In DASH 2 BPs were compared on control diet or DASH combination (extra fruits and vegetables, low fat dairy) at three different levels of salt intake (for one month in each subject in random order).[25] As before BPs were lower on the DASH combination diet. Reduction from usual Na (143 mmol/day) to intermediate (105 mmol/day) they averaged 2.1 and 1.3 mm systolic on control and DASH diets. Between intermediate and low sodium (65 mmol/day) systolic BPs were $-4.6$ and $-1.7$ mmHg respectively. Black people with mild hypertension showed the largest falls of BP.

---

### Magnesium distribution in foods

*Magnesium* is distributed in foods somewhat similarly to potassium. Bran, wholegrain cereals, and legumes are the richest sources. Most vegetables contain similar moderate amounts to meat.

---

### From management guidelines of the British Hypertension Society[22]

Non-pharmacological measures ... should be offered to all hypertensive patients whether taking drugs or not. This advice should also be offered to people with a strong family history of hypertension. In mild hypertension non-pharmacological measures may obviate the need for drugs.

- Reduce energy intake to achieve ideal weight.
- Alcohol <21 units/week in men and <14 units per week in women. One or two days/week no alcohol.
- Reduce salt intake.
- Regular physical exercise and improve level of fitness.

And to reduce the risk of cardiovascular disease stop smoking and reduce saturated fat intake.

---

## References

1 Page LB, Damon A, Moellering RC Jr. Antecedents of cardiovascular disease in six Solomon Islands societies. *Circulation* 1974; **49**: 1132-45.
2 Truswell AS, Kennelly BM, Hansen JDL, Lee RB. Blood pressure of Kung Bushmen in northern Botswana. *Am Heart J* 1972; **84**: 5-12.
3 Intersalt Cooperative Research Group. Intersalt: an international study of electrolyte excretion and blood pressure. Results for 24-hour urinary sodium and potassium excretion. *BMJ* 1988; **297**: 319-28.
4 Frost CD, Law MR, Wald NJ. By how much does dietary salt reduction lower blood pressure? II. Analysis of observational data within populations. *BMJ* 1991; **302**: 815-18.
5 Morimoto A, Uzu T, Fujii T *et al*. Sodium sensitivity and cardiovascular events in patients with essential hypertension. *Lancet* 1997; **350**: 1734-7.
6 Beard TC, Blizzard L, O'Brien DJ, Dwyer T. Association between blood pressure and dietary factors in the dietary and nutritional survey of British adults. *Arch Intern Med* 1997; **157**: 234-8.
7 Tuomilehto J, Jousilahti P, Rastenyte D *et al*. Urinary sodium excretion and cardiovascular mortality in Finland: a prospective study. *Lancet* 2001; **357**: 848-51.
8 Elliott P, Stamler J, Nichols R *et al*. Intersalt revisited: further analyses of 24-hour sodium excretion and blood pressure within and across populations. *BMJ* 1996; **312**: 1249-53.
9 Department of Health. *Dietary reference values for food energy and nutrients for the United Kingdom. Report of the Panel of the Committee on Medical Aspects of Food Policy.* London: HMSO, 1991, pp 152-5.
10 Denton D, Weisinger R, Mundy NI *et al*. The effect of increased salt intake on blood pressure of chimpanzees. *Nature Med* 1995; **1**: 1009-16.
11 Department of Health. *Nutritional aspects of cardiovascular disease. Report of the Cardiovascular Review Group Committee on Medical Aspects of Food Policy.* London: HMSO, 1994.
12 Law MR, Frost CD, Wald NJ. By how much does dietary salt reduction lower blood pressure? III. Analysis of data from trials of salt reduction. *BMJ* 1991; **302**: 819-24.
13 Beard TC, Cooke HM, Gray WR, Barge R. Randomised controlled trial of a no-added-sodium diet for mild hypertension. *Lancet* 1982; **ii**: 455-8.
14 Edwards DG, Kaye AE, Druce E. Sources and intakes of sodium in the United Kingdom diet. *Eur J Clin Nutr* 1989; **43**: 855-61.
15 McMahon SW, Macdonald GJ, Bernstein L, Andrews G, Blacket RB. Comparison of weight reduction with metaprolol in treatment of hypertension in young overweight patients. *Lancet* 1985; **i**: 1233-5.
16 Larsson B, Björntorp P, Tibblin G. The health consequences of moderate obesity. *Int J Obesity* 1981; **5**: 97-116.
17 Saunders JB, Beevers DG, Paton A. Alcohol-induced hypertension. *Lancet* 1981; **ii**: 653-6.
18 Puddey IB, Beilin LJ, Vandongen R. Regular alcohol use raises blood pressure in treated hypertensive subjects. *Lancet* 1987; **i**: 647-50.
19 Smith SJ, Markandu MD, Sagnella GA, MacGregor GA. Moderate potassium chloride supplementation in essential hypertension: is it additive to moderate sodium restriction? *BMJ* 1985; **290**: 110-13.
20 Ministry of Agriculture, Fisheries and Food. *The Dietary and Nutritional Survey of British Adults—Further Analysis.* London: HMSO, 1994.
21 Bucher HC, Cook RJ, Guyatt GH *et al*. Effects of dietary calcium supplementation on blood pressure. A meta-analysis of randomised controlled trials. *JAMA* 1996; **275**: 1016-22.

22 Sever P, Beevers G, Bulpitt C *et al.* Management guidelines in essential hypertension: report of the second working party of the British Hypertension Society. *BMJ* 1993; **306**: 983-7.

23 Rouse IL, Beilin LJ, Armstrong BK, Vandongen R. Blood pressure-lowering effect of a vegetarian diet: controlled trial in normotensive subjects. *Lancet* 1983; **i**: 5-10.

24 Appel LJ, Moore TJ, Obarzanek E. A clinical trial of the effects of dietary patterns on blood pressure. *N Engl J Med* 1997; **336**: 1117-24.

25 Sacks FM, Svetkey LP, Vollmer WM *et al.* Effects on blood pressure of reduced dietary sodium and the Dietary Approaches to Stop Hypertension (DASH) diet. *N Engl J Med* 2001; **344**: 3-10.

**Further reading**

Scientific Advisory Committee on Nutrition. *Salt & Health.* London: Stationery Office, 2003.

# 3   Nutritional advice for some other chronic diseases

## Dental caries

Dental caries affects people predominantly in the first 25 years of life. Dental enamel is the hardest material in the body. Its weakness is that, because it is basically calcium phosphate, it is dissolved by acid. Three factors together contribute to caries.

### Infection

A specific species of viridans streptococci, *Streptococcus mutans*, metabolises sugars to lactic acid and also polymerises sugars to a layer of covering polysaccharide in which the bacteria are shielded from saliva and the tongue. Some people harbour more of these bacteria than others.

### Substrate

Most sugars serve as substrate—sucrose, glucose, fructose, and lactose (not sorbitol or xylitol). Starches too, if they stay in the mouth, are split to sugars by salivary amylase. Consumption of sugary foods between meals, especially if they are sticky and consumption is repeated, favours the development of caries. Brushing the teeth and flossing between them after meals reduces the likelihood of caries.

### Resistance of the teeth

Caries is more likely in fissures. In older people the "mature" enamel is more resistant. An intake of 1-3 mg/day of fluoride—as occurs, for example, if drinking water is fluoridated at a concentration of 1 mg/l—increases the enamel's resistance, especially if taken while enamel is being laid down before the tooth erupts.

The cariostatic effect of fluoride in natural water was noticed in Maldon, Essex in 1933, and confirmed by comparing children's teeth and water fluoride across the United States in the early 1940s. Water fluoridation is widespread in the United States, Australia and New Zealand but still unusual in Scandinavia and The Netherlands. In Britain only about 10% of the population receive fluoridated water. Dental caries has nevertheless become less prevalent in most industrialised countries. Most toothpastes now contain fluoride and this, rather than any change in children's sugar consumption, seems the main reason for the decline where water is not fluoridated. A controlled study in the north of England found 44% less caries in 5 year olds in 1991-94 in towns with a fluoridated water supply.[2]

Mottling of the (anterior permanent) teeth occurs if the fluoride intake is too high in the first eight years of life. Young children should either be persuaded not to swallow their toothpaste or be provided with a "junior" product with half-strength fluoride.

## Gallstones

Most gallstones are composed mainly (about 85%) of crystallised cholesterol with small proportions of calcium carbonate, palmitate, and phosphate. Cholesterol, which is excreted by the liver into the bile, would be completely insoluble in an aqueous fluid like bile if it were not kept in micelle microemulsion by the combined detergent action of the bile salts and phospholipids (chiefly lecithin) in bile.

Non-dietary risk factors include female sex, pregnancy, oral contraceptives, age, ileal disease, clofibrate therapy, and certain

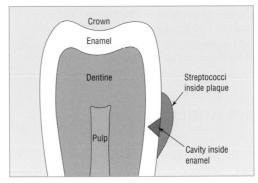

Dental caries

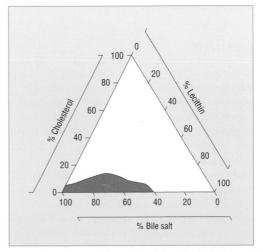

The shaded bars show what happened to the number of decayed temporary teeth in Kilmarnock after fluoridation of water, which started in 1956 and was discontinued in 1962. Unshaded bars are findings in Ayr, which never had fluoridated water.[1] Figures for children aged 5 years

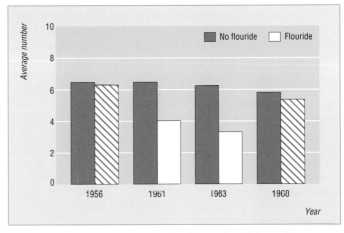

Three major components of bile (bile salts, lecithin, and cholesterol) on triangular coordinates. Each component is expressed as percentage moles of total bile salt, lecithin, and cholesterol. The shaded area shows conditions required for cholesterol to be soluble in micellar form. If the concentration of cholesterol goes up or bile acids or lecithin go down then cholesterol is likely to precipitate out[3]

ethnic groups—for example, Pima Amerindians have a high incidence of gallstones.

In obesity and during dieting (with rapid weight loss) cholesterol secretion into bile tends to increase. During fasting and on total parenteral nutrition the gall bladder does not contract normally. In people on vegetarian and high cereal fibre diets the pattern of biliary bile acids change favourably, with less deoxycholate and more chenodeoxycholate.[4] Moderate alcohol intake appears to be protective; decreased cholesterol saturation of bile has been reported. Regular exercise also appears to protect against gallstones [5]

These associations do not apply to the less common pigment stones.

---

**Gallstone formation**

Gallstones are more likely to form if:
- biliary cholesterol is increased, *or*
- biliary bile acids are reduced, *or*
- the gall bladder is less motile, *or*
- factors in the bile favour nucleation of cholesterol crystals.

---

# Urinary tract stones

## Calcium stones

Dietary factors which tend to increase urinary calcium or have been associated with stones are high intakes of protein, sodium, refined carbohydrate, vitamin D, calcium (spread over the day), alcohol, curry, spicy foods, and Worcester sauce, and low intakes of cereal fibre and water. Since most patients with hypercalciuria have intestinal hyperabsorption of calcium it has been common to recommend a low calcium diet or phytic acid or a resin to reduce calcium absorption. Long term trials have been lacking. Now a diet providing usual calcium intake (1200 mg/day) but very low salt (50 mmol Na/day) and reduced animal protein (50 g/day) has reduced calcium stone recurrences significantly over five years compared with a low calcium diet (400 mg/day).[6] The normal calcium, low protein, low salt diet reduced urinary excretion of both calcium and oxalate.

## Oxalate stones

Associated dietary factors are high intakes of oxalate or vitamin C and low water intake.

---

**Foods rich in oxalate**

**Spinach, rhubarb, beetroots, cocoa, chocolate, currants, dried figs, tea, swiss chard, blackberries, oranges, turnip greens.**

---

## Uric acid stones

Uric acid stones are associated with an acid urine, a high purine diet, and low water consumption.

The one common dietary association with all the common types of stone—and with the rare ones also—is a low water intake. Drinking plenty of water is an important habit for anyone liable to stones, especially if the weather is hot. Last thing at night is the important time to take water.

---

**Uric acid stones**

- One dietary cause of acid urine is a high protein intake. The amino acids methionine and cystine are metabolised to urinary sulphuric acid.
- Foods traditionally rich in purines include liver, kidneys, sweetbreads, sardines, anchovies, fish roes, and yeast extracts, but there are no modern tables and dietary RNA may raise plasma urate more than DNA.

---

# Diabetes mellitus

Insulin-dependent diabetes (Type 1) is usually caused by autoimmune damage to the $\beta$-cells in the pancreatic islets, which lose their ability to secrete enough insulin. This type of diabetes typically starts in adolescents or younger adults. Several epidemiological studies have reported that patients with type 1 diabetes were less often exclusively breast fed for the first 3-4 months of life than unaffected controls.

The prevalence of non-insulin dependent diabetes (Type 2) increases with age; overall it is about six times more common than Type 1. This type 2 diabetes is closely associated with overweight or obesity and with lack of exercise. Beyond Europe and Anglo-Celtic north Americans there is almost a pandemic of type 2 diabetes occurring in some communities that may have earlier experienced undernutrition but are now sedentary and eating refined, high energy "Western" foods. The thrifty genotype hypothesis attempts to explain this phenomenon, which is especially affecting people of south Asian descent in

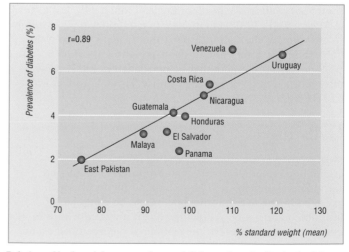

Relation of body weight to prevalence of diabetes (standardised criteria) between countries[7]

Britain and elsewhere, Pacific islanders, and north American and Australian aboriginals.[8]

Looked at another way, diabetes is the complication of **obesity** whose incidence goes up at the steepest gradient with degree of overweight. The risk of developing diabetes is greater in people whose obesity is mainly intra-abdominal rather than on the hips or buttocks (subcutaneous)—people with a high ratio of waist:hip circumferences.[9]

Diabetes is a multifactorial disease. There is a strong family influence, though this may be partly because eating habits and body weight are influenced by family behaviour. But a **genetic** factor is clear in some groups: the Pima Amerindians in North America and Micronesians in Nauru. When these people are obese (which most of them are these days) the incidence of diabetes (in older life) is over 50%.

The popular belief that eating a lot of sugar predisposes to diabetes is not confirmed by several epidemiological and prospective studies. High fat intake is more likely to lead to diabetes, a hypothesis first put forward in Britain in 1935 by Sir Harold Himsworth. High total carbohydrate (mostly starch) and high fibre intakes are characteristic of peasant communities, in which type 2 diabetes is uncommon.

In a **prospective study** of 7735 middle-aged men, drawn from group practices in 24 towns in England, Wales, and Scotland and followed for 12 years, the incidence was 2 per 1000 person years.[11] The risk of developing diabetes increased exponentially with increasing body mass index (BMI). It was 11 times higher in the upper fifth of BMI ($>28\,kg/m^2$). Men with moderate physical activity had less than half the risk. Moderate drinkers also developed less diabetes. On average those who developed diabetes had higher plasma triglycerides, higher blood pressures and higher casual blood glucose. Another finding in people who will later develop type 2 diabetes has been an increased fasting insulin and/or insulin response to standard glycaemic stimulus, due to insulin resistance.

Diets for managing established diabetes are discussed in chapter 13.

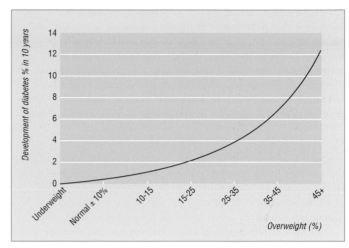

Relation of body weight to subsequent development of diabetes in 10 years[10]

Two large *randomised controlled trials*, one in 27 centres in the United States,[12] the other in five cities in Finland[13] have both shown that lifestyle intervention can halve the incidence of type 2 diabetes in middle-aged, overweight, sedentary people with impaired glucose tolerance. In the US trial lifestyle intervention was weight reduction averaging 6 kg and increased physical activity. This was more effective in preventing diabetes than metformin. In Finland the subjects were also asked to reduce saturated fat and increase whole grain foods.

# Alcoholic liver disease

Countries with high alcohol consumption per head have high mortalities from cirrhosis. These have fallen when there has been a reduction in the supply of alcohol—for example, during prohibition in the United States and during the two world wars in Europe. Correlation of alcohol consumption and deaths from cirrhosis between countries is close, but there are deviations. Britain has a lower incidence of cirrhosis than might be expected from the rate of alcohol consumption but mortality from cirrhosis has doubled here since 1970. Where alcohol consumption is high most cases of cirrhosis are due to alcohol. Other causes—for example, viral hepatitis B or C, account for important proportions of cases.

In heavy drinkers pre-cirrhotic liver disease—fatty liver or alcoholic hepatitis—is more common than cirrhosis. A fourth condition, primary liver cell cancer, is a complication of alcoholic cirrhosis.

Within countries the risk of developing cirrhosis is related to the dose and duration of alcohol intake. Daily heavy drinking for years is the typical pattern—80 g (eight drinks) a day in men, and usually well over this. In a large Italian study, cirrhosis appeared to be less likely in those who drank only with meals.[15]

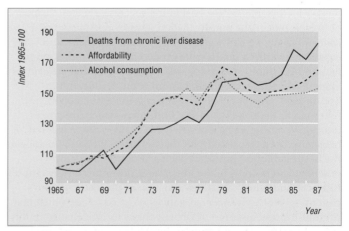

Alcohol affordability and consumption and deaths from cirrhosis in the United Kingdom, 1965-87. As alcohol became more affordable, consumption of alcohol and harm related to alcohol increased[14]

The essential treatment of alcoholic liver disease is complete and permanent abstinence from alcohol. Although alcoholics may become deficient in nutrients, those who develop cirrhosis are often socially organised and well nourished. There is no evidence that a high protein diet or choline can prevent alcoholic cirrhosis in man. Even when cirrhosis is established, an improved clinical state and prognosis may be expected in those who manage to abstain completely.

> No precise safe level of alcohol intake can be given—only a clinical impression—because people who drink heavily underestimate their consumption when asked about it, and no prospective epidemiological study has been done. Women are more susceptible to hepatic damage from alcohol because they have smaller livers (where most metabolism of alcohol occurs) and also lower rates of gastric (first pass) oxidation of alcohol than men.[16] Only a minority of heavy drinkers get cirrhosis; there is presumably a synergy between alcohol and hepatitis viruses.

## Some types of cancer[17]

Differences in diets are thought to account for more variation in the incidence of all cancers than any other factor (with smoking in second order).[18] The big questions are which dietary components are active, and how do they work? Our bodies have three routes of entry for foreign compounds: the skin, lungs, and intestines. As a function of surface area the chances of absorption are skin 1, lungs 1000, and intestines 1 000 000. There are countless natural non-nutrient substances in foods and several are mutagens. The fact that they can induce mutations in a standard bacterial culture does not, however, establish that they are dangerous to man: there are many available protective mechanisms.

Poor diet may have a more decisive effect by weakening defence mechanisms than by supplying potent carcinogens. Epidemiologists estimate that synthetic chemical additives in food account for under 1% of all cancers.[18] The cancers most clearly related to habitual diet are oesophageal, gastric, and large intestinal cancers.

### Oesophagus

In the Chinese focus of oesophageal cancer, nitrosamines have been found in mouldy food and there is a deficiency of molybdenum. Domestic fowl are affected too. In the Iranian focus there are some vitamin deficiencies and people may take opium by mouth. In the Transkei researchers think that fusarium mycotoxins, together with deficiencies of niacin, zinc, and other micronutrients, are responsible for the epidemic of oesophageal cancer. In Europe alcohol, especially that derived from apples, and tobacco are associated factors.

### Stomach

From present epidemiological data protective factors are fruits and vegetables, refrigeration of foods and vitamin C intake. Apparent causative factors are intake of salt, pickled and salted foods, *Helicobacter pylori* infection, and smoking.

### Large intestine

Cancer of the large intestine usually arises in a polyp. Different dietary factors may be involved in the successive stages: formation of polyps; malignant transformation; growth and spread of a cancer. Having a halfway stage of polyps should make study of causative factors easier. In some epidemiological studies animal fat and meat have emerged as risk factors. But in the majority of epidemiological studies meat has not been significantly associated.[20] One possible mechanism is the formation of heterocyclic amines (1Q, MelQ, PhIP, etc.), which are potent mutagens, on the surface of well-cooked meat. Some types of beer have been associated with rectal cancer. Wheat fibre appears the best established protective factor. It dilutes and moves on potential carcinogens in the lumen and promotes fermentation. Brassicas and other vegetables also appear protective; they contain several anticancer substances and also folate, which may prevent hypomethylation of DNA, a characteristic change in this cancer. In a trial wheat bran plus low fat prevented polyp development. $\beta$-Carotene or vitamin E ($\alpha$-tocopherol) have been ineffective; other prevention trials are underway.

---

**Oesophageal cancer**

- 300× range in incidence
- Highest rates: Linxian, People's Republic of China; East Mazandaran, Iran; and Transkei, South Africa.
- In Europe there are moderately high rates in NW France and in Switzerland.

---

**Gastric cancer**

- Incidence in Britain has spontaneously fallen to half in the past 25 years.
- There have been similar reductions in many developed countries.[19]
- Highest rates, in Japan, are three times those in England and Wales, 10 times those in the United States of America, 20 times those in countries with the lowest rate, for example Gambia and Kuwait.
- Chronic atrophic gastritis is a precancerous state.

---

**Cancer of the large bowel**

- Fourth largest cause of death from cancer in Britain (after lung cancer, breast cancer in women, and prostate cancer in men).
- Ten times more common in developed Western countries such as Britain and USA than in the Third World.
- Rates in Scotland have been among the highest in world
- Epidemiology of rectal cancer shows some minor differences from the larger group of colon cancer.
- Left side of the large bowel is usually affected.

## Breast

Between-country comparisons and animal experiments suggest that high fat intake increases the risk of breast cancer but prospective and case-control epidemiological studies have not confirmed a role for fat, unless it operates in childhood or adolescence. Weight gain in adult life increases the risk of postmenopausal breast cancer. Adipose tissue is a major source of oestrogen after the menopause. Alcohol consumption also shows some association but this is not dose related. Plant foods appear protective. The two most promising of these are wheat fibre (which can bind oestrogens in the bowel, reducing reabsorption) and soya (which contains phytoestrogens, isoflavones).

### Breast cancer

In countries with a high incidence the majority of cases are postmenopausal. Incidences are four times higher in western Europe and North America than in East Asia. Early menarche and/or late menopause increase the risk; bilateral oophorectomy protects, and endogenous plasma oestrogens are higher in patients with postmenopausal breast cancer.

## References

1 Department of Health & Social Security. *The fluoridation studies in the United Kingdom and the results achieved after eleven years.* London: HMSO, 1969 (Reports on Public Health & Medical Subjects no 122).

2 Jones CM, Taylor GO, Whittle JG, Evans D, Trotter DP. Water fluoridation, tooth decay in 5 year olds, and social deprivation measured by the Jarman score: analysis of data from British dental surveys. *BMJ* 1997; **315**: 514-17.

3 Small DM. Gallstones. *N Engl J Med* 1968; **279**: 588-93.

4 Low-Beer TS. How the colon begets gallstones. *Lancet* 1998; **351**: 612-13.

5 Vega KJ, Johnston DE. Exercise and the gallbladder. *N Engl J Med* 1999; **341**: 836-7.

6 Borghi L, Schianchi T, Meschi T *et al.* Comparison of two diets for the prevention of recurrent stones in idiopathic hypercalciuria. *N Engl J Med* 2002; **346**: 77-84.

7 West KM, Kalbfleisch JM. Influence of nutritional factors on prevalence of diabetes. *Diabetes* 1971; **20**: 99-108.

8 Report of a WHO Study Group. *Prevention of diabetes mellitus.* WHO Tech Rep Ser 844. Geneva: WHO, 1994.

9 Ohlson LO, Larsson B, Svarsudd K *et al.* The influence of body fat distribution on the incidence of diabetes mellitus. 13.5 years of follow up of the participants in the study of men born in 1913. *Diabetes* 1985; **34**: 1055-8.

10 Westlund K, Nicolayson R. Ten year mortality and morbidity related to serum cholesterol. *Scand J Clin Lab Invest* 1972; **30**: 3-24.

11 Perry IJ, Wannamethee SG, Walker MK, Thomson AG, Whincup PH, Shaper AG. Prospective study of risk factors for development of non-insulin dependent diabetes in middle aged British men. *BMJ* 1995; **310**: 560-4.

12 Diabetes Prevention Program Research Group. Reduction in the incidence of type 2 diabetes with lifestyle intervention or metformin. *N Engl J Med* 2002; **346**: 393-403.

13 Tuomilehto J, Lindström J, Eriksson JG *et al.* Prevention of type 2 diabetes mellitus by changes in lifestyle among subjects with impaired glucose tolerance. *N Engl J Med* 2001; **344**: 1343-50.

14 Department of Health. *On the state of the public health for the year 1988.* London: HMSO, 1989, fig 2.1.

15 Bellantani S, Saccoccio G, Costa G *et al.* Drinking habits as cofactors of risk for alcohol induced liver damage. *Gut* 1997; **41**: 845-50.

16 Frezza M, di Padova C, Pozzato G. High blood alcohol levels in women. The role of decreased alcohol dehydrogenase activity and first pass metabolism. *N Engl J Med* 1990; **322**: 95-9.

17 Department of Health. Nutritional aspects of the development of cancer. *Report of the Working Group on Diet and Cancer of the Committee on Medical Aspects of Food and Nutrition Policy.* The Stationery Office, 1998.

18 Doll R, Peto R. The causes of cancer: qualitative estimates of avoidable risks of cancer in the United States today. *J Natl Cancer Inst* 1981; **66**: 1191-308.

19 Howson CD, Jiyama T, Wynder EL. The decline in gastric cancer: epidemiology of an unplanned triumph. *Epidemiol Rev* 1986; **8**: 1-27.

20 Truswell AS. Meat consumption and cancer of the large bowel. *Eur J Clin Nutr* 2002; **56** suppl 1: 19-24S.

# 4 Nutrition for pregnancy

Pregnancy is a time when appetite is altered and nutritional needs change. What the expectant mother eats or drinks can affect her baby's health and her own comfort. In pregnancy women develop a new interest in the consequences for health of what they eat. They are entitled to advice from their doctors.

The first advice should ideally be communicated before pregnancy, when a woman decides to try to have a baby. Pregnancies in women who are overweight, have anorexia nervosa, or whose growth is not completed are more difficult, and these women need extra nutritional care.

A good intake of folate is important in preventing neural tube defects and some other malformations in the fetus of a minority of women. The stage when this vitamin is most needed is the first 28 days after conception so supplementation or high folate diet has to be periconceptional. The supplement dose is 400 or 500 µg/day. Likewise, it is the early weeks when excess alcohol intake may lead to malformations.

During pregnancy extra nutrients are required, especially from 20 weeks, for the growing fetus and for the placenta. Tissue is also laid down in the uterus and breasts, blood volume is increased, and, in healthy women with adequate food, adipose tissue increases by around 2.7 kg. This fat is deposited more on the hips and thighs.

## Folate and neural tube defects

- Folate is the most important nutrient for replication of DNA in cell division. Evidence for the role of folic acid in preventing neural tube defects (NTDs) has been accumulating for 50 years. The folate antagonist aminopterin, taken in pregnancy, led to NTDs.
- Lower biochemical folate levels in women who gave birth to babies with NTD were reported in 1975 and 1976. The first secondary prevention trials (reported in 1980) were encouraging but not randomised. So the MRC conducted a large randomised double-blind trial in seven countries and found that folic acid could prevent three-quarters of recurrences.[2] Other epidemiological studies are supportive and so is a primary prevention trial in Hungary.[3] Evidently at the time of closure of the neural tube there is extra demand for folate for cell division and in some pregnancies on ordinary diets the level of folate at the site is inadequate.

## Nutrition for pregnancy

The extra energy need for a pregnancy can be calculated as about 250 MJ (60 000 kcal).[6] This includes energy stored in fetal fat and protein, and in maternal reproductive tissues and adipose tissue. It takes account of the mother's increased basal metabolic rate and the energy needed to move a heavier body. This corresponds to 1 MJ (240 kcal) a day (excluding the first month, for 250 days), and in Britain the recommended daily intake of energy during pregnancy (10 MJ, 2400 kcal) until 1991 was 1 MJ (240 kcal) above the non-pregnant amount (9 MJ or 2150 kcal). When actual food intakes are carefully measured, however, little indication exists of extra energy intake in Western women. This was found in careful intake measurements in London, Cambridge, Aberdeen, Glasgow,[7] Wageningen, and Sydney. In all these centres women ate an average of almost 9 MJ (2150 kcal) per day. The extra energy need is probably balanced by decreased exercise and increased

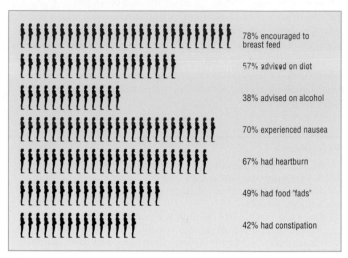

BBC television survey of 6000 women, 1982[1]

## Alcohol in pregnancy[4]

- Heavy drinkers have a greatly increased risk of inducing the fetal alcohol syndrome—characteristic underdevelopment of the mid face, small size, and mental retardation.
- Women who intend to become pregnant should not sit drinking whatever the occasion: they could be two or three weeks pregnant.
- Once pregnancy is established the rule should be no more than one alcoholic drink a day to be sure of preventing minor effects, chiefly growth retardation.

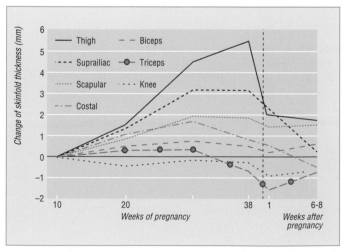

Changes in skinfold thickness at different sites during pregnancy[5]

efficiency of metabolism. Pregnant women seem to reduce their exercise if they can. Postprandial cholecystokinin concentrations increase, which enhances nutrient absorption and the anabolic actions of insulin.[8] So it is not true that a pregnant woman has to eat calories for two, but a few nutrients should be substantially increased. In 1991 the Department of Health revised the estimated average extra requirement of energy in pregnancy to 0.8 MJ (200 kcal) a day and this is only for the third trimester.[9] However, in a developing country like rural Thailand,[6] where pre-pregnant food intake may be marginally adequate and women are involved in agricultural labour, food intake may—and should—increase in pregnancy.

The amounts of different nutrients which the mother has to put into her fetus by the time of delivery have been worked out by chemical analysis of stillbirths. These can be estimated more accurately for stable inorganic elements than for the vitamins. From these figures for nutrients accumulated and from information on whether there is any change in their absorption and turnover, the extra requirements for pregnancy can be estimated.

The metabolism of protein is more efficient and so is the absorption of iron in pregnancy. For most nutrients like **protein** the small extra amounts required are covered adequately by a normal diet. But intakes are more critical for the other five nutrients in the table showing recommended daily intakes.

### Recommended daily intakes* for six critical nutrients in pregnancy[10]

| | Addition for pregnancy | Non-pregnant women | Total |
|---|---|---|---|
| Protein (g) | +10 | 50 | 60 |
| Folate (µg total folate) | +220 | 180 | 400 |
| Calcium (mg) | +400 | 800 | 1200 |
| Iron (mg) | +15 | 15 | 30 |
| Zinc (mg) | +3 | 12 | 15 |
| Iodine (µg) | +25 | 150 | 175 |

*United States recommended dietary allowances, 1989

**Folate** is the only vitamin, and iron the only nutrient element whose requirements double in pregnancy. Extra folate is needed for the first month and again for the last trimester. Serum and red cell folate concentrations decline in pregnancy and, if looked for, some degree of megaloblastic change can be found in substantial minorities of women in late pregnancy. Such changes have been reported in 6-25% of women not taking supplements in Britain. The word folate comes from the Latin *folia* (leaf) because it was first found in spinach, but food sources are not the same as for vitamin C. Whole grain cereals, nuts, and legumes are good sources of folate. The folate content of vegetables varies from about 10 µg/100 g in potatoes and carrots up to 155 µg in asparagus, averaging round 50 µg per 100 g. Fruits average round 5 µg per 100, citrus and blackberries higher. The vitamin is largely destroyed by prolonged boiling.

The **iron** content of the fetus (about 300 mg), placenta (50 mg), and average postpartum blood loss (200 mg) add up to some 550 mg. The red cell mass also increases after 12 weeks by an amount which corresponds to about another 500 mg of iron, but this is a temporary internal borrowing from stores and causes no extra demand provided the stores are sufficient. Against these extra needs there is the saving from no menstruation (some 200 mg) and improved intestinal absorption. Maternal haemoglobin concentration declines by about 10% because of physiological haemodilution; and serum

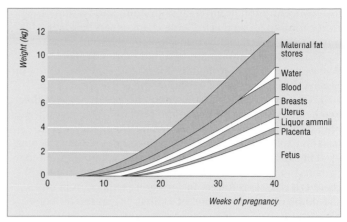

Contributions to weight gain in average pregnancy

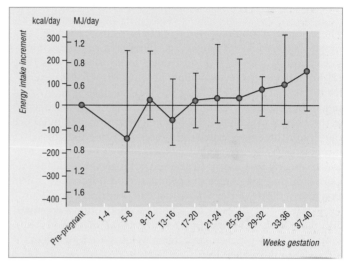

Energy intake increments (and confidence limits) for 71 Glasgow women throughout pregnancy[7]

### Contribution of food groups to total folate content per head, Great Britain 1998[3]

- Vegetables 32%, of which potatoes 10%
- Cereals 32%, of which bread 11%*, breakfast cereals 14%*
- Milk and products 10%
- Fruit 7%
- Meat 5%
- Tea 4%
- Eggs 2%

*A significant proportion of the folate from cereals comes from fortification. In general the folic acid used for food fortification is more biologically available than naturally occurring folate.

### Iron in pregnancy

There is no universal policy. Some doctors are more interventionist than others. Iron tablets can cause indigestion or constipation. The following is generally agreed.

- Women should be advised to eat meat regularly (unless vegetarian). This is the best absorbed source of iron in the diet.
- A woman with a history of anaemia, menorrhagia, poor diet, or repeated pregnancies should be given iron supplements or an iron-folate preparation.
- Haemoglobin should be checked and iron given if it is below 110 g/l (with a low mean cell volume).
- For prophylactic purposes one iron tablet a day is adequate.
- With the smaller dose of iron, side effects are fewer and compliance should be better.

iron concentration, transferrin saturation, and ferritin concentration all go down. These changes can be partly—but only partly—prevented by iron supplementation.

With **calcium**, absorption becomes more efficient.[11] Without any change of vitamin D intake or exposure to the sun, plasma concentrations of calcitriol (the active form of the vitamin converted in the kidney) are increased. Some of this extra conversion takes place in the placenta. The easiest way of obtaining the extra calcium needed for pregnancy and lactation is from milk; 0.5 litre supplies about 600 mg calcium.

The increased need for **iodine** may be taken for granted in Britain, but in areas where goitre is endemic (see chapter 8) there is a risk of cretinism. In such areas expectant mothers should be given an injection of iodised oil, preferably before conception.

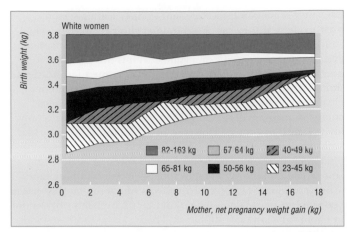

Birth weight is related positively to amount of maternal weight gain and to pre-pregnancy weight of the mother[13]

## Weight gain

The amount of weight gained from before conception to shortly before delivery ranges considerably in normal women—from about 6 to 24 kg. A good average to try to achieve is 12 kg (26 lb). This might be made up of about 115 g (1/4 lb)/week for the first 10 weeks and 300 g (2/3 lb)/week for the remaining 30 weeks. A mother's height, her weight for height at the start of pregnancy, and her weight gain can all influence the size of the fetus. Birth weights are lower in babies of mothers who choose (against medical advice) to continue to smoke during pregnancy. In affluent countries the body fat gained during pregnancy can persist after childbirth. Pregnancy is one of the factors that can predispose to obesity.[12]

In Third World countries, where mothers often start small and thin and gain little weight because of restricted and bulky food, and heavy physical work, birth weights are lower than in affluent communities. They have been increased, in controlled trials, by providing food (energy) supplements during pregnancy. Average gains of birth weight in eight different trials have been from 40 to 300 g.

Obesity in pregnancy increases the chances of a heavier and fatter baby and also of hypertension and gestational diabetes. Since 3 to 4 kg of the usual 12 kg weight gain is fat, overweight women should try to put on only 7 to 8 kg overall during their pregnancy.

## Hypertension and "toxaemia"

In pregnancy-induced hypertension (toxaemia) no excess of sodium is retained. It is proportional to the fluid retained. No evidence exists that either a high or a low salt diet predisposes to pregnancy-induced hypertension or that any other dietary component—energy, protein, or any micronutrient—is directly responsible, except perhaps calcium deficiency.[14]

## Diet and discomforts of pregnancy

**Nausea and vomiting of pregnancy** (NVP) is not confined to the mornings (so "morning sickness" is a misleading name). It is probably due to rising levels of pregnancy-associated hormones and often accompanied by increased olfactory sensitivity and aversion to strongly flavoured food and drink. In developed countries normal NVP appears to be beneficial, not detrimental to the fetus.[19] There has been no controlled trial of simple management. One opinion is that it is related to a low blood glucose concentration and that a dry biscuit or similar light snack before getting up may help. It now seems

### The Barker hypothesis

- Professor David Barker (Southampton) found very good birth weight records in Hertfordshire for 1911-30 and was able to trace health records of most of this cohort in later life. Coronary heart disease (CHD) mortality was higher in those who had had low birth weights (at term).[15]
- The large US Nurses prospective study provides good supportive evidence (birth weights here were by recall).[16] Low birth weight, reflecting subnormal intrauterine growth, can only influence CHD incidence if there are risk factors for CHD in adult life (chapter 1). Low birth weights have also been reported to be followed in middle age by hypertension and type 2 diabetes.
- All these discoveries emphasise the importance of good nutrition in young women before and during pregnancy. But this does **not** mean that women who enter pregnancy with a body mass index over 26 need to "eat for two"![17]
- In Britain little or no relation has been found between nutrient intakes in pregnancy and birth weight.[18]

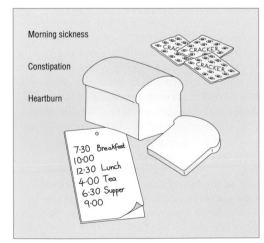

Diet and discomforts of pregnancy

possible that the increased cholecystokinin concentration could explain the symptoms. Unlike other conditions that cause nausea, women tend to put on weight during the phase of morning sickness.[8] Severe, persistent NVP, hyperemesis gravidarum is uncommon. When it occurs, note that thiamin is the most critical micronutrient.[20]

**Constipation** and its complication haemorrhoids are very common in pregnancy. All pregnant women should be advised to eat more wholemeal bread, bran, or bran cereals to loosen and increase the bulk of their faeces.

**Heartburn** should improve if the woman eats smaller meals and avoids foods which she finds indigestible. The common meal pattern of tiny breakfast, small lunch, and large dinner becomes unsuitable in late pregnancy. It is a good plan for her to have four, five, or even six small meals throughout the day. This also helps NVP.

**Cravings and aversions**—at some stage in pregnancy most women experience a distortion of their usual range of likes and dislikes of foods. Women may develop a nine-month aversion to foods they usually like—for example, fried foods, coffee, tea. Contrariwise and at the same time they may experience a craving for certain foods. These are often sweet foods, such as fruits and chocolate ice cream, and sometimes salty, but some remarkable non-foods—coal, soap, soil—have been recorded.

**Vegetarians** who are pregnant may need extra dietary advice. There are several types of vegetarian (chapter 7). Those most at risk are vegans. It is essential for them to take a supplement of vitamin B-12 for normal cerebral development of the fetus. Other lacto-ovo vegetarians, especially if they are prosperous and belong to a traditional vegetarian group, usually manage well enough but may want or need advice to optimise their protein and iron intakes. Legumes and nuts are an important part of a balanced vegetarian diet.

---

**Food safety in pregnancy**

- Avoid unpasteurised milk, soft cheeses and paté, raw eggs—danger of listeria and salmonella infection is more serious in pregnancy.
- Pre-cooked foods (for example, pies) should be thoroughly re-heated before eating.
- Avoid extra vitamin A, in the form of supplements or multivitamins containing vitamin A, or liver more than occasionally in early pregnancy. Retinoic acid is involved in normal morphogenesis and excess can be teratogenic.

---

**What are pregnant women thinking about their food?**

- "Eating the right foods", for example plenty of meat, fish, eggs, milk and fresh vegetables
- "Watching weight", taking care how much weight is gained
- "Eating for two", a largely outmoded idea

Based on Baric and MacArthur, cited by Anderson[21]

---

## References

1 Boyd C, Sellars L. *The British way of birth*. London: Pan, 1982.
2 MRC Vitamin Study Research Group. Prevention of neural tube defects: results of Medical Research Council vitamin study. *Lancet* 1991; **338**: 131-7.
3 Department of Health. *Folic Acid and the prevention of disease*. Report of the Committee on Medical Aspects of Food and Nutrition Policy. London: Stationery Office, 2000.
4 Forrest F, Florey du VC. The relation between maternal alcohol consumption and child development: the epidemiological evidence. *J Publ Health Med* 1991; **13**: 247-55. [Review by members of the Dundee prospective team.]
5 Taggart NR, Holliday RM, Billewicz WZ, Hytten FE, Thomson AM. Changes in skinfolds during pregnancy. *Br J Nutr* 1967; **21**: 439-51.
6 Durnin JVGA. Energy requirements of pregnancy: an integration of the longitudinal data from the five country study. *Lancet* 1987; **ii**: 1131-3.
7 Durnin JVGA, McKillop FM, Grant S, Fitzgerald G. Energy requirements of pregnancy in Scotland. *Lancet* 1987; **ii**: 897-900.
8 Unväs-Moberg K. The gastrointestinal tract in growth and reproduction. *Sci Am* 1989; **July**: 60-5.
9 Department of Health. *Dietary Reference Values for Food Energy and Nutrients for the United Kingdom*. Report of the Panel on Dietary Reference Values of the Committee on Medical Aspects of Food Policy. London: HMSO, 1991.
10 Subcommittee on the 10th edition of the Recommended Dietary Allowances, Food and Nutrition Board, National Research Council. *Recommended dietary allowances*. 10th edn. Washington, DC: National Academy Press, 1989.
11 Prentice A. Calcium in pregnancy and lactation. *Annu Rev Nutr* 2000; **20**: 249-72.
12 Harris HE, Ellison GTH. Do the changes in energy balance that occur during pregnancy predispose parous women to obesity? *Nutr Res Rev* 1997; **10**: 57-81.
13 Naeye RL. In: Dobbing J, ed. *Maternal nutrition: eating for two?* London: Academic, 1981.
14 Bucher HC, Guyatt GH, Cook RJ *et al.* Effect of calcium supplementation on pregnancy induced hypertension and pre-eclampsia: a meta-analysis of randomised controlled trials. *JAMA* 1996; **275**: 7113-17.
15 Barker DJP. *Mothers, Babies and Diseases in Later Life*. London: BMJ Books, 1994.
16 Rich-Edwards JW, Stampfer MJ, Manson JAE *et al.* Birth weight and risk of cardiovascular disease in a cohort of women followed up since 1976. *BMJ* 1997; **315**: 396-400.
17 Fraser R, Cresswell J. What should obstetricians be doing about the Barker hypothesis? *Br J Obstet Gynecol* 1997; **104**: 645-7.
18 Matthews F, Yudkin P, Neil A. Influence of maternal nutrition on outcome of pregnancy: prospective cohort study. *BMJ* 1999; **319**: 339-43, and subsequent correspondence 2000, **320**: 941-2.
19 Pirisi A. Meaning of morning sickness still unsettled. *Lancet* 2001; **357**: 1272.
20 Tesfaye S, Achari V, Yang YC, Harding S, Bowden A, Vora JP. Pregnant, vomiting and going blind. *Lancet* 1998; **352**: 1594.
21 Anderson AS. Pregnancy as a time for dietary change? *Proc Nutrition Soc* 2001; **60**: 497-504.

# 5 Infant feeding

Infant feeding is the dominant nutritional interest in less affluent countries and it gets much attention in Western countries because infants depend on others to feed them. For their first few months babies are fed only one food, so its composition is much more critical than the compositions of the many different foods in a mixed diet. Babies cannot eat ordinary adult food or say how they feel after the feed. Though there are still many questions, scientific knowledge is perhaps fuller about nutrition for this age of man than any other.

## Breast or bottle?

For the first 4-6 months of life the infant should be fed either by breast feeding or on a formula based on cows' milk modified to make its composition suitable for infants—that is, more like breast milk. The decision on which method to use should be made well before delivery, and it should be made by the mother. The doctor's role is to give advice to help her make up her mind and then, whichever method she wants to use, to provide support and arrange instruction.

### Advantages of breast feeding

- Breast feeding is natural and may confer advantages that science has not yet discovered.
- Breast milk is microbiologically clean.
- Breast milk's nutrient composition is the standard against which infant formulas for bottle feeding must be judged. Many of the differences between cows' and human milk have been minimised in modern infant formulas, but by no means all and some nutrients such as iron and zinc are known to be better absorbed from human milk.
- Only breast milk provides a complex range of anti-infective components: macrophages, lymphocytes, immunoglobulins (especially IgA), lactoferrin, lysozyme, complement, interferon, oligosaccharides (for example, bifidus factor), sialic acid, xanthine oxidase, gangliosides, glycoconjugates, growth factors, and enzymes.
- Breast feeding reduces the risk of gastrointestinal, respiratory and other infections (otitis media, meningitis, urinary tract infections), SIDS, childhood lymphomas, early allergic diseases, and type 1 diabetes.
- For most women breast feeding is a satisfying, convenient and enjoyable experience that is beneficial to the mother-child relationship.
- Mothers' milk is always at the right temperature.
- A mother can always change from breast to bottle feeding but not the other way round.

Breast feeding is recommended by the UK Department of Health, the WHO, the American Academy of Pediatrics and all authorities. The organisation of maternity wards (encouraged by UNICEF's Baby Friendly Hospital Initiative), control of advertising watched by WHO's Code of Marketing Breast Milk Substitutes, and change of social attitudes all make it easier than it used to be. On the other hand, modern technology makes bottle feeding easy and safe in developed countries and the newer infant formulas are closer to breast milk in nutrient composition.

> Breastfeeding from a woman who is in good health and nutritional status provides a complete food, which is unique to the species. There is no better nutrition for healthy infants at term and during the early months of life.... Breast feeding is preferable to feeding with infant formulas and should be encouraged.
> DHSS[5]

**Composition of cows' milk compared with human milk and a modified infant formula (breast milk substitute) (All per 100 ml)**

| | Human* (mature)[1,2] | Cows' (full cream) (unfortified) | A modified milk formula† (powder diluted as directed) |
|---|---|---|---|
| Energy (kcal) | 70 | 67 | 67 |
| Protein (total) (g) | 1.1 | 3.5 | 1.5 |
| Casein (% protein) | 40% | 80% | 40% |
| Carbohydrate (g) | 7.4 | 5.0 | 7.2 |
| Fat (total) (g) | 4.2 | 3.7 | 3.6 |
| Saturated fat (% fat) | 46% | 66% | 44% |
| Linoleic (% fat) | 7-11% | 3% | 17% |
| Sodium (mmol) | 0.6 | 2.2 | 0.71 |
| Calcium (mg) | 35 | 120 | 49 |
| Phosphorus (mg) | 15 | 95 | 28 |
| Iron (mg) | 0.075 | 0.050 | 0.8 |
| Vitamin C (mg) | 3.8 | 1.5 | 6.9 |
| Vitamin D ($\mu$g) | 0.8 | 0.15 | 1.1 |

\* The composition of breast milk varies considerably with stage of lactation, between individuals, and with maternal nutrition
† Mean of Cow and Gate Premium and SMA Gold Cap

> In Third World countries breast feeding unquestionably reduces infant mortality.
>
> In affluent countries, however, epidemiologists have difficulty in showing an appreciable reduction in mortality when confounding factors are taken into account. Mothers who breast feed tend to have higher educational and income levels. A well designed study in Dundee seems to have corrected for all such confounding variables. It showed that breast feeding for the first three months of life confers a protection against gastrointestinal illness, which persists beyond the period of breast feeding itself.[3,4]

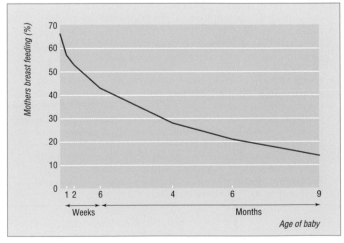

Prevalence of breast feeding in Great Britain, 1995[6]

### Two examples of ongoing research about human milk

*Docosahexaenoic acid (DHA)*

The brain grows rapidly in infancy, from 350 g at birth to 1000 g at 12 months. Sixty per cent of its solids are lipids and two very long chain polyunsaturated fatty acids are more abundant here and in the photoreceptors of the retina than elsewhere—DHA (22:6, ω-3) and AA (arachidonic, 20:4, ω-6). DHA is present in human, not cows' milk. It is synthesised in the body from α-linolenic (18:3, ω-3) but probably not fast enough for the brain's requirements especially in premature babies. Young infants fed on standard formulas had lower DHA concentration in red cells and brain (SIDS post-mortem) than breast fed infants.[7]

*Oligosaccharides*

Lactose is not the only sugar in human milk. The concentration of oligosaccharides is higher than the protein! Over 100 of these oligosaccharides have been chemically defined—all made up of five monosaccharides: fucose, galactose, glucose, *N*-acetylglucosamine, and sialic acid (NANA) and ranging from three to ten residues in length. Cows' milk, and infant formulas, contain only trace amounts. These human milk oligosaccharides (HMOs) are not digested in the small intestine. Small amounts are absorbed and found in the urinary tract. Most passes to the large intestine where it acts like dietary fibre.[9] Oligosaccharides containing N-acetylglucosamine promote the growth of bifidobacteria, which are the dominant colonic bacteria in breast fed infants.

Micro-organisms and their toxins gain entry to cells by attaching to specific sugars on the cell surface. Oligosaccharides in mucus and in human milk include particular sugars that can act as decoys for many specific micro-organisms and so prevent their access to the body. HMOs have been shown to include receptors for *E. coli*, *E. coli* toxins, Campylobacter, Candida, Rotavirus and *Strep pneumoniae*.[10]

## How to manage breast feeding

Knowing how to establish breast feeding is no longer instinctive in the women of our complex industrial societies. Some take to it naturally but others will not do well without guidance and a sympathetic environment.

- The mother should be adequately nourished during pregnancy.
- She should have watched others breast feeding and talked about it.
- She needs to involve and consider her partner. There can be sexual implications in breast feeding. His support (or opposition) is important.
- The National Childbirth Trust or La Lèche League or the Association of Breastfeeding Mothers can help to provide information and support (for addresses see end of this chapter).
- The baby should be put to the breast as soon as possible after delivery.
- The midwife can play an important part, giving advice on positioning the baby, and encouragement in the first few days.[11]
- Frequent suckling stimulates prolactin secretion. Suckling more than six times a day maintains high basal prolactin as well as initiating prolactin surges with feeding.
- Feeding should be on demand or baby-led.
- After delivery the baby should be in a crib next to its mother all or most of the time and suckled whenever it seems to be hungry. Colostrum is a concentrated anti-infective fluid.
- Relaxation and privacy are needed.

Randomised controlled trials have found better eye function in pre-term infants who were breast fed or given formula enriched with DHA and AA than in babies fed on standard formulas. In full term infants a few (not all) trials have had similar results.[8] It is not known whether there will be benefits beyond infancy. Socio-economic and psychological confounding factors will make interpretation of brain function tests difficult. Some manufacturers now add DHA and AA to premium infant formulas.

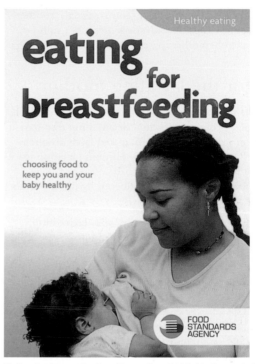

*Eating for breast feeding. Reproduced with kind permission from the Food Standards Agency*

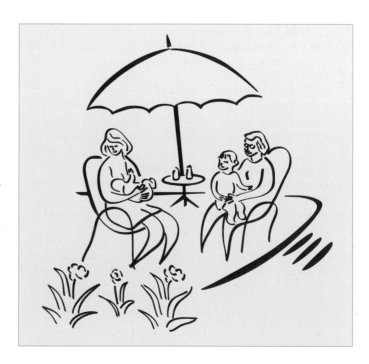

- The baby should not be given other complementary milk or juice—only water if necessary.
- The baby should feed from both breasts each time and start the feed with the breast used last.
- Advice may be needed about sore nipples or breasts, oversupply, or undersupply.
- In developed countries rates of breast feeding are lower in younger, less educated mothers in less skilled occupations, and in single mothers.

Obstacles to initiation and continuation of breast feeding are listed in the box alongside.

**Contraindications** to breast feeding are rare: galactosaemia in the infant; mother uses illegal drugs; mother has active untreated tuberculosis; mother has HIV infection (controversial); mother has to take therapeutic drugs that adversely affect her milk— radioisotopes, cancer chemotherapy, etc.

## Nutrition for the lactating mother

Except in malnourished communities, there is little evidence that dietary calories, protein, fat, water, or anything else have a consistent effect on milk volume. Regular and fairly frequent suckling is the well established stimulus. Human lactation works more by pull than by push.

Some constituents in the milk are affected by the mother's intake.

(1) Fatty acid pattern, vitamin A, thiamin, riboflavin, biotin, folate, vitamin B-12, and vitamin C are affected, especially downwards if the mother's diet is deficient.
(2) Zinc, iron, fluoride, and vitamin D may be responsive in some circumstances, but more research is needed.
(3) Protein, lactose, total fat content, calcium—that is, the major proximate constituents of milk—do not appear to be affected.
(4) Specific proteins in the mother's diet might be excreted intact in small amounts and an allergic (IgE) reaction occasionally occurs in the baby.
(5) The amount of caffeine in the milk after a cup of coffee is only about 2% of the maternal dose. Likewise, the alcohol concentration of breast milk is about the same as that of plasma so single drinks of coffee or alcohol, well spaced out, are harmless, but the babies of alcoholics can be affected. Beer stimulates prolactin secretion (at least in non-lactating women) and so might increase lactation. Milk production is reduced in heavy smokers.
(6) The fat-soluble environmental contaminants, polychlorinated biphenyls, dry cleaning solvents, and organochlorine insecticides (DDT, etc), are stored in adipose tissue and excreted in the cream of breast milk (though the DDT group is fairly innocuous in man).

### The mother's need for extra nutrients

A good average production of breast milk is 800 ml/day, and the mother's extra nutritional requirements are calculated from this and the average composition of milk, taking into account the available information about efficiency of absorption. The gross energy value of average human milk is 280 kJ/100 g and efficiency of conversion from maternal dietary energy to milk energy is assumed to be 80%. Hence the energy lost in exclusive breast feeding in the first three months is:

$$800 \text{ ml} \times 280 \text{ kJ} \times 100/80 = 2.8 \text{ MJ (675 kcal).}[13]$$

If, as is usual, the mother does not eat the full amount of this extra energy she will lose some of the body fat put on during

---

**Obstacles to breast feeding**[12]

- Doctor's apathy and misinformation
- Insufficient prenatal education in breast feeding
- Disruptive hospital policies
- Inappropriate interruption of breast feeding
- Early hospital discharge
- Lack of regular home health visits, post-partum
- Maternal employment (especially if no workplace facilities or support for breast feeding)
- Lack of broad societal support
- Portrayal by media of bottle feeding as normative
- Commercial promotion of infant formula, for example distribution of hospital discharge packs

**Drugs and lactation**

- For most drugs the concentration in human milk is of the same order of magnitude as the plasma concentration or in some cases less. The infant would thus receive around 1% of the maternal dose. But the milk/plasma ratio is 12 for propylthiouracil and 25 for iodine-131.
- Other drugs are contraindicated if they are radioactive, can cause allergy, agranulocytosis or bleeding disorders, or are poorly metabolised in the newborn, or can suppress lactation. These include chloramphenicol, indomethacin, diazepam, reserpine, anti-cancer drugs, lithium, and some others.
- Tetrahydrocannabinol is concentrated in the milk of cannabis smokers, as are opiate narcotics in the milk of those taking them.
- The *British National Formulary* has an appendix on prescribing during breast feeding.

**Constituents of milk affected by mother's intake**

- Fatty acid pattern, vitamin A, thiamin, riboflavin, biotin, folate, vitamin B-12 and vitamin C
- Possibly zinc, iron, fluoride and vitamin D
- Protein, lactose, total fat content, calcium
- Some proteins in mother's diet
- Caffeine in milk after coffee, alcohol after alcohol consumption (only in large doses)
- Environmental contaminants

pregnancy. When the infant is getting other foods the energy expenditure on breast milk usually declines.

Most of the nutrients come along with the extra calories; lactating women usually have a good appetite and if this is satisfied by a mixed diet the nutrients that need watching (because there is little excess in the diets of non-lactating women) are calcium, iron, folate, and vitamin D. The extra **calcium** can come from a pint of milk or two cartons of yoghurt. Calcium metabolism changes during lactation. There is some loss of bone density, which is apparently not prevented by calcium supplements. These changes are reversed when lactation ceases.[14] There is no evidence that women who have breast fed have increased incidence of osteoporosis. **Iron** supplements may be advisable, and **vitamin D** supplements are recommended for any mother whose vitamin D status is in doubt (such as Asian mothers eating a wholly vegetarian diet). **Folate** deficiency incurred during pregnancy may first show as anaemia in the puerperium. **Zinc** is secreted in the milk but staple isotope studies show increased zinc absorption during lactation.

**Mothers return to pre-pregnant weight?**
Mothers are more likely to lose the fat stores put on during pregnancy if they choose to breast feed. The energy lost in lactation is usually more than the mother's increased food intake over her non-pregnant, non-lactating level. DHSS estimated an average energy deficit of 0.5 MJ (120 kcal) per day, which corresponds to a fat loss of 0.5 kg per month (14.5 MJ).[13] But in fact appetite and weight loss during lactation is highly variable.[15] Obviously lactation cannot contribute to worthwhile weight loss if it is only brief. The question arises whether milk production will suffer if the mother deliberately restricts her food intake. Lovelady et al. tested this out in a randomised controlled trial in overweight (not obese) women. (BMI 25-30).[16] They lost approximately 0.5 kg per week between 4 and 14 weeks post partum from moderate food restriction and exercise: their infants gained the same weight and length as the controls, but some of the control mothers put on weight.

**Ending lactation**
In an industrial population the prevalence of breast feeding goes down with infant's age in a curve reminiscent of first order elimination kinetics. A few mothers continue breast feeding towards or beyond 12 months. In a British national sample the major reasons for stopping in the first six weeks were insufficient milk (54%) and painful breasts or painful or inverted nipples (18%); the commonest reason for stopping between 6 and 16 weeks was also insufficient milk (66%). Those with insufficient milk early on never got lactation well established. Those with insufficient milk later may have had normal volume production but the baby's energy needs started to outgrow this.

**Complementary and supplementary bottles of milk**
Complementary bottle feeds are used to finish off a breast feed and supplementary bottle feeds replace a breast feed. The occasional bottle feed once a day or less is convenient if the mother has to leave the baby with a friend, but regular topping up of the baby's intake with bottle milk is likely to reduce sucking and breast milk production. Some mothers produce less milk than others, however, and if the baby is not gaining, and hungry on pure breast feeding with good technique, extra bottle feeding may be necessary.

# Bottle feeding

Some mothers choose to bottle feed from the start and others will change over from breast to bottle feeding after weeks or months, so they need practical advice.

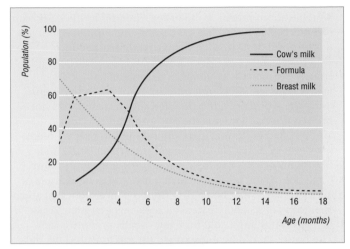

Mean consumption of different types of milk in normal Canadian infants[17]

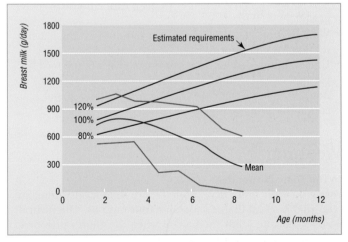

Measured breast milk intakes of Cambridge infants. Mean and ranges against estimated requirements[18]

- A cows' milk formula specially modified for infants should be used in which the protein has been reduced, the casein partly replaced by whey protein, the fat made more unsaturated, the lactose increased, sodium and calcium reduced, and enough of all the essential micronutrients added.
- Bottles and teats should be washed in water and detergent (the bottle brush used only for this), rinsed and sterilised by boiling in water or by standing covered in sterilising solution (usually hypochlorite) in a plastic container. It saves time to prepare several bottles at once. Empty the water out of each bottle, without touching the inside, then fill to the mark with recently boiled water that has cooled some minutes, not too hot or it will destroy some vitamins and may produce clumping.
- Exactly the amount of power in the manufacturer's instructions should be put into the (wide mouthed) bottle, using the scoop provided (levelled with a clean knife, not pressed down). "One for the pot" can lead to obesity. Mothers and even nurses are often found to prepare feeds inaccurately. Screw on the cap and shake the bottle well. Bottles may be kept in the refrigerator for up to 24 hours.
- If the hole in the teat is too small it can lead to aerophagia or underfeeding. Milk should drip from the inverted teat at about one drop per second. Teats need replacing every few weeks.
- Babies do not mind cold milk but usually prefer it warm. The bottle should be not warmed for too long and the milk's temperature should be checked by dropping some on the parent's skin. Infant feed should be not warmed in a microwave oven once it is in the feeding bottle. Very hot fluid at the centre of the bottle may be missed and may scald the baby.[5] For about the first eight weeks of life babies need to be fed every three to four hours, including the small hours of the morning. (Fathers can bottle feed as well as mothers.) By the end of the first week most babies are taking 120-200 ml/kg per day (160 ml/kg corresponds to the old $2\frac{1}{2}$ fluid ounces per lb bodyweight).
- Cereals or rusks should not be added to milk in the bottle and babies should not be left to sleep with a bottle in their mouth.
- Vitamin drops, fruit juices, are not required as supplements to modern infant formulas.
- Uncles, grannies, and baby sitters can give a bottle feed but parents should feed their infant themselves as much as possible with the same sort of closeness, cuddling, and communication as in breast feeding.

# Weaning[19]

### In the first six months

Young infants cannot deal properly with solid foods (in reality semisolid foods at first) for the first four months. The natural time for starting solids (beikost) is when the energy provided by well established breast feeding starts to become insufficient. The Department of Health and other authorities advise that the introduction of any food to the baby, other than milk, should be unnecessary before the age of 4 months, but mothers may be tempted to jump the gun. Most babies should start a mixed diet not later than the age of 6 months.

Weight in the lower half of the standard percentiles without other symptoms is not an indication to augment breast feeding. Breast fed babies tend to put on weight (and length) a little more slowly than bottle fed infants. Indeed, the standard percentiles, derived mostly from bottle fed babies, may not be ideal. The time to start thinking about adding solids is when the infant still seems hungry after a good milk feed. But by

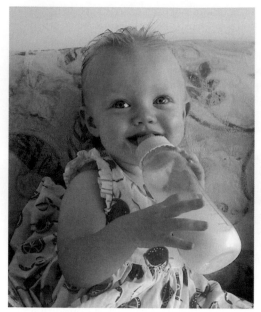

Fifteen month old child bottle feeding. (Courtesy of Mr PM Whitfield, reproduced with permission)

---

**Babies cannot cope with solid food in the first few months because:**

- the extrusion reflex prevents spoon feeding
- they cannot swallow solids
- pancreatic amylase is not produced for the first three months
- pancreatic lipase is absent for the first month (fat digestion in breast milk is facilitated by the bile salt-activated lipase it contains)
- there is an increased likelihood of absorption of intact foreign (food) proteins.

---

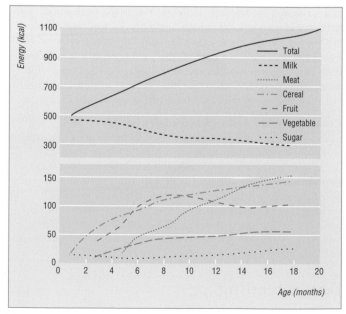

Mean consumption of energy from different foods in normal Canadian infants[17]

six months body stores of several nutrients, such as iron, zinc, and vitamin C, are often falling in exclusively milk fed infants, whether from breast or bottle.

When solids are introduced, single ingredient foods should be used and started one at a time at half weekly intervals so that there is time to recognise allergy or other intolerance to each food. A little of the food on the tip of a teaspoon is enough at first, given after a milk feed when the baby is wide awake.

Infant cereals (usually enriched with iron) are traditional foods to start with; rice is better before wheat. They can be thinned with baby's usual milk (mother's or formula) or water. Thereafter different soft foods can be added: mashed potato; soft porridges; puréed fruit and vegetables, meat, or chicken. Foods should be semisolid—sieved or blended or commercial baby food. It is nutritionally sensible to give a balance of foods from the four major food groups: cereals, vegetables/fruit, dairy products, and meats/fish. Combination foods should not be given until tolerance to their individual components is established. Egg should not be started before six months because of the chance of allergic reactions, and then it is best to begin with a small amount of cooked yolk. Spinach, turnip, and beets can contain enough nitrate to cause methaemoglobinaemia in young infants. Coffee and tea should not be given. Babies should not be left alone while they are eating.

## In the second six months

In the second six months other liquids can be given from a cup, especially citrus fruit juices. Untreated cows' milk can sometimes cause gastrointestinal bleeding from irritation by the bovine serum albumin. This does not happen with boiled milk or infant formulas (which have been heat treated). Iron-fortified infant formula contributes to iron intake, which is critical in the second six months of life. It is wrong to add any salt to the foods given to infants. A fully breast fed infant receives only about one-twentieth of the sodium in a typical British adult diet. There has been a quiet revolution in commercial baby foods; most contain no added salt or colours and only up to 4% sugar (needed with sour fruits). Infants' sodium intakes have been found to shoot up after six months but more from home prepared rather than commercial baby foods.

An increasing range of foods is given in the second six months. Variety is likely to cover the needs for most nutrients and provide a basis for healthy food habits. Some fruits or vegetables should be given each day, but the most critical nutrients at this stage are protein and iron: finely minced beef and legumes should be given regularly and the protein in cereal foods should not usually be diluted by refining or by added fat or sugar. Foods should become progressively more chewy and fibrous and include rusks and other finger foods like bread or cheese. Babies do not usually like strongly flavoured foods like pickled onions. Nuts, popcorn, raw peas, and similar small hard foods should be avoided; they can be breathed in accidentally. Commercial baby food manufacturers offer a succession of "strained", "junior", and "toddler" foods for maturing babies, and similar meals are usually made at home. Some cookbooks for babies are more sensible than others.

Milk continues to be the main source of calories but a diminishing one. Sweetened fruit juices should be given by cup not bottle because the latter can promote dental caries. Infantile obesity is probably becoming less common in the United Kingdom now that people are aware of it. It is not usually caused by bottle feeding or early introduction of solids in themselves, but by more concentrated feeds, by pushing food at mealtimes, or by snacks in between. Between feeds, water for thirst and a minimum of snacks or sweets are good general rules.

### A suggested timetable for the introduction of solid foods

- 1-4 months     Breast milk only
- 4-6 months     Cereal(s) added
- 6-7 months     Vegetables (puréed) added
- 8-9 months     Start finger foods (rusk, banana) and chopped (junior) foods
- 9 months     Meat, citrus juice (from a cup)
- 10 months     Egg yolk (cooked), bite-sized cooked foods
- 12 months     Whole egg, most table foods
                        No peanuts or hard particles of similar size

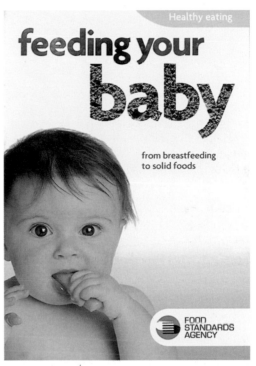

Feeding your baby (from breast feeding to solid foods). Reproduced with kind permission from the Food Standards Agency

In a survey for MAFF of food and nutrient intakes of British infants aged 6-12 months,[20] the percentage contribution of food types to energy intake were:

- *In infants 6-9 months old (median energy 792 kcal)*, family foods 30%, infant formula 23%, infant foods 23%, cows' milk 18%, breast milk 6%
- *In infants 9-12 months old (median energy 894 kcal)*, family foods 53%, cows' milk 28%, infant foods 11%, infant formula 7%, breast milk 1%.

Two other nutrients are not adequately supplied in all mixed diets. In communities where rickets occurs—for example, among Asian babies in northern cities—a supplement of vitamin D 10 $\mu$g (400 IU) a day is good insurance. Bottle fed infants who are consuming 500 ml infant formula as follow on formula a day do not need vitamin supplementation because these manufactured products are fortified with vitamin D. In areas where the drinking water is not fluoridated, sodium fluoride prophylactic tablets or drops (0.25 mg/day) should be considered.

**Useful addresses for help with breast feeding**

- Association of Breast Feeding Mothers, PO Box 207, Bridgewater, Somerset, TA6 7YF http://home.clara.net/abm, (0)20 7813 1481.
- La Lèche League, PO Box BM 3424, London WC1N 3XX. http://www.laleche.org.uk, (0)20 7242 1278.
- National Childbirth Trust, Alexandra House, Oldham Terrace, Acton, London W3 6NH. http://www.nctpregnancyand babycare.com, 0870 770 3236.

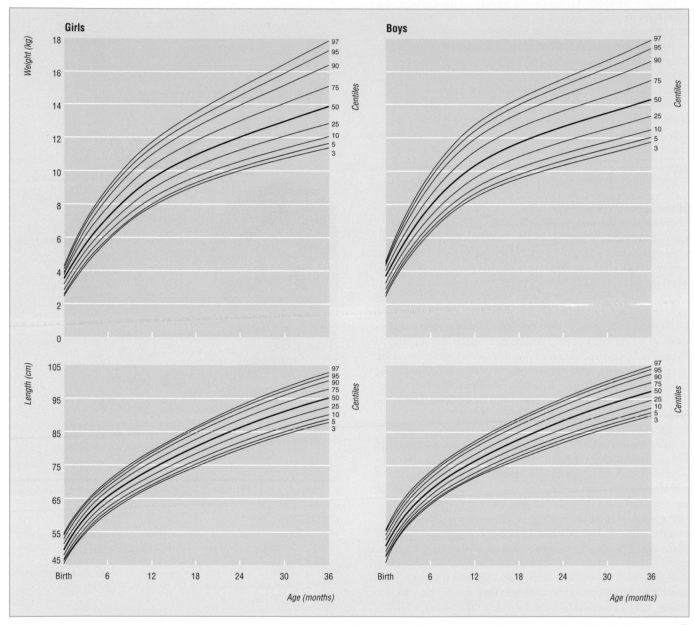

Center for Health Statistics graph of percentile weights and heights for girls and boys from birth to 36 months, adopted by the World Health Organization[21]

## References

1 Department of Health & Social Security. *The Composition of Mature Human Milk*. (Report on Health & Social Subjects no 12.) London: HMSO, 1977.

2 Reeve LE, Chesney RW, de Luca HF. Vitamin D of human milk: identification of biologically active forms. *Am J Clin Nutr* 1982; **36**: 122-6.

3 Howie PW, Forsyth JS, Ogston SA, Clark A, Florey C du V. Protective effect of breast feeding against infection. *BMJ* 1990; **300**: 11-16.

4 Wilson AC, Forsyth JS, Greene SA, Irvine L, Hau C, Howie PW. Relation of infant diet to childhood health: seven year follow up of cohort of children in Dundee infant feeding study. *BMJ* 1998; **316**: 21-5.

5 Department of Health & Social Security. *Present Day Practice in Infant Feeding: Third Report*. (Report on Health and Social Studies no 32.) London: HMSO, 1988.

6 Foster K, Lader D, Cheesbrough S. *Infant feeding 1995*. London: HMSO, 1997.

7 Farquharson J, Jamieson EC, Abbasi JA, Patrick WJA, Logan RW, Cockburn F. Effect of diet on the fatty acid composition of the major phospholipids of infant cerebral cortex. *Arch Dis Childhood* 1995; **72**: 198-203.

8 Gibson RA. Long chain polyunsaturated fatty acids and infant development. *Lancet* 1999; **354**: 1919-20.

9 Brand-Miller JC, McVeigh P, McNeil Y, Messer M. Digestion of human milk oligosaccharides by healthy infants evaluated by the lactulose hydrogen breath test. *J Pediatr* 1998; **133**: 95-8.

10 Newburg DS, Street JM. Bioactive materials in human milk. Milk sugars sweeten the argument for breast-feeding. *Nutr Today* 1997; **32**: 191-201.

11 Anonymous. *Successful breastfeeding. A practical guide for mothers and midwives and others supporting breastfeeding mothers*. London: Royal College of Midwives, 1989.

12 American Academy of Pediatrics: Work Group on Breast feeding. Breast feeding and the use of human milk. *Pediatrics* 1997; **100**: 1035-9.

13 Department of Health. *Dietary reference values for food energy and nutrients for the United Kingdom. Report of the Panel of the Committee on Medical Aspects of Food Policy*. London: HMSO, 1991.

14 Prentice A. Calcium in pregnancy and lactation. *Annu Rev Nutr* 2000; **20**: 249-72.

15 Butte NF, Hopkinson JM. Body composition changes during lactation are highly variable among women. *J Nutr* 1998; **128 Suppl**: 381S-385S.

16 Lovelady CA, Garner KE, Moreno KL, Williams JP. The effect of weight loss in overweight, lactating women on the growth of their infants. *N Engl J Med* 2000; **342**: 449-53.

17 Yeung DL. *Infant nutrition. A study of feeding practices and growth from birth to 18 months*. Ottawa: Canadian Public Health Association, 1983.

18 Whitehead RG, Paul A, Rowland MGM. Lactation in Cambridge and in the Gambia. In: Wharton BA (ed) *Topics in paediatrics 2*. Tunbridge Wells: Pitman (for the Royal College of Physicians), 1980.

19 Department of Health. *Weaning and the weaning diet. Report of the Working Group on the Weaning Diet of the Committee on Medical Aspects of Food Policy*. (Report on Health & Social Subjects no 45.) London: HMSO, 1994.

20 Mills A, Tyler H (Ministry of Agriculture, Fisheries & Food). *Food and nutrient intakes of British infants aged 6-12 months*. London: HMSO, 1992.

21 National Center for Health Statistics/National Center for Chronic Disease Prevention and Health Promotion. New childhood growth charts, 2000. http://www.cdc.goc/growthcharts

# 6  Children and adolescents

## Pre-school children (1-5 years of age)

What children eat between being weaned and starting school is important. Food habits are established in this phase of life. They are less under parental control than they used to be. Mothers often go out to work, the toddler eats at a child care centre or pre-school. Food companies make some products specially for this age group and young children are targeted by advertisements on television. Young children have different taste perception from adults. They prefer sweeter foods, dislike bitter tastes, and often object to vegetables of the cabbage family.

Young children's eating is still mostly controlled by their mothers. Four simple principles should help them.

(1) Eat from each of the **four basic groups** every day (the fifth will accompany the basic four). These four basic food groups contain all the essential nutrients between them.

(2) Aim for **variety** within each food group—for example not always the same vegetable. The modern child should be prepared to eat food from other cultures. Food neophobia is a social handicap in later life. Young children should be able to eat most of the same food as the rest of the family.

(3) To minimise **dental caries**, sweets and other sugary foods should be rationed and not eaten between meals as a rule.

(4) The most likely **nutrient deficiency** in Britain is a low iron status with mild anaemia.[2] The easiest way to prevent this is for the child to be given meat, chicken or fish regularly, which provide haem iron.

Rickets in the northern winter, though now uncommon, is prevented by children getting out of doors regularly, eating plenty of the foods that contain some vitamin D and, in vulnerable groups, taking BNF vitamin capsules or children's vitamins drops (contains $7.5\,\mu g$ vitamin D) during the winter. In a sample of Asian children, $1\frac{1}{2}$-$2\frac{1}{2}$ years old in England, 20-34% had 25-OH vitamin D levels under $25\,nmol/l$.[3] Low vitamin D status tended to be associated with low haemoglobin and serum iron.

### Overweight increasing

Health visitors in the Wirral, NW England weigh and measure pre-school children regularly. Records from over 28 000 children show that the percentage overweight (>85% of the British growth reference BMI) rose from 14.7% in 1989 to 23.6% in 1998.[4] What has changed since the 1980s? The *Lancet* asked:

> Children's leisure activities have shifted from active outdoors play—often because of parents' perception that neighbourhoods are unsafe—to television watching and computer games. Cars are used even for short distance journeys. And children's diets including school meals, commonly consist of fast food with high fat and sugar contents. Many parents, especially when overweight themselves, do not recognise obesity in their children.[5]

### Faddy toddlers

After having a reliable appetite for their first twelve months, some children aged 1-3 go through a phase of poor eating, which can make parents anxious or even exasperated. Children are less enthusiastic about eating and refuse foods that the rest of the family eat, especially vegetables.

---

**Food groups for nutrition**[1]

(1) Bread, other cereals and potatoes
(2) Fruits and vegetables
(3) Milk and dairy foods
(4) Meat, fish, and alternatives
(5) Foods containing fat
     Foods containing sugar

1-4 are the basic four food groups. The fifth group includes foods low in nutrient density that should be used sparingly or enjoyed as treats.

---

**Foods that contain some vitamin D**

- Milk, eggs, cheese, butter, liver, all contain some.
- Fatty fish (herring, mackerel, sardines, pilchards, tuna, and salmon) contain more.
- Infant milks, infant cereals, margarines, some breakfast cereals, some yoghurts, and branded food drinks have vitamin D added during manufacture.

---

**Favourite foods**

- In the 1992-93 survey of British children aged $1\frac{1}{2}$-$4\frac{1}{2}$ years[2] the foods or drinks most frequently recorded over 4 days were (in descending order): biscuits (88%); white bread (86%); non-diet soft drinks (86%); whole milk (83%); savoury snacks (potato crisps or cereal-based) (78%); boiled, mashed or jacket potatoes (77%); chocolate confectionery (75%); potato chips (71%); chicken (70%); breakfast cereals (66%); cheese (59%); sugar confectionery (58%); buns, cakes and pastries (55%); sausages (53%); beef dishes (47%); pasta (51%); carrots (54%); peas (53%); baked beans (49%); apples & pears (50%); bananas (46%); fruit juice (36%); eggs (46%); yoghurt (40%); coated and fried white fish (36%); leafy green vegetables (39%).
- Many of the top half of items in this frequency list are high in fat, added sugar or salt. It would be preferable if the lower half of the list had been at the top.

One reason for this is that growth slows at around twelve months. This can be seen in the changes in gradient of normal weight for age, and height for age curves. It is even more obvious in weight and height velocity curves, which descend to about a quarter and a half, respectively, of the values in early infancy. Energy intake can be very variable from time to time in toddlers.

Other things are also happening. Children are discovering their independence and testing their choice in food selection. Once they have some control over what is offered, foods that they find unattractive are displaced by those they think delicious: cakes, biscuits, chocolate, crisps, ice cream, etc.

# Schoolchildren

In developed countries undernutrition is exceptional nowadays—a big advance from Dickens' time. Children are growing taller than ever.[8] Deficiency is limited to a few micronutrients and usually subclinical. Iron nutrition is low in a minority of older girls (their requirements increased by menstruation) and plasma 25-OH vitamin D is low in some susceptible children.

The main nutritional concerns in schoolchildren are:

- the increasing percentage who are overweight, even obese
- whether the most frequently consumed foods are healthiest in the long term? Vegetable, fruit and whole grain consumptions are often below dietary guideline recommendations (see chapter 7)
- the continuing opportunity to minimise dental caries by reducing the time that teeth are exposed to acid-producing carbohydrates in the mouth
- diets of socially deprived children can be of poorer quality.[9]

## Overweight
It is now agreed that overweight can be diagnosed with body mass index $(kg/m^2)$ using reference curves worked out for children's different ages. There are BMI reference curves for the United Kingdom (1995) and for the United States (2000). The cut offs shown on page 34[11] were calculated by Cole et al. for international use, based on data from Brazil, Great Britain, Hong Kong, the Netherlands, Singapore and the USA.

The role of high fat foods in the epidemic of overweight is generally known, and realised among schoolchildren themselves, though cheese or biscuits may not be recognised as high fat. Another contributor to overweight, more recently revealed, is the widespread consumption of sugar-sweetened soft drinks.[12] It is sometimes hard to visualise how much sugar and calories are in these liquids. In the NDNS survey[8] 76% of 4-18 year olds consumed "carbonated soft drinks, not low calorie" over seven days while only 61% drank tap water!

Energy expenditure has fallen in young people. Many do not participate in sport, are driven to school and spend hours everyday looking at television or a personal computer. Children who watch more TV have higher BMIs[13] and most of the food adverts they see are for fast foods, high in fat, sugar or salt.

## How could schools help?
(Suppose a local doctor is on the school board.)

Much could be done (though nutrition is low priority at present for management, teachers, and pupils), including:

- there needs to be modernised food education across the years
- ALL pupils should get regular physical exercise; there is too much emphasis on competitive sport
- foods served in and around the school should help children eat a varied and nutritious diet

## Advice for parents of faddy toddlers[6,7]
- Most toddlers will eat some form of bread, cereals, meat, milk, and some fruits and fruit juices. The fibre foregone in vegetables can be replaced by breads and the vitamins by fruits and juices.
- Do not have battles over foods. Do not use bribes or force. Try to avoid tension at meal times.
- Keep meal preparation for toddlers easy and quick, so you can accept it without anger if they will not eat what you have made for them.
- Make eating fun—for example, cut sandwiches, pieces of fruit, cheese into patterns. Let toddlers eat at a small table, etc.
- When it is clear that they will not eat any more, let them leave the table. Do not insist on clean plates; serve a little less next time. With proper education, parents may be led to understand that a "good" eater is not a big eater but a moderate eater.
- Rejection of new foods is usually a transitory phenomenon which can be reduced by repeated exposure to small quantities without undue coercion (followed by praise if the child eats some). Parents should not interpret initial rejection to mean the child has an immutable distaste for the food.
- Children are more likely to try new foods offered in small amounts at the start of meals when they are hungry. If they help preparing (or even growing) vegetable foods (for example, shelling peas or making a salad) they may like to taste them.
- Do not give delicious (for them) high fat and sugar foods (cake or chocolate) before a meal **or** if they will not eat their main meals.
- Many toddlers cannot adjust to their parents' three meals but will eat nutritious foods as snacks.

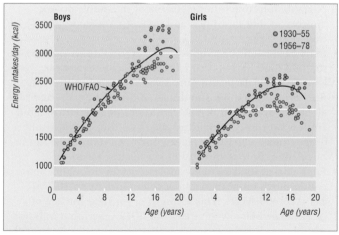

Mean energy intakes of boys and girls studied in 1930-55 compared with more recent studies in relation to WHO/FAO (1973) recommendations[10]

## National Diet & Nutrition Survey, Great Britain[8]
- Young people, aged 4-18 years from 1700 weighed dietary records.
- Most frequently consumed (% consuming over 7 days): White bread (95), milk (93), potato chips (89), biscuits (84), chocolate confectionery (82), other potato dishes (82), carbonated drinks (76), cakes (74), chicken (74).
- But consumption frequency was lower for: sausages (64), baked beans (60), apples, pears (54), beef, veal (51), peas (50), fruit juice (49), fried coated fish (46), pizza (45), green vegetables (39), bananas (38), citrus fruits (26).
- Average fat intake total 35.5% of energy, saturated 14.25% of energy, polyunsaturated 5% of energy.

- resist sponsorship by food companies and vending machines
- all children's weights and heights should be measured at school once a year.

James and McColl have written a paper for government departments setting out the justification for **schools that promote a healthy lifestyle** and how changes can be made.[14]

## Adolescents

> Teenagers are not fed; they eat. For the first time in their lives they assume responsibility for their own food intakes. At the same time they are intensely involved in day-to-day life with their peers, and preparation for their future lives as adults. Social pressures thrust choices at them: to drink or not to drink, to smoke or not to smoke, to develop their bodies to meet sometimes extreme ideals of slimness or athletic prowess. Few become interested in foods and nutrition except as part of a cult or fad such as vegetarianism or crash dieting.[15]

Several facets of eating behaviour are different or more pronounced in adolescents than in other people and each may cause concern in the older generation.

- **Missing meals**, especially breakfast. This does not usually affect classroom performance, partly because of—
- **Eating snacks** and confectionery. The major snack is usually in the afternoon, after school. Snacks tend to be high in "empty calories"—fat, sugar, and alcohol—but some provide calcium (for example milk) or vitamin C (fruit).
- **"Fast", take-away, or carry-out foods**. These provide some nutritious portions, but adolescents may not choose balanced meals from what is offered. There is not enough accessible information about the nutrient composition of fast foods.
- **Unconventional meals** may be eaten in combinations and permutations that other members of the family do not approve of, but they often add up to an adequate nutritional mix.
- **Start of alcohol consumption.** This is the most dangerous of the new food habits. Alcohol-related accidents are the leading cause of death in the 15-24 year age group.
- **Soft drinks and other fun drinks.** If they are an alternative to alcoholic drinks soft drinks should not be discouraged, but (unless sweetened with aspartame, etc) they provide only empty calories and by replacing milk can reduce the intake of calcium. Bottled pure water is a healthy trend.
- **High energy intakes.** Many adolescents go through a phase of eating much more than adults, sometimes up to 16.7 MJ per day (4000 kcal). This seems to occur near the age of peak height velocity in girls (around 12 years), but in boys may come later than the age of peak height velocity (usually 14 years). Presumably the larger, more muscular male adolescent is expending more energy at this stage.
- **Low levels of some nutrients.** Iron deficiency is quite common in adolescent girls who are menstruating, still growing, and often restricting their food intake. It may sometimes occur in boys too. Calcium accretion in the skeleton can be as much as 100 g/year at peak height velocity. Around 20% is absorbed so that about 500 grams per year are needed in the diet—that is, 1370 mg/day.
- **Adolescent dieters.** There are two aspects to this: overweight/obesity and social dieting. Obese adolescents are usually inactive and tend to have low socio-economic status. Dietary management should aim to hold the weight constant while the young person continues to grow and so thins out. Increased exercise should be emphasised and anorectic drugs should not be used.

**Body Mass Index international cut off points for overweight (≡25 kg/m² in adults) and obesity (≡30 kg/m² in adults)[11]**

| Age (years) | Overweight | | Obese | |
|---|---|---|---|---|
| | Boys | Girls | Boys | Girls |
| 2 | 18.4 | 18.0 | 20.1 | 20.1 |
| 3 | 17.9 | 17.6 | 19.6 | 19.4 |
| 4 | 17.6 | 17.3 | 19.3 | 19.1 |
| 5 | 17.4 | 17.1 | 19.3 | 19.2 |
| 6 | 17.6 | 17.3 | 19.8 | 19.7 |
| 7 | 17.9 | 17.8 | 20.6 | 20.5 |
| 8 | 18.4 | 18.3 | 21.6 | 21.6 |
| 9 | 19.1 | 19.1 | 22.8 | 22.8 |
| 10 | 19.8 | 19.9 | 24.0 | 24.1 |
| 11 | 20.6 | 20.7 | 25.1 | 25.4 |
| 12 | 21.2 | 21.7 | 26.0 | 26.7 |
| 13 | 21.9 | 22.6 | 26.8 | 27.8 |
| 14 | 22.6 | 23.3 | 27.6 | 28.6 |
| 15 | 23.3 | 23.9 | 28.3 | 29.1 |
| 16 | 23.9 | 24.4 | 28.9 | 29.4 |
| 17 | 24.5 | 24.7 | 29.4 | 29.7 |
| 18 | 25 | 25 | 30 | 30 |

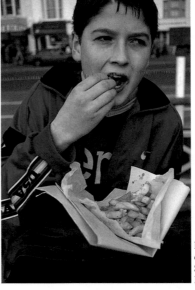

Reproduced courtesy of Steve Parry/Impact

**Percentage of daily nutrients provided by different meals among 290 school students (boys and girls) aged 16-17 in Sydney, Australia (based on 4-day records and interviews)[16]**

| | Breakfast | Lunch | Dinner | Snacks |
|---|---|---|---|---|
| Energy | 16.7 | 23.8 | 33.0 | 26.1 |
| Protein | 16 | 25 | 41 | 18 |
| Fat | 15 | 25 | 37 | 23 |
| Carbohydrate | 20 | 23 | 27 | 31 |
| Alcohol | 0 | 14 | 36 | 50 |
| Calcium | 26 | 19 | 26 | 28 |
| Iron | 23 | 23 | 37 | 9 |
| Vitamin A | 18 | 26 | 36 | 21 |
| Thiamin | 28 | 22 | 28 | 20 |
| Riboflavin | 27 | 17 | 26 | 18 |
| Vitamin C | 14 | 19 | 27 | 27 |

As well as overweight youngsters there are adolescent girls of normal weight modifying their diet because they are not as thin as they or their peers think they should be. Some may fast and binge alternately. With a smaller energy intake they are more likely not to reach their requirements for iron and other essential nutrients. In a small minority this social dieting goes on to anorexia nervosa (incidence in some places as high as 1% of middle class girls aged 15-25) or bulimia. Treatment of anorexia nervosa is best handled by a specialised team of psychiatrist and dietitian. The general practitioner's main role is to recognise the early case. The longer the duration the worse the prognosis. A young woman whose weight goes below a body mass index (weight (kg)/height(m)$^2$) of 17 should be warned, with her parents, that her thinness is unhealthy and referred for treatment if she cannot put on weight. (See page 56 for more on eating disorders.) By contrast, adolescent boys are more likely to worry that they are not growing tall enough or not developing enough muscles.

### Does diet affect acne?

The popular belief is that chocolate, fatty foods, soft drinks, and beer can all aggravate acne vulgaris. This is not surprising since 85% of people have acne at some time during adolescence and most adolescents eat and enjoy these foods.

Controlled trials—for example, of chocolate—have proved negative but their design can be criticised. It is very difficult to produce double blind conditions. Individual cases appear to respond to cutting down confectionery, fatty foods, or alcoholic drinks and there are other reasons to recommend such a dietary change. Zinc, polyunsaturated fats, and vitamin A are reported to improve acne, and adolescents can be advised to eat foods that are good sources of each: meat and wholemeal bread (zinc), polyunsaturated margarine or cooking oil, and (for vitamin A) carrots or liver.

### Perspective

Patience, and a sense of humour help in watching and advising on adolescent food habits. The serious concerns are drinking with driving, usually in boys, and excessive slimming, usually in girls.

No young person wants to lose their teeth and spoil their good looks. As in children, sticky sugary foods should not be eaten between meals, or if they are, the teeth should be thoroughly brushed afterwards.

Parents have more influence than they may think. They can choose which foods and drinks they buy and prepare and keep in the refrigerator. The adolescent's food habits are laid down in the family and the family remains one influence. The other three are the peer group, the need to develop an independent personality, and society in general.

Adolescence is a transitional stage when the structure of food habits is loosened. In a few years the young person will usually get married, work out a compromise set of food habits with the spouse or partner,[17] and settle down to re-establish the eating behaviour of a new family. It is here, in preparing for and starting marriage that nutrition education should probably focus more.

Between the ages of 10 and 20 years:

- **lean body mass** goes from (average) 25 to 63 kg in boys, 22 to 42 kg in girls
- **body fat** goes from (average) 7 to 9 kg in boys, 5 to 14 kg in girls
- **triceps skinfolds (subcutaneous fat)** in boys stay at about 9 mm with a dip at year 15; in girls they climb steadily from 11 to 16 mm.

**Too thin: entering anorexia nervosa range, BMI=17**

| Height (no shoes) | | Weight (min clothes) |
|---|---|---|
| Metres | Ft/inches | kg |
| 1.45 | 4, 9 | 36 |
| 1.48 | 4, 10 | 37 |
| 1.50 | 4, 11 | 38.5 |
| 1.52 | 5, 0 | 39.5 |
| 1.54 | 5, 1 | 40.5 |
| 1.56 | 5, 1 | 41.5 |
| 1.58 | 5, 2 | 42.5 |
| 1.60 | 5, 3 | 43.5 |
| 1.62 | 5, 4 | 44.5 |
| 1.64 | 5, 5 | 45.7 |
| 1.66 | 5, 5 | 47 |
| 1.68 | 5, 6 | 48 |
| 1.70 | 5, 7 | 49 |
| 1.72 | 5, 8 | 50.3 |

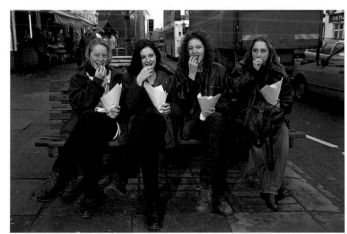

Reproduced courtesy of Bruce Stephens/Impact

## References

1 Health Education Authority. *Enjoy healthy eating*. London: Health Education Authority, 1995.

2 Gregory JR, Collins DL, Davies PSW, Hughes JM, Clarke PC. *National Diet and Nutrition Survey: children aged 1½ to 4½ years, vol 1. Report of the diet and nutrition survey*. London: HMSO, 1995.

3 Lawson M, Thomas M. Vitamin D concentrations in Asian children aged 2 years living in England: population survey. *BMJ* 1999; **318**: 28.

4 Bundred P, Kitchiner D, Buchan I. Prevalence of overweight and obese children between 1989 and 1998: population based series of cross sectional studies. *BMJ* 2001; **322**: 326-8.

5 Editorial. Childhood obesity: an emerging public-health problem. *Lancet* 2001; **357**: 1989.

6 Skuse D. Identification and management of problem eaters. *Arch Dis Childh* 1993; **69**: 604-8.

7 Green C. *Toddler training. A parents' guide to surviving the first four years*. Sydney: Doubleday, 1986.

8 Gregory J, Lowe S, Bates CH *et al. National Diet and Nutrition Survey. Young people aged 4 to 18 years, Vol 1. Report of the Diet and Nutrition Survey*. London: Stationery Office, 2000.

9 Nelson M. Childhood nutrition and poverty. *Proc Nutrition Soc* 2000; **59**: 307-15.

10 Whitehead RG, Paul AA, Cole TJ. Trends in food energy intakes throughout childhood from one to 18 years. *Hum Nutr Appl Nutr* 1982; **36A**: 57-62.

11 Cole TJ, Bellizzi MC, Flegal KM, Dietz WH. Establishing a standard definition for child overweight and obesity worldwide: international survey. *BMJ* 2000; **320**: 1240-3.

12 Ludwig DS, Peterson KE, Gortmaker SL. Relation between consumption of sugar-sweetened drinks and childhood obesity: a prospective, observational analysis. *Lancet* 2001; **357**: 505-8.

13 Anderson RE, Crespo CJ, Bartlett SJ, Cheskin LJ, Pratt M. Relationship of physical activity and television watching with body weight and level of fatness among children. *JAMA* 1998; **279**: 938-42.

14 James WPT, McColl KA. *Healthy English schoolchildren: a new approach to physical activity and food*. Aberdeen: Rowett Research Institute, 1997.

15 Hamilton EMN, Whitney EN. *Nutrition: concepts and controversies*. St Paul, MN: West Publishing, 1979.

16 Truswell AS, Darnton Hill I. Food habits of adolescents. *Nutr Rev* 1981; **39**: 73-88.

17 Craig P, Truswell AS. Dynamics of food habits in newly married couples: who makes changes in the food consumed? *J Hum Nutr Diet* 1994; **7**: 347-61.

# 7 Adults young and old

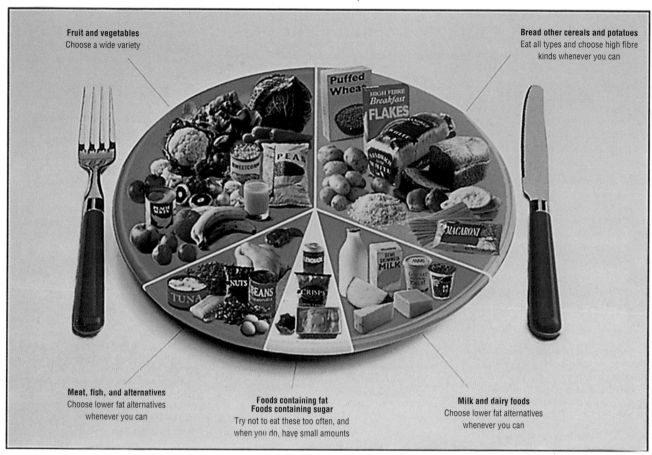

**Fruit and vegetables**
Choose a wide variety

**Bread other cereals and potatoes**
Eat all types and choose high fibre kinds whenever you can

**Meat, fish, and alternatives**
Choose lower fat alternatives whenever you can

**Foods containing fat**
**Foods containing sugar**
Try not to eat these too often, and when you do, have small amounts

**Milk and dairy foods**
Choose lower fat alternatives whenever you can

UK food guide plate[1]

## Most adults

Adults should eat enough of the essential nutrients by eating a healthy varied diet. This is more difficult to achieve if people have a low energy intake and if much of their diet consists of fats, alcohol, and sugar, which provide empty calories but little or no protein, or micronutrients.

### Food guides

The food guide plate, with pictures of real foods, shows the four groups of foods that should between them provide enough of all the essential nutrients and the fifth group that provides mostly energy. (The plate picture makes a good poster for the waiting room.) The areas indicate relative amounts, so that people can see they should eat plenty of vegetables and fruit, plenty of cereal foods, and potatoes; moderate amounts of meat, fish and alternatives, and of dairy foods. The fifth group, "fatty and sugary foods", are foods and drinks on which to go easy. Other countries have food guides rather like this but use different shapes. The United States and Australia use (different) pyramids. Canada has a quarter rainbow.

It becomes complicated to specify amounts (in grammes or servings) because there is a big range of energy intake from small old ladies to large male athletes. UK health authorities, however, do recommend that adults aim to eat five (or more) servings of vegetables or fruit each day.[2]

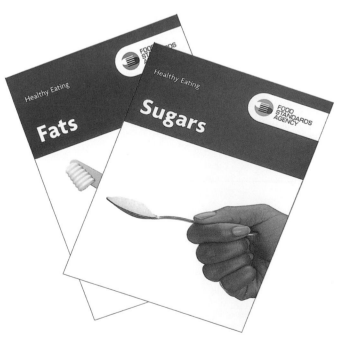

Fats and Sugars leaflets. Reproduced with kind permission from the Food Standards Agency

### HEA/MAFF/DoH eight guidelines for a healthy diet[3]

(1) *Enjoy your food*
No food needs to be excluded from the diet—except occasionally for special medical reasons. There is enough stress in life already without adding to it by worrying unnecessarily about food. It is good to be a little adventurous too with foods that have not previously been tried.

(2) *Eat a variety of different foods*
The food plate guide shows the types and proportions. Under this heading is a note on **salt:** eating too much can contribute to high blood pressure. Most people eat more salt than they need.

(3) *Eat the right amount to be a healthy weight*
Fat has more than twice as many calories as the same weight of starch or protein. Exercise does not have to be strenuous. Lots of small changes like walking … and using the stairs … can add up.

(4) *Eat plenty of foods rich in starch and fibre*
Foods like bread, other cereals (rice and pasta) and potatoes and legumes. Cooking potatoes in oil or fat greatly increases their calorie content.

(5) *Eat plenty of fruit and vegetables*
There are many biologically active substances in fruit and vegetables, as well as essential nutrients, that may help to reduce the risk of chronic diseases.

(6) *Don't eat too many foods that contain a lot of fat*
It is best to cut down on saturates as much as possible.

(7) *Don't have sugary foods and drinks too often*
Eating sugary foods frequently is the main cause of tooth decay. Children's teeth are the most susceptible.

(8) *If you drink alcohol, drink sensibly*
Up to 3-4 units* a day for men; 2-3 units* for women (except in pregnancy) will not significantly increase the risk to health over time.

*British units are 8 g of alcohol; US units are approximately 12 g of alcohol

### US National Research Council 1989[4]

Reduce total fat to 30% or less of calories and saturated fat to less than 10% of calories and dietary cholesterol to less than 300 mg/day. Polyunsaturated fatty acid optimal intake 7% to 8% of calories (not over 10%). $\omega$-3-polyunsaturates from regular fish consumption. (Concentrated fish oil supplements not recommended for general public).

Eat five or more servings of vegetables or fruits daily, especially green and yellow vegetables and citrus fruits, and six or more daily servings of bread, cereals, and legumes. Do not increase intake of added sugars.

Maintain a moderate protein intake, not more than twice the RDA.

Balance food intake and physical activity to maintain appropriate body weight.

If you drink alcohol limit it to no more than two standard drinks a day. Women who are pregnant or attempting to conceive should avoid alcoholic beverages.

Limit total salt intake to 6 g a day sodium chloride.

Maintain adequate calcium intake.

Avoid eating nutrient supplements with dose above the RDA (that is, avoid megavitamin supplements).

Maintain an optimal intake of fluoride, particularly during the years of primary and secondary tooth formation and growth.

RDA = recommended dietary allowance

### Dietary guidelines for Americans[5]

- *Aim for a healthy weight.* If you are at a healthy weight aim to avoid weight gain. If you are already overweight (BMI > 25 kg/m²) first aim to prevent further weight gain, and then lose weight to improve your health.

- *Be physically active each day.* Choose activities that you enjoy and that you can do regularly. Be physically active for at least 30 minutes most days of the week. You can do it all at once or spread it over two or three times during the day.

- *Let the pyramid guide your food choices.* That is eat most bread, cereal, rice and pasta; next level (not so much) vegetable group (including potatoes) and fruit group; next level (less again) milk, yoghurt, cheese group and meat, poultry, fish, dry beans, eggs, nuts group. The smallest group (use sparingly) is fats, oils and sweets.

- *Choose a variety of grains daily, especially whole grains.*

- *Choose a variety of fruits and vegetables daily.*

- *Keep food safe to eat.* Safe means that the food poses little risk of foodborne illness from harmful bacteria, toxins, parasites, viruses or chemical contaminants.

- *Choose a diet that is low in saturated fat and moderate in total fat.* Use moderate amounts of food high in unsaturated fat, taking care to avoid excess calories.

- *Choose beverages and foods to moderate your intake of sugars.* In the United States the number one source of added sugar is non-diet soft drinks (soda or pop)… Drink water often.

- *Choose and prepare foods with less salt.* Many people can reduce their chance of developing high blood pressure by consuming less salt… Most of the salt you eat comes from foods that have salt added during food processing.

- *If you drink alcoholic beverages, do so in moderation.* Moderation here is defined as no more than one drink per day in women (that is, 12 g alcohol) and no more than two drinks per day in men (that is, 24 g alcohol).

## Dietary guidelines

The box on page 38 shows three sets of dietary guidelines. These mostly give advice about how the part of the diet that provides energy—fats, carbohydrate, protein, etc,—should be made up. They are expressed in terms of averages. The average person, eating the average amount of (say) fat, should reduce this by or to a new national average. The advice has to be modified for individuals: Jack Spratt should not reduce fat intake as much as his wife. Recommendations from the US National Research Council use some numbers and technical terms. They need to be translated by health professionals for most consumers. The UK and US guidelines are written in non-technical language. The box shows the headings. There are more details in the booklets.[3-5]

## Other aspects

Other aspects of a healthy diet, sometimes taken for granted, are that food should be wholesome and not contaminated with pathogenic micro-organsims or their toxins or with other toxins (chapter 14). Some of our foods are routinely enriched with micronutrients—for example, B vitamins and iron in white flour, vitamins A and D in margarine.

The municipal drinking water should likewise be nearly chemically pure. Calcium, magnesium, sodium, and fluoride concentrations in it vary from place to place. There is suggestive—but not conclusive—evidence that hard water (more calcium or magnesium, or both), is associated with lower cardiovascular mortality. Fluoridation at 1 ppm is recommended by all orthodox medical and dental authorities.

# Vegetarianism

Are vegetarians more healthy or less? The answer depends first on the degree of vegetarianism.

**Vegans**, who eat no animal products, are at risk of vitamin B-12 deficiency. Supplements are essential during pregnancy and for infants of vegans. Vegans lack the best dietary sources of calcium—milk, yoghurt, and cheese.

**Lacto-ovo-vegetarians** have no absolute nutritional risk. They miss the best absorbed form of iron in the diet, haem iron, but may largely compensate because ascorbic acid enhances the absorption of non-haem iron.

The other determinant is the reason for the vegetarianism. People belonging to long traditions of vegetarianism have the necessary recipes to prepare vegetarian centres for their dishes, using legumes (including soya) and nuts, and so have a good protein intake. It is new vegetarians, some of whom simply remove meat from the centre of the plate, who may eat inadequately.

On the whole vegetarians appear to have lower risk of obesity, coronary heart disease,[7] hypertension, and possibly some cancers. However, many of the figures come from well documented groups such as Seventh Day Adventists, who have a more healthy lifestyle than average in other ways—for example, they do not smoke or drink alcohol.

# Nutrition and poverty in industrialised countries

In different countries of the EU between 4% and 25% of people live below the poverty line (50% of the national average household expenditure, adjusted for family size).[8] In these subcultures of otherwise rich societies people are deprived of jobs, education, security, family support, adequate housing, transport, and/or language skills. The food and nutrients they eat and resulting nutritional status contribute to inequalities of health.[9]

## Five grades of vegetarianism

- Do not eat meat of some animals (for example, horse) or some organs (for example, brain). *This is the norm for omnivorous humans except in a disaster.*
- Do not eat meat but eat fish (and dairy produce). *Very little nutritional risk.*
- Do not eat meat or fish but eat milk and eggs = lacto-ovo-vegetarian. *This is the most common degree of vegetarianism. The only nutritional risk is of iron deficiency.*
- Do not eat any animal products = vegan. *Vitamin B-12 deficiency is likely and can be very serious in infants.[6] Adequate protein can be ensured with regular legume products and nuts. Calcium, iron, and zinc nutrition should be watched.*
- Do not eat anything but fruit = fruitarian. *Unlike some primates, people cannot usually manage on such a diet for long and seldom try to. It is inadequate in protein (unless nuts are included) and even in sodium as well as the nutrients above.*

## Supplements

- Most people do not need nutritional supplements, but women with high menstrual losses may benefit from iron supplements.
- Women who are, or who are planning to become, pregnant are advised to take 0.4 or 0.5 mg of folic acid each day and to eat folate-rich foods (chapter 4).
- Older house-bound people, or people who wear enveloping clothes out of doors all year round, do not make enough vitamin D for their needs by the action of sunlight on their skin and should take 7-10 $\mu$g of vitamin D daily.
- Vitamin drops are available for young children below the age of 5.
- Before starting to take a dietary supplement it is advisable for people to consult a medical practitioner.
- Someone drinking alcohol too heavily can at least prevent Wernicke's encephalopathy by taking thiamin (or vitamin B Co) tablets.

## Sports nutrition[10]

- Dietary guidelines are the foundation of nutritional health, and competitive athletes are motivated to take their health seriously. There are no magic foods, no supplements which will improve sports performance on their own. Body weight and build differ for the various sports and events. Marathon runners are lightly built with little body fat. Champion weight lifters have a BMI in the "obese" range but this is due to an unusual amount of muscle, not fat. Athletes in regular training use and need more energy than sedentary folk. Compared with an average energy intake of around 10 MJ/day (2500 kcal), competitors during the Tour de France use a very high average of 33.7 MJ/day (8000 kcal).
- Athletes take various regimes of high carbohydrate intakes before major events to maximise muscle glycogen content and hence extend the duration of top performance. During long events, drinks similar to oral rehydration fluid (chapter 8) (with glucose, NaCl, and potassium) may sustain performance and prevent dehydration. Different sports drinks and schedules have their devotees.
- Two conditions are important in female athletes, including ballet dancers: mild iron deficiency anaemia, which limits performance, and osteopenia associated with amenorrhoea. For the latter, reduced training and/or increased body fat to restore menstruation, and calcium supplements are advised.

Low birth weight, lower rates of breast feeding, shorter children and overweight adults are more common in these people.

People in this group have to pay more for their food because they lack transport and funds to shop in large supermarkets. They consume less lean meat, fresh fruit and vegetables, and wholemeal bread than average. They suffer food insecurity at times. Their intake of micronutrients is lower, they are liable to anaemia, and their plasma lipids are higher than the average of the country. The Rome Declaration of World Food Security (1996) stated: "Governments will implement cost-effective public works, programmes for unemployed (and) develop social welfare and nutrition safety nets to meet the needs of the food insecure". In Britain the Low Income Project Team of the Nutrition Taskforce has published a report with far-ranging recommendations.[11] This problem of poor nutrition in deprived sections of prosperous countries is a failure of present capitalism and all who are trying to alleviate it deserve our support.

# Older people

In developing countries children suffer most of the malnutrition. In developed countries it is the elderly who are most at risk of nutritional deficiency, though this is usually mild or subclinical and often associated with other disease(s). But it is very misleading to lump everyone over 65 together and expect them all to show the same problems and diseases. Healthy older people who are socially integrated are no more likely to get into nutritional trouble than anyone else.

For the majority people most of their life after 65 should be healthy and enjoyable. This "third age" is a time when people want to look after their health. They can now give more attention, time and money to getting and keeping healthy. They can take plenty of gentle exercise, have none of the stress of the workplace, few deadlines, and plenty of rest, and have time to choose food carefully and prepare it nicely. The dietary guidelines for younger adults all apply after retirement.

### Dietary guidelines after retirement age

- A nutritious diet from a variety of foods is more important than when people are younger because the total energy intake is usually smaller than in young adults. The number of calories needed is less but not the requirements for most essential nutrients.
- To be light in weight eases the load on osteoarthritic joints and ageing heart and lungs and reduces the risk of accidents. Judicious regular exercise is much better than food restriction.
- Cut down on fat, especially saturated fat. Fat supplies more empty calories than any other dietary component. It predisposes to thrombosis, raised plasma cholesterol, and atherogenesis.
- Eat plenty of bread and cereals (preferably wholegrain) and vegetables and fruits; older people are liable to constipation, and a good intake of fibre will help to control this.
- Limit alcohol consumption. The smaller liver cannot metabolise as much alcohol as in young adults and the consequences of falls or accidents are more serious. No more than one or two drinks a day.
- Cut down on salt and salty foods. They tend to raise blood pressure; salt sensitivity increases with age and hypertension predisposes to strokes.
- Avoid too much sugar because of the empty calories, but dental caries is less troublesome in surviving mature teeth.

It is wrong, however, to use these guidelines for people who are declining in health (the "fourth age"); and some doubt even exists about whether low serum cholesterol concentration or body weight give any survival advantage to very old people.

---

**Eating for the environment**

People may rightly choose foods because the environment was considered in their production, for example more humane housing of hens and chickens (free-range eggs), fish nets that do not catch dolphins, or organic farming. The basis for preferring such produce has to be environmental rather than nutritional. Analysis of all the nutrients in foods adds up to be very expensive and no one can guarantee an overall nutritional advantage.[12]

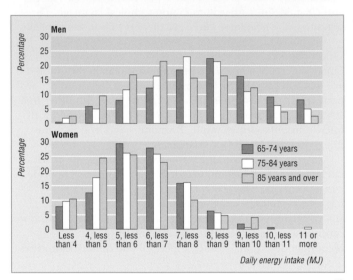

Average daily intakes of 1275 free living older people in Britain (age 65-97)[13]

---

**With ageing (from 20-30 to over 70 years):**

- average body weight goes down after middle age (partly because of selective mortality of obese people)
- lean body mass declines from average 60 to 50 kg in men and 40 to 35 kg in women
- there is a loss of height and of mass of the skeleton
- muscle mass declines from about 450 g/kg to 300 g/kg
- body density goes down from 1.072 to 1.041 in men and from 1.040 to 1.016 in women
- body fat (as % of body weight) increases from about 20% to 30% in men and from 27% to 40% in women. It becomes more central and internal
- liver weight falls from about 25 g to 20 g/kg body weight
- basal metabolic rate goes down proportionally with lean body mass.

---

**Diet and longevity 1**[14]

- McCay in 1931, and others since, have found that rats and mice live longer if their diet is restricted to 60% of ad libitum intake long term. This is not because one type of food, fat or protein, is restricted and the effect still occurs after growth is completed. A favoured explanation is reduced exposure to reactive oxygen species from lower metabolic activity. Rats usually live about two years. Dietary restriction experiments have not yet been completed in larger animals. Whenever humans have been subjected to undernutrition they have usually been in an unhealthy environment with heavy exposure to infections but the diet-restricted rodents were kept away from pathogens. It is unlikely that a sufficiently long and controlled human experiment could ever be carried out.
- Humans are in any case an unusually long-lived species. We live twice as long as great apes. This may be because several antioxidant systems are unusually well developed in our species.[15]

## Risk factors for impaired nutrition in older people

### Social risk factors

- Loneliness
- Isolation
- Immobility (no transport)
- Poverty
- Ignorance (the widower who cannot cook)
- Bereavement
- Alcoholism
- Dependence
- Regression

### Medical risk factors

- Cancer and radiotherapy
- Depression
- Chronic bronchitis and emphysema
- Anorexia
- Cardiac failure
- Angina
- Insomnia
- Blindness
- Deafness
- Paralysis
- Arthritis
- Dementia
- Gastrectomy
- Sjörgen's syndrome
- Diverticulitis
- No teeth
- Frailty

### Some common drugs that can lead to malnutrition

- Aspirin and NSAIDs → blood loss, so iron deficiency
- Digoxin → lowers appetite
- Purgatives → potassium loss
- Cancer chemotherapy → anorexia
- Many diuretics → potassium loss
- Metformin → vitamin B-12 malabsorption
- Co-trimoxazole → can antagonise folate

NSAIDs = non-steroidal anti-inflammatory drugs

## Some suggested extra dietary guidelines for older people

- Women especially should keep up a good intake of calcium from (low fat) milk or cheese, or both. This may help to delay osteoporosis.
- Those who are housebound or do not get out regularly should take small prophylactic doses of vitamin D (5-10 µg/day).
- Elderly people should avoid big meals, as Hippocrates, Galen, and Avicenna all advised. On the other hand, they should not miss any of the three main daily meals.

> Old men have little warmth and they need little food which produces warmth; too much only extinguishes the warmth they have.
>
> Hippocrates, *Aphorisms* 1, 14

- Coffee or tea in the evening may contribute to insomnia.
- There is a place for fatty fish or small amounts of fish oils containing fatty acids like eicosapentaenoic acid (20:5, ω-3), which can reduce the risk of thrombosis.

## Assessment of nutritional status

There have been several studies of the nutrition of elderly people in Britain and similar countries. Findings have differed, partly because different sectors of the elderly population have been sampled, partly because different parts of the range of possible biochemical tests have been done. Nutritional deficiency is nearly always secondary to a social problem or to disease. The first step in diagnosing malnutrition is to recognise one or more **risk factors**. The chances of risk factors and of nutritional deficiencies in elderly people increase progressively from those at normal risk (the healthy and socially integrated), through those who have one or more chronic illnesses but are nevertheless socially organised, and the housebound, to those at high risk—the institutionalised.

Assessment of nutritional status can be difficult in old people. The history of food intake may be unreliable because of poor memory. We are not yet sure whether the recommended intakes of some nutrients should be adjusted downward or upward, or by how much. Height (stature) may be impossible to measure exactly because of deformities.

## Nutrients most likely to be deficient in old people are (roughly in order of importance):

- total energy—thinness, wasting, undernutrition
- potassium—deficiency can present with confusion, constipation, cardiac arrhythmias, muscle weakness, etc
- folate—deficiency can present with anaemia or with confusion
- vitamin B-12—because of gastric atrophy. Serum methylmalonate may be elevated before vitamin B-12 is low
- vitamin D—deficiency can present with fractures or bone pains of osteomalacia
- water—frail old people may not drink enough, which can lead to urinary tract infection or dehydration
- dietary fibre—deficiency leads to constipation
- vitamin C—low plasma concentration, haemorrhages
- iron—anaemia, koilonychia
- protein—low plasma albumin, oedema
- calcium—low intake; decreased bone density
- zinc—low plasma concentration
- thiamin—biochemical features of deficiency (red cell transketolase)
- magnesium—low plasma concentration
- pyridoxine—biochemical features of deficiency.

## Knee height (from heel to top of patella with the knee flexed) can be used to estimate stature in centimetres

- **for men** stature = 2.02 KH − (0.04 × age, y) + 64.2
- **for women** stature = 1.83 KH − (0.24 × age, y) + 84.9.

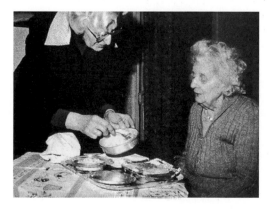

Weight-for-height standards (for younger adults) are not strictly applicable because of the decline in lean body mass. Some recent anthropometric data on 200 people over 75 living independently in two general practices are provided by Bannerman et al.[16]

Clinical examination is complicated by the presence of other diseases. Oedema is usually due to cardiovascular disease, loss of ankle jerks to ageing nerves rather than nutritional deficiency. For several biochemical tests we are not quite sure what the normal range is in old people.

### Preventive measures

Only rarely are low intakes of nutrients and abnormal laboratory findings associated with a disturbance of function that would support the diagnosis of clinical malnutrition. The usual finding can best be called subclinical deficiency, and we are often not sure of its clinical importance. It is prudent to attempt to raise the level of nutrients to make people with subclinical deficiency more resistant to the effects of stress caused by non-nutritional diseases, which become increasingly common with advancing years.

General practitioners, with the younger family members or a friend, district nurse, or social worker can improve an old person's nutrition in several ways:

- suggest cooking lessons for retired men
- arrange help for partly disabled people to adapt cooking techniques
- organise delivery of heavy shopping
- suggest (where one is absent) buying a refrigerator or freezer
- ensure that every elderly person or couple has an emergency food store
- suggest that a younger relative helps with shopping and invites the elderly person for a regular good meal
- arrange for him or her to attend a lunch club
- arrange for meals on wheels
- possibly prescribe micronutrient supplements, but some multivitamin tablets do not contain them all (some miss folic acid) and there may be more need for potassium
- build on established eating patterns when advising about changing food consumption; drastic changes are likely to confuse
- warn that reduced sense of smell and sight make it hard to detect food that is no longer wholesome.

## Nutrition in institutions

In nursing homes, practices that contribute to poor nutrition include:

- lack of communication between nursing and kitchen staff
- disregarding residents' suggestions about menus
- ignoring residents' requirements for special diets
- offering no choice of portion size or second helping
- monotonous menus
- not noting food left or residents not eating
- not weighing residents regularly
- little or no homestyle cooking
- inadequate help with feeding frail residents
- cooks that lack basic knowledge of nutrition
- meals rushed or served too early
- no facilities for residents to make hot drinks for themselves
- low fibre diets.

More details for those inspecting or advising on nutrition in nursing homes can be found in *Eating well for older people*.[18]

---

### Diet and longevity: 2

- Claims that people live longer than usual in parts of Georgia (Europe), or in Vilcabamba in Ecuador have proved dubious on investigation. There were no birth certificates.
- The food that our centenarians ate when young they say was less processed and simpler than contemporary food patterns. Of course it was. That was what ordinary people ate in 1903.
- No special food emerged when a sample of centenarians recalled their lifestyles to the US House of Representatives Select Committee on Aging.

---

"Food, like sex, is one of the pleasures that stays with us all our lives" (as Alex Comfort put it).[17] When life is limited because of disabilities and loss of social and environmental stimulation, it is very important for the morale and well being of elderly people in institutions that their food is what they like, and is served with courtesy, and that they have at least some control over it. We younger adults are always making compromises between ideal nutrition and a little of what we fancy, and we must allow and help elderly people in nursing homes to do the same—by offering them a glass of sherry or beer, a favourite dessert, or a piece of confectionery.

---

### References

1 Health Education Authority. *The balance of good health. Introducing the national food guide.* London: Health Education Authority, 1994.
2 National Heart Forum. *At least five a day. Strategies to increase vegetable and fruit consumption.* London: Stationery Office, 1997.
3 HEA/MAFF/DoH. *Eight guidelines for a healthy diet. A guide for nutrition educators,* Abingdon, Oxon: HEA Customer Services, 1997.
4 Committee on Diet and Health, Food and Nutrition Board, National Research Council. *Diet and health. Implications for reducing chronic disease risk.* Washington, DC: National Academy Press, 1989.
5 USDA, USDHHS. *Dietary guidelines for Americans.* Washington, DC: US Department of Agriculture, 2000.
6 Wighton MC, Manson JI, Speed I *et al.* Brain damage in infancy and dietary vitamin B-12 deficiency. *Med J Aust* 1979; **2**: 1-3.
7 Thorogood M, Mann JI, Appleby P, McPherson K. Risk of death from cancer and ischaemic heart disease in meat and non-meat eaters. *BMJ* 1994; **308**: 1667-71.
8 Dowler EA, Dobson BM. Nutrition and poverty in Europe: an overview. *Proc Nutr Soc* 1997; **56**: 51-62.
9 James WPT, Nelson M, Ralph A, Leather S. The contribution of nutrition to inequalities in health. *BMJ* 1997; **314**: 1545-9.
10 Burke L, Deakin V (eds). *Clinical sports nutrition,* 2nd edn. Sydney: McGraw Hill, 2000.
11 Department of Health. *Low income, food, nutrition and health: strategies for improvement.* Wetherby: Department of Health, 1996.
12 Williams CM. Nutritional quality of organic food: shades of grey or shades of green. *Proc Nutr Soc* 2002; **61**: 19-24.
13 Finch S, Doyle W, Lowe C *et al. National Diet and Nutrition Survey: People aged 65 years and over. Vol 1. Report of the diet and nutrition survey.* London: Stationery Office, 1998.
14 Masoro EJ. McCay's hypothesis: undernutrition and longevity. *Proc Nutr Soc* 1995; **54**: 657-64.
15 Cutler RG. Antioxidants and aging. *Am J Clin Nutr* 1991; **53**: 373-79S.
16 Bannerman E, Reilly JJ, MacLennan WJ, Kirk T, Pender F. Evaluation of validity of British anthropometric reference data for assessing nutritional state of elderly people in Edinburgh: cross sectional study. *BMJ* 1997; **315**: 338-41.
17 Comfort A. *A good age.* London: Mitchell Beazley, 1977.
18 Report of an Expert Working Group. *Eating well for older people. Practical and nutritional guidelines for food in residential and nursing homes and for community meals.* London: The Caroline Walker Trust, 1995.

# 8 Malnutrition in developing countries

Some former "developing countries" really have been developing, and as a byproduct malnutrition has largely disappeared. Other countries have been static or lost ground. A country can become poorer from reduced income, reduced gross national product (GNP) per head (caused by bad climate, economic mismanagement, or war) or from population growth faster than economic growth, or both. Many of the poorest countries have suffered civil wars.

About two-thirds of the world's six million people live in countries with low and lower middle incomes (on the current lists of the United Nations). In most of these countries people are very poor; the population is young and growing fast; there is no welfare state and little mechanisation. Food at an affordable price cannot be taken for granted; nor can clean drinking water. Tropical infections are an additional burden.

Public health indicators do not correlate closely with national income. Vietnam is an outstanding example of a poor country which nevertheless has enough food to go round, and health statistics better than that, for example, of South Africa, whose GNP/head is 10 times higher. Economic development is thus only one factor—an important one— that reduces malnutrition. But even if a country's income stays low there are things that doctors, nurses, agriculturists, administrators, and politicians can do to combat malnutrition.

Diagnosis and management of malnutrition in developing countries have to be mostly a public health operation. Many of the malnourished live in slums, shanty towns, or remote rural areas. They cannot be brought to a central teaching hospital. There are fewer doctors—in some countries only 1 for 50 000 people—so they have to work through teams of community health workers, who should be trained to recognise and cope with the common diseases, including malnutrition and the closely related infections.

## Protein-energy malnutrition[3,4]

What is described here is malnutrition in young children. They are dependent on adults for their food and are therefore especially vulnerable where there is food insecurity. They have high food energy needs for their size (kg body weight) and because of higher protein requirements per calorie (or kJ) they are more at risk of protein deficiency than adults.

The prevalence of protein-energy malnutrition (PEM) in its various forms is high in South and South-East Asia, in Africa and the Middle East, in some Caribbean islands, and in Central and South America. Severe forms affect around 2% and mild to moderate PEM affects around 20% of young children (in many places more) in developing countries. WHO has estimated that about 200 million children in the world at any time have moderate or severe PEM. Although it affects only some children in each community, it is a larger and more intractable problem than famines.

### Severe PEM
**Nutritional marasmus** is the commonest severe reform of protein-energy malnutrition, the childhood version of starvation. It usually occurs at a younger age than kwashiorkor. The cause is a diet very low in both calories and protein— caused, for example, by early weaning then feeding dilute food because of poverty or ignorance. Poor hygiene leads to

| 1998 Figures | 39 Poorest countries | Vietnam | United Kingdom |
|---|---|---|---|
| GNP/head (US$) | 110 to 390 | 310 | 20 870 |
| Population growth % | −0.7 to 4.7 | 1.9 | 0.2 |
| Infant mortality Rate/1000 | 31 to 182 | 31 | 6 |
| Under 5 mortality Rate/1000 | 42 to 316 | 42 | 6 |
| Life expectancy at birth (years) | 38 to 68 | 68 | 77 |

Data from *The State of the World's Children* 2000[1]

### From the first three paragraphs of the World Declaration on Nutrition, 1992[2]

- We, the Ministers and Plenipotentiaries representing 159 states and the EEC ... declare our determination to eliminate hunger and to reduce all forms of malnutrition. Hunger and malnutrition are unacceptable in a world that has both the knowledge and the resources to end this human catastrophe ...
- ... We all view with the deepest concern the unacceptable fact that about 780 million people in developing countries—20% of their combined population—still do not have access to enough food to meet their basic daily needs for nutritional well-being.
- We are especially distressed by the high prevalence and increasing numbers of malnourished children under five years of age in parts of Africa, Asia and Latin America and the Caribbean. Moreover, more than 2000 million people, mostly women and children, are deficient in one or more micronutrients: babies continue to be born mentally retarded as a result of iodine deficiency; children go blind and die of vitamin A deficiency; and enormous numbers of women and children are adversely affected by iron deficiency...

| Protein-energy malnutrition | Bodyweight as % of standard | Oedema | Deficit in weight for height |
|---|---|---|---|
| Marasmus | 60 | 0 | ++ |
| Marasmic kwashiorkor | 60 | + | ++ |
| Kwashiorkor | 80-60* | + | + |
| Nutritional dwarf | 60 | 0 | minimal |
| Underweight child | 80-60 | 0 | + |

*Occasional cases are not underweight at the oedematous stage

gastroenteritis and a vicious circle starts. Diarrhoea leads to poor appetite and more dilute foods. In turn further depletion leads to intestinal atrophy and more susceptibility to diarrhoea.

**Kwashiorkor** in its full blown form is less common than marasmus. It is most common in poor rural children, displaced from the breast by the next child and given a very low protein starchy porridge—for example, made with cassava or plantain. There have been several hypotheses about the antecedent diet because it is very difficult to reconstruct the exact dietary history of a malnourished child. But careful studies by Whitehead's group[5] of pre-kwashiorkor in Uganda compared with pre-marasmus in the Gambia, and other information support the classical hypothesis of protein deficiency with relatively adequate carbohydrate intake. Pure cases of kwashiorkor can develop in a few weeks and the patients sometimes have normal weight for age.

The pathogenesis of kwashiorkor appears to be: very low protein intake with more dietary carbohydrate leads to insulin secretion being maintained (unlike marasmus). Insulin spares muscle protein when there is shortage of amino acids, but there is loss of liver protein. So synthesis is reduced of two proteins made in the liver: (*a*) plasma albumin, hence oedema (potassium depletion makes it more likely), and (*b*) low density lipoproteins, hence lipids accumulate in the liver. Some of the features of kwashiorkor may be due to associated zinc deficiency.

**Marasmic kwashiorkor** has some features of both conditions. Severe protein-energy malnutrition can be thought of as a spectrum from marasmus to kwashiorkor. Most affected children have some skin lesions, hair changes, and fatty liver (as in kwashiorkor) together with the wasting of marasmus.

Malnourished children are likely to be depleted in other nutrients (see box opposite).

### Treatment

Management of severe protein-energy malnutrition is in three phases.[6]

(1) **Resuscitation**
Correction of dehydration, electrolyte disturbances, acidosis, hypoglycaemia, hypothermia, and treatment of infections.

(2) **Start of cure**
Refeeding, gradually working up the calories (from 100 to 150 kcal (420-630 kJ) per kg) and protein (to about 1.5 g per kg). There may be anorexia, and children often have to be hand fed, preferably in the lap of their mother or a nurse they know. Potassium, magnesium, zinc, and a multivitamin mixture are needed but iron should not be given for the first week.

(3) **Nutritional rehabilitation**
After about three weeks if all goes well the child has lost oedema and the skin is healed. The child is no longer ill and has a good appetite but is still underweight for age. It takes many weeks of good feeding for catch up growth to be complete. During this stage the child should be looked after in a convalescent home or by its mother, who should if possible have been educated about nutrition and provided with extra food. Locally available foods are best.

### Mild and moderate protein-energy malnutrition

This is much more common than the obvious severe forms. Outside observers, even the mothers themselves, do not notice most of these cases because the children are similar in size and vitality to some of the other children of the same age. The condition is like an iceberg. For every severe case there are likely to be seven to 10 in the community with lesser degrees of malnutrition. These latter children do not grow normally and

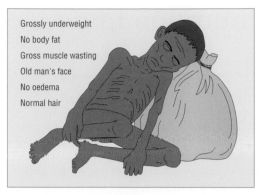

Grossly underweight
No body fat
Gross muscle wasting
Old man's face
No oedema
Normal hair

Marasmus

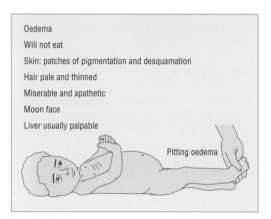

Oedema
Will not eat
Skin: patches of pigmentation and desquamation
Hair pale and thinned
Miserable and apathetic
Moon face
Liver usually palpable

Pitting oedema

Kwashiorkor

### Other nutrients deficient in protein-energy malnutrition

*Usually:*
• Potassium
• Magnesium
• Zinc
• Vitamin A
• Iron
• Folate

*In some areas:*
• Thiamin—Thailand
• Riboflavin—Thailand
• Niacin—southern Africa
• Iodine—areas of endemic goitre
• Selenium

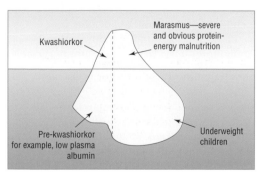

Kwashiorkor

Marasmus—severe and obvious protein-energy malnutrition

Pre-kwashiorkor for example, low plasma albumin

Underweight children

The iceberg of malnutrition

are at increased risk of infection. They may also have more difficulty learning motor and cognitive skills.

### National statistics used to indicate nutrition[1]
**Underweight** can be due to either wasting or stunting. **Wasting** is a fairly direct indication of undernutrition but the causes of **stunting** are complex. The NCHS anthropometric references used by WHO for international comparisons are based on large samples of US children measured in the 1960s and 1970s. A high percentage of stunted children means that they are short by US standards. The causes can be genetic, or intra-uterine growth retardation, or delayed growth from multiple infectious diseases, or insufficient nutrition. Small size is an adaptation. It cannot be equated with malnutrition.[7]

Most children with mild protein-energy malnutrition are thin and underweight. Because scales are difficult to carry children who are malnourished may be identified in the field by measuring the mid-upper arm circumference. From 12 to 60 months of age over 13.5 cm is a normal circumference; 12.5 to 13.5 cm suggests mild malnutrition and under 12.5 cm indicates definite malnutrition. The normal circumference stays the same for these four years.

Sometimes a child is seen who has adapted to chronic inadequate feeding by reduced linear growth but looks like a normal child a year or two younger—this is **nutritional stunting**.

### Prevention of protein-energy malnutrition
Five measures to prevent protein-energy malnutrition are being actively promoted round the world.

**Growth monitoring.** The WHO has devised a simple growth chart—the Road to Health card. The mother (not the clinic) should keep the card in a cellophane envelope and bring the child (plus card) to the nearest clinic regularly for weighing and advice.

**Oral rehydration.** The UNICEF formula is saving many lives from gastroenteritis: NaCl 3.5 g, $NaHCO_3$ 2.5 g, KCl 1.5 g, glucose 20 g (or sucrose 40 g) and clean water to 1 litre.

**Breast feeding** is a matter of life and death in a poor community with no facilities for hygiene. Additional food, prepared from locally available products, is needed from four to six months of age.

**Immunisation** should be done against measles, tetanus, pertussis, diphtheria, polio, and tuberculosis.

**Family planning** advice and inexpensive or free contraception should be readily available.

# Starvation and famine

When there is not enough food for an entire community children stop growing, and children and adults lose weight. The symptoms include craving for food, thirst, weakness, feeling cold, nocturia, amenorrhoea, and impotence.

The face at first looks younger but later becomes old and withered and expressionless; pupils react poorly to light. The skin is lax, pale, and dry and may show pigmented patches. Hair becomes thinned or lost except in adolescents. The extremities are cold and cyanosed. There may be pressure sores. Subcutaneous fat disappears, skin turgor is lost, and muscles waste. The arm circumference is subnormal. Oedema may be present; in adults this is famine oedema, which is not always associated with hypoalbuminaemia. Temperature is subnormal. The pulse is slow, blood pressure low, and the heart small with muffled sounds. The abdomen is distended. Diarrhoea is common, often associated with blood. Muscles are weak and tendon jerks diminished. Psychologically, starving

---

### Underweight, wasting and stunting, defined by WHO

- Underweight is moderate if 2 to 3 standard deviations below the median NCHS **weight for age** (see page 30) and severe if more than 3 SDs below the reference.
- Wasting is moderate if 2 to 3 standard deviations (79-70%) below the median NCHS **weight for height** and severe if more than 3 SDs (<70%) below the reference.
- Stunting is moderate if 2 to 3 standard deviations (89-85%) below the NCHS median **height for age** and severe if more than 3 SDs (<85%) below the reference.

The standard deviation score is also called the "z score".

---

### Percentage of children under 5 with moderate or severe underweight, wasting or stunting

|  | Under weight | Wasting | Stunting |
|---|---|---|---|
| Sub Saharan Africa | 32 | 9 | 41 |
| Middle East and North Africa | 18 | 8 | 25 |
| South Asia | 51 | 18 | 52 |
| Latin America and Caribbean | 10 | 3 | 18 |
| USA | 1 | 1 | 2 |

From UNICEF *State of the World's Children* 2000[1]

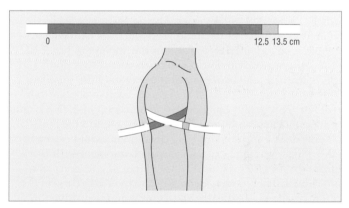

Measuring circumference of mid-upper arm

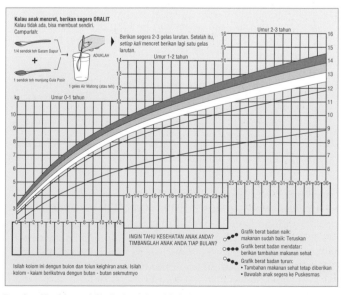

Road to Health card for Indonesia with instructions for making oral rehydration fluid. Numbers along the base are months

people lose initiative; they are apathetic, depressed, and introverted but become aggressive if food is nearby.

Infections are to be expected, especially gastrointestinal infections, pneumonia, typhus, and tuberculosis. The usual signs of infection (pyrexia, leucocytosis) may not appear. Delayed skin sensitivity with recall antigens—for example, tuberculin—are falsely negative. But the erythrocyte sedimentation rate is normal unless there is infection. In advanced starvation patients become completely inactive and may assume a flexed, fetal position. Death comes quietly and often quite suddenly in the late stage of starvation. The very young and the very old are most vulnerable.

Inside the body plasma free fatty acids are increased; there is ketosis and may be a mild metabolic acidosis. Plasma glucose is low but albumin concentration is often normal. Insulin secretion is diminished, reverse triiodothyronine replaces normal T3, and glucagon and cortisol concentrations tend to increase. The resting metabolic rate goes down considerably; oxygen consumption per person goes down more than when expressed per kg body weight. The urine has a fixed specific gravity, and creatinine excretion becomes as low as 300 mg/day. There may be a mild anaemia, leucopenia, and thrombocytopenia. The electrocardiogram shows sinus brachycardia and low voltages. All the organs are atrophied and have subnormal weights at necropsy except the brain, which tends to maintain its weight.

Much the same clinical and metabolic features of starvation are seen in hunger strikers as in the much more common situation in a famine, but in the latter intercurrent infections usually compound the disorder. The problem in a famine is not so much loss of food availability as loss of food entitlement. People have to sell all their assets in the attempt to buy food. Practically all social and economic structures break down and there may as a last resort be mass migration of the sufferers. The worst famines of recent times have been in areas torn by civil war. This greatly hampers communication of early warning of food shortage and transport of relief food into the area.

Any doctor involved in relief operations should expect to have a mainly administrative and organisational role. It is impossible to give most time to treatment of a few very sick individuals. Therapeutic feeding is not an effective use of resources. Field workers have three options for distribution of food where supplies are insufficient to provide the minimum requirements of 1900 kcal (8MJ)/person/day:

(1) where community and family structure is still intact and community representatives can be identified, let the community decide how the limited food should be distributed
    *or*
(2) where community structures have been disrupted field workers distribute food selectively to those at highest risk of mortality
    *or*
(3) the third alternative is equitable distribution of the same basic ration to all members of the affected population with selection of particularly vulnerable members.[9]

Each option has its unsatisfactory aspects and work is easier when and if enough food is shipped in for all. The standard rations usually consist of cereals, legumes, and some oil. If the cereal is wholegrain, milling equipment is needed. Milk powder is used for malnourished children. Care must be taken that the population is getting the critical micronutrients, for example, vitamin C, potassium.[10]

To assess the degree of undernutrition in individuals two measures are used: mid-upper arm circumference (MUAC) and

### Famine is different from endemic undernutrition

Because present-day famines strike in developing countries where malnutrition is endemic, there is an unfortunate tendency to blur the differences between endemic malnutrition and famine-induced malnutrition, to treat the latter as if it were simply the former writ large …

Famines are distinct … They are different not only in severity, but in kind. This is because the famine year is neither characterised by poverty, nor even death, but by social disruption. Miserable though it is, chronic poverty in traditional societies is a situation to which considerable social, psychological and physiological adaptation has occurred. Only when these mechanisms of cultural homoeostasis are unable to cope does the situation shift into famine …

What distinguishes famine-induced malnutrition is not that it is *acute*, but that it is *extensive*.

Rivers JPW, in Harrison[8]

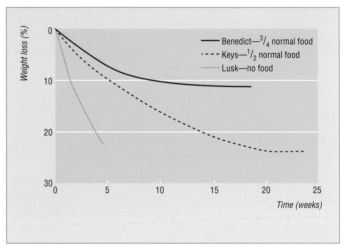

Body weight loss during fasting. (Adapted from Payne[7])

### Degrees of underweight in adults at different heights

| Height (m) | Weight (kg) | |
| --- | --- | --- |
| | 80% of standard* | 70% of standard |
| 1.45 | 38 | 33 |
| 1.48 | 39.5 | 34.5 |
| 1.50 | 40.5 | 35 |
| 1.52 | 41.5 | 36 |
| 1.54 | 42.5 | 37 |
| 1.56 | 44 | 38.5 |
| 1.58 | 45 | 39 |
| 1.60 | 46 | 40 |
| 1.62 | 47 | 41 |
| 1.64 | 48.5 | 42 |
| 1.66 | 49.5 | 43 |
| 1.68 | 50.5 | 44 |
| 1.70 | 52 | 45.5 |
| 1.72 | 53 | 47 |
| 1.74 | 54.5 | 48 |
| 1.76 | 56 | 49 |
| 1.78 | 57 | 50 |
| 1.80 | 58 | 51 |
| 1.82 | 60 | 52 |
| 1.84 | 61 | 53.5 |
| 1.86 | 62 | 54 |
| 1.88 | 63.5 | 55.5 |
| 1.90 | 65 | 57 |

*Standard weight = W/H² 22.5. 80% standard = BMI 18
70% standard = BMI 16

weight for height in children or BMI (kg/m$^2$) in adults. MUAC is obviously quicker and a tape measure more portable, but in children low MUAC tends to select younger children as malnourished and miss older children with low weight for height.[11] In adults MUAC and BMI appear to correlate fairly well. A MUAC of 220 mm in men or 210 mm in women corresponds approximately to a critical BMI of 16 kg/m$^2$.[12] As a general rule **moderate starvation**=weight for height 80-71% of standard (BMI 18-16 kg/m$^2$) and **severe starvation**=weight for height ≤70% of standard (BMI ≤ 15.7).

Circumstances and resources are different in every famine. The problems are mainly non-medical: organising transport and repair of trucks and shelters, coordinating relief from different organisations, reconciling international workers with local politicians and administrators, arranging security of food stores, seeing that food is distributed on the basis of need, trying to procure the right food and the appropriate medical supplies. Civil disturbances do not occur during severe famine. They may happen at an early stage (food riots) or afterwards (revolution). Meanwhile, the future has to be planned for; agricultural workers are going to be needed with enough strength to plough and plant the next crop when the rains return.

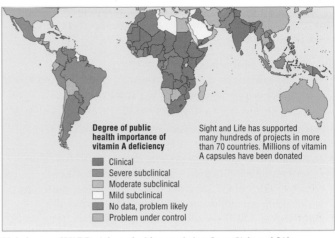

Global map of VADD. Adapted with permission from *Sight and Life* (http://www.sightandlife.org)

# Vitamin A deficiency and xerophthalmia

In 1857 David Livingstone first suggested that eye lesions in some African natives were caused by nutritional deficiency: "The eyes became affected as in the case of animals fed pure gluten or starch." The antixerophthalmia factor was the first of the vitamins to be isolated, in 1915 by McCollum in the USA. Xerophthalmia is a late manifestation of vitamin A deficiency. Its global incidence has been estimated at some 500 000 new cases a year, half of which lead to blindness. Because of its social consequences vitamin A deficiency is given priority by the WHO for prevention programmes. The highest incidence is in South and South-East Asia—for example, India, Bangladesh, and the Philippines. It also occurs in some underdeveloped parts of Africa and Central and South America.

Vitamin A is not only the antixerophthalmia vitamin. It has also been called the "**anti-infective vitamin**" because rats with experimental deficiency had multiple infections. Children with full-blown xerophthalmia have high mortality. The importance of vitamin A for humans broadened when a longitudinal survey in Java showed that even mild forms of xerophthalmia were associated with a four-fold risk of death, often from respiratory or intestinal infections. Sommer's group[13] went on to a large randomised controlled trial in an area where cases of xerophthalmia occur. Children of 1-5 years given vitamin A capsules (one single capsule of 200 000 IU, repeated after six months) had a 34% lower mortality than untreated children in adjacent villages.[13] Subsequently similar prevention trials have been completed in several developing countries. Most reported significant benefits from vitamin A supplementation; the overall average reduction of death rate was 23%. By 1996, 40 developing countries had programmes for giving routine vitamin A supplements to young children.[1]

There is a strong synergistic association of measles and vitamin A deficiency. Measles can precipitate xerophthalmia and leads to low plasma vitamin A even in developed countries. In Cape Town (where clinical xerophthalmia is rare) a controlled trial in black children hospitalised with measles showed a strikingly better outcome in those given vitamin A (200 000 IU once on admission and repeated the next day).

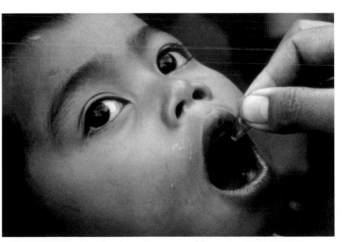

Child receiving vitamin A capsule. Reproduced with permission from *Sight and Life*

47

Vitamin A should be given to any child with severe measles or from a deprived background.[14] With the new broader concepts of subclinical vitamin A deficiency, over 200 million young children have been estimated to be at risk and three million clinically affected.[15]

## Stages of xerophthalmia

Severe xerophthalmia is virtually confined to infants and young children and usually associated with protein-energy malnutrition. The stages are classified by the WHO as follows.

- **Night blindness** (XIN) is the earliest symptom but not elicited in infants.
- In **conjunctival xerosis** (XIA) one or more patches of dry non-wettable conjunctiva emerge "like sand banks at receding tide" when the child ceases to cry. It is caused by keratinising squamous metaphasia of the conjunctiva.
- **Bitot's spots** (XIB) are glistening white plaques formed of desquamated thickened epithelium, usually triangular and firmly adherent to the underlying conjunctiva.
- **Corneal xerosis** (X2) is a haziness or a granular pebbly dryness of the cornea on routine light examination, beginning in the inferior cornea.
- **Corneal ulceration** (X3A) **or keratomalacia** (X3B). A punched out ulcer may occur or, in a severe case, colliquative necrosis of the cornea (keratomalacia). If promptly treated a small ulcer usually heals, leaving some vision. Large ulcers and keratomalacia usually result in an opaque cornea (X5) or perforation and phthisis bulbae.

## Pathogenesis of xerophthalmia

In countries where xerophthalmia occurs, adults have much lower vitamin A stores in their livers than in well-fed people. Women start with low stores and throughout pregnancy have low intakes of vitamin A and carotene. Newborn babies have only one-fifth the liver vitamin A concentration of their mothers, even in well-fed communities, because vitamin A transport across the placenta is limited. Since the mother has low intakes and stores, her breast milk contains low concentrations of vitamin A and carotene. If the child has protein-energy malnutrition this impairs absorption and transport of vitamin A. Then a severe infection can precipitate clinical deficiency by increasing urinary loss of the vitamin and reducing hepatic synthesis of retinol binding protein.

The symptomatology of vitamin A deficiency can be explained by several functions of the vitamin. Retinaldehyde (retinal) is needed for the response of rods in the retina to light. Retinoic acid is needed to maintain differentiation of epithelia (for example, conjunctiva, respiratory), secretion of mucus, and tear production. In vitamin A deficiency cell-mediated immunity is impaired.

## Diagnosis and treatment

Xerophthalmia is rare in Britain. It is seen occasionally in patients with chronic jaundice or small bowel resection or very restricted diets. A British doctor going to work in a developing country should familiarise themself with the early features of xerophthalmia from colour photographs. (An excellent set is obtainable from American Foundation for Overseas Blind, 22 West 17th St, New York, NY 10011, USA. Or see a recent WHO publication on diagnosis and management of xerophthalmia.)

Treatment of xerophthalmia is urgent. The differential diagnosis includes smoke exposure, trauma, bacterial infections, measles, and trachoma. The child often has some other illness at the time like gastroenteritis, kwashiorkor, measles, or respiratory infection, which can distract attention from the eyes unless they are examined systematically. If in doubt a dose of vitamin A

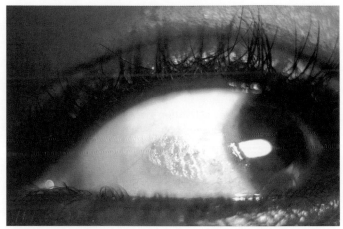

Bitot's spot. Reproduced with permission from *Sight and Life*

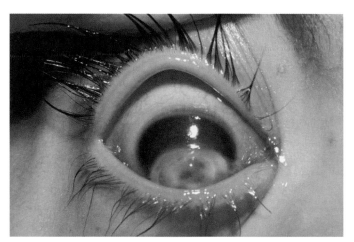

Colliquative necrosis of lower 2/3 of the cornea (Keratomalacia). Reproduced with permission from *Sight and Life*

In Britain conscientious objectors volunteered for a classic vitamin A depletion experiment in Sheffield during the Second World War. There were no features of deficiency until they were into the second year of a diet lacking vitamin A and carotene, and even then the symptoms were minor (night blindness and follicular hyperkeratosis). In well-nourished countries adults have enough vitamin A stored in their liver to last over a year of deprivation.

should be given. It can do no harm. The immediate treatment is 110 mg retinol palmitate or 66 mg retinol acetate (200 000 IU) orally or (if there is repeated vomiting or severe diarrhoea) 55 mg retinol palmitate (100 000 IU) **water soluble** preparation intramuscularly. For the next few days repeat the oral dose.

### Prevention

There are four strategies for prevention. In some countries two or more are being used side by side.

(1) **Nutrition education**

This emphasises garden cultivation and regular consumption of locally grown plant sources of β-carotene (pro-vitamin A). The best sources include mango, papaya, pumpkin, yellow sweet potatoes, carrots and palm oil, as well as eggs and liver. Dark green leafy vegetables, formerly encouraged, contain useful amounts of β-carotene but this was found to be poorly absorbed (and converted to vitamin A) with traditional cooking methods. β-Carotene in plant leaves is mostly in the chloroplasts, which are not well digested. The carotene in fruits that contain it are more available[16] and absorption of β-carotene is improved if there is oil or fat in the meal.

(2) **Vitamin A for mothers**

The vitamin may be given to pregnant women, but it must not exceed 3300 IU (1 mg retinol) per day (or 23 300 IU once a week) because more vitamin A can be teratogenic. After delivery large single oral doses (200 000 IU) can be given to them in the first month. It should not be given later in case they become pregnant again.

(3) **Periodic dosing of young children**

This should be done in areas of high incidence with capsules of 110 mg retinol palmitate or 66 mg retinol acetate (200 000 IU) at six monthly intervals. Doses must be smaller in infancy.

(4) **Fortification of staple foods with vitamin A**

In industrialised countries vitamin A is added to margarines to the level found in summer butter (2500 IU or 0.75 mg retinol per 100 g). In Central America sugar is fortified; the World Food Programme requires dried skim milk used in its aid schemes to be fortified with vitamin A.

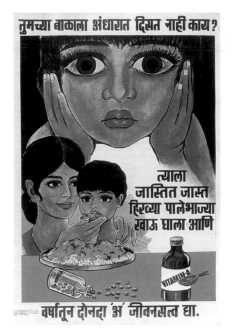

Indian education poster (the plate contains green vegetables and orange-coloured fruits in additions to the staple, rice)

# Iodine deficiency disorders (IDDs)[17]

Iodine deficiency disorders are also given priority by WHO for preventive efforts among nutritional diseases because of their extent—about 1500 million people live in iodine-deficient environments—and feasibility of prevention. Their social importance is greater than was formerly realised. In the major inland mountainous areas of the world, especially the Himalayas, the Alps, the Andes, inland mountainous areas of China and Africa, Indonesia and Papua New Guinea, the soil has had its original iodine leached out of it by heavy rainfall or glaciation, so that the human diet is lacking in iodine if people rely on locally grown foods. When the iodine intake is below the minimum (about 50-75 μg/day) required to replace the turnover of thyroid hormones, pituitary thyrotrophin secretion increases and the thyroid takes up more than its usual 50% of absorbed iodine. Hypertrophy of the gland develops—a goitre. The prevalence of goitre was estimated at about 200 million people worldwide in the early 1990s.

When just visible goitres occur in at least 5% of adolescents this is defined as **endemic goitre**. It usually shows first at puberty, and women are more affected than men. In some areas the iodine intake, indicated by the 24-hourly urinary iodine, is not very low and endemic goitre is attributed partly to thyroid antagonists such as glucosinolates or thiocyanate in certain brassicas or in cassava or soya beans.

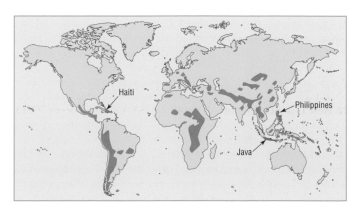

Areas of endemic goitre

When endemic goitre occurs in almost all the women a small percentage of babies, 1% up to 5%, are born with **cretinism**. There are two types. In nervous cretinism there is mental deficiency, deaf mutism, spasticity, and ataxia but features of hypothyroidism are hard to find. In myxoedematous cretinism there are dwarfism, signs of myxoedema, and no goitre. The nervous type predominates in Papua New Guinea and parts of the Andes, while the myxoedematous type is seen in Zaire.

Endemic goitre has by now almost disappeared from the low iodine regions of developed, industrial areas like Derbyshire, the North American middle west, Switzerland, New Zealand, and Tasmania because much or all the salt that people eat is iodised; foods come in to the area that were grown or reared on soils with normal iodine; iodophors used as disinfectants in dairies get into the milk; dairy cows' winter rations have added iodine; and iodate may be used as a bread additive.

But in many remote, inaccessible parts of developing countries, endemic goitre and cretinism persist. Iodine status can be surveyed in such places by collecting single urine samples. Where goitre is common iodine excretions are all low and average less than $25\,\mu g/1\,g$ creatinine; the whole community is deficient. Endemic goitre was thought to be unaccompanied by functional effects (except for occasional local retrosternal pressure).

But in the 1980s it was recognised that "normal" people in goitrous districts (not diagnosed as cretins) have among them higher prevalences of deafness, slower reflexes, features of hypothyroidism, poorer learning ability, more stillbirths and malformed babies, and subnormal plasma thyroxines compared with control communities.[19] Any cretinism is thus the tip of the iceberg and the whole community on very low iodine intakes has a burden of miscellaneous impairments, iodine deficiency disorders (IDD), which reduce its capacity for productive work and development.

The collaboration of WHO, UNICEF, and ICCIDD (the International Council for Control of IDD) has achieved remarkable progress in reducing IDD during the 1990s. The major preventative measure is for governments of countries at risk to make iodisation of salt mandatory—and most of these countries have now done this, with particular success in South America. Where communities are isolated, away from the market economy the first line of prevention is to give all women of childbearing age 1 ml of iodised oil (rapeseed or poppy seed). In original trials this was injected but an oral capsule is nearly as effective and more convenient. UNICEF estimates that the number of children born with cretinism has been halved from the 1990 estimates of 120 000 worldwide. Doctors interested in activities towards IDD elimination can keep informed with the IDD Newsletter (obtainable free from the Editor, Dr J T Dunn, Box 800746, University of Virginia Medical Center, Charlottesville VA 22908, USA, email: jtd@virginia.edu).

## Other types of malnutrition

### Nutritional anaemia
The other WHO priority is nutritional anaemia. The commonest cause is iron deficiency, with folate deficiency second but well behind. Iron deficiency is probably the commonest of all nutritional deficiencies. WHO estimates more than 2 billion people—principally women and children—are iron deficient. It occurs in developed as well as developing countries and will be considered in the next chapter.

---

### Iodine deficiency disorders (IDDs)
**Endemic goitre**—just visible goitre in at least 5% of adolescents
When nearly all mothers have endemic goitre 1%-5% of babies are born with one of two types of **cretinism:**

- *Nervous cretinism*

  mental deficiency
  deaf mutism
  spasticity
  ataxia, squint
  (features of hypothyroidism hard to find)

- *Myxoedematous cretinism*

  dwarfism
  signs of myxoedema
  mental deficiency
  (no goitre)

"Normal" people (not cretins) in goitrous districts, when compared with control communities have:

  higher incidence of deafness
  slower reflexes
  more pronounced features of hypothyroidism
  poorer learning ability

---

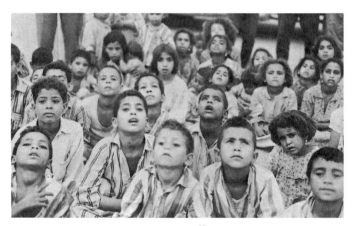
Boys at an oasis in Egypt. Most have goitres[18]

---

### Distribution of other types of malnutrition
- Anaemia—common world wide
- Pellagra—seasonal in some developing countries in maize eaters —florid form rare
- Beriberi—occasional in infants in parts of South-East Asia

## Pellagra

This is still seen in parts of Africa where people subsist on maize, in black people in rural areas of southern Africa, and in Egypt. Most of the niacin in maize is bound and not bioavailable. It is also poorer than other cereals in tryptophan, which can be partly converted to niacin in the liver. Clinical pellagra is seasonal and the florid form is no longer common anywhere in the world. Pellagra is also reported from Hyderabad, India, in people whose staple diet is sorghum. Sorghum eaters elsewhere in the world do not seem to be vulnerable. In Central America the staple food is maize (American corn), but pellagra is rare. This is because treating maize meal with lime ($Ca(OH)_2$) water, a traditional preliminary step in making tortillas, makes the bound niacin in cereals bioavailable. In developed countries, maize meal is fortified with niacin (as in the United States) or maize has been largely replaced by wheat in the diet.

## Beriberi

In adults beriberi has almost disappeared but infantile beriberi is still occasionally seen in some underdeveloped rural areas of South-East Asia.

## References

1 UNICEF. *The State of the World's Children 2000.* Oxford: Oxford University Press, 2000.
2 World Declaration on Nutrition. *Plan of action for nutrition. Adopted by the International Conference on Nutrition, jointly sponsored by FAO and WHO on 11 December 1992.* Geneva: WHO Division of Food & Nutrition.
3 Waterlow JC. *Protein energy malnutrition.* London: Edward Arnold, 1992.
4 Torun B, Chew F. Protein-energy malnutrition. In: Shils ME, Olson JA, Shike M, Ross AC (eds). *Modern Nutrition in Health and Disease,* 9th edn. Baltimore: Williams & Wilkins, 1999.
5 Whitehead RG, Coward WA, Lunn PG *et al.* A comparison of the pathogenesis of protein energy malnutrition in Uganda and the Gambia. *Trans R Soc Trop Med Hyg* 1977; **71**: 189-95.
6 World Health Organization. *Management of severe malnutrition: a manual for physicians and other senior health workers.* Geneva: WHO, 1999.
7 Payne P. Not enough food: malnutrition and famine. In: Harris-White B, Hoffenberg R (eds). *Food, multidisciplinary perspectives.* Oxford: Blackwell, 1994.
8 Harrison GE (ed). *Famine. (Biosocial Society Series no 1.)* Oxford: Oxford University Press, 1988.
9 Nutrition in times of disaster. *United Nations SCN News* 1989 no 3: 11-13.
10 Toole MJ. Micronutrient deficiencies in refugees. *Lancet* 1992; **339**: 1214-16.
11 Bern C, Lathanail L. Is mid-upper-arm circumference a useful tool for screening in emergency settings? *Lancet* 1995; **345**:631-3.
12 Ferro Luzzi A, James WPT. Adult malnutrition: simple assessment techniques for use in emergencies. *Br J Nutr* 1996; **75**: 3-10.
13 Sommer A, Tarwotjo I, Djunaedi E, West KP, Loeden AA, Tilden R. Impact of vitamin A supplementation on childhood mortality. A randomised controlled community trial. *Lancet* 1986; **i**: 1169-73.
14 American Academy of Pediatrics: Committee on Infectious Diseases. Vitamin A treatment of measles. *Pediatrics* 1993; **91**: 1014-15.
15 McLaren DS, Frigg N. *Sight and Life Manual on Vitamin A Deficiency Disorders (VADD),* 2nd edn. Basel: Sight and Life, 2001.
16 de Pee S, West CE, Permaesih D, *et al.* Orange fruit is more effective than are dark-green leafy vegetables in increasing serum concentrations of retinol and $\beta$-carotene in schoolchildren in Indonesia. *Am J Clin Nutr* 1998; **68**: 1058-7.
17 Hetzel BS, Dunn JT, Stanburg JB (eds). *The prevention and control of iodine deficiency disorders.* Amsterdam: Elsevier, 1987.
18 Davidson S, Passmore R, Brock JF, Truswell AS. *Human nutrition and dietetics,* 7th edn. Edinburgh: Churchill Livingstone, 1979.
19 Hetzel BS. Iodine deficiency disorders (IDD) and their eradication. *Lancet* 1983; **2**: 1126-9.

# 9 Other nutritional deficiencies in affluent communities

Protein-energy malnutrition in Britain and other Western industrial countries is almost always secondary to disease—for example, it may be due to diseases of the gastrointestinal tract (persistent vomiting, dysphagia, upper intestinal obstruction, malabsorption) or wasting diseases (some cancers, HIV infection, metabolic disorders) or to radiotherapy. It is briefly described in chapter 17 (enteral and parenteral nutrition management to prevent or treat malnutrition in hospital). How to assess the degree of malnutrition is dealt with in chapter 12 (Measuring nutrition). For a background, famine and childhood protein malnutrition are described in chapter 8 (Malnutrition in developing countries).

In Britain vitamin D deficiency is still a public health issue, requiring preventive measures, though rickets is not common now. Its pathogenesis is discussed in chapter 10 (Vitamins). Among hospital patients in developed countries, however, the most common vitamin deficiency is probably folate deficiency, of which there is an account in chapter 10. The most serious nutritional deficiency in alcoholics is the complex of Wernicke's encephalopathy and Korsakoff's psychosis, which is summarised under thiamin in chapter 10. The following nutritional problems have not been discussed anywhere else in this book.

## Iron deficiency

Iron deficiency is probably the commonest micronutrient deficiency in the world. Over 400 million women are estimated to have subnormal haemoglobins and over one billion people to have iron deficiency.[1] People in industrialised countries are affected as well as those in developing countries, especially women aged 15 to 50. In a survey in Vanuatu, however, most people with hypochromic anaemia were found to have normal plasma ferritin but, by DNA analysis, a unsuspectedly high prevalence of $\alpha$-thalassaemias.[2] Hypochromic anaemias in other tropical countries cannot all be assumed to be due to iron deficiency unless biochemical studies of iron status are done. In Britain 33% of women had serum ferritin under $25\,\mu g/l$, indicating low stores and 14% had very low ferritins (below $13\,\mu g/l$). In the same survey only 4% of women had haemoglobins below $11\,g/dl$.[3] In British children serum ferritins are more likely to be low in youngest boys (13% were $<20\,\mu g/l$) and in adolescent girls (27% were $15\,\mu g/l$).[4]

Iron is the second most abundant metal in the earth's crust but it is virtually insoluble in the complexes of ferric iron usual in foods at neutral pH, and absorption is difficult. There is no physiological mechanism for secretion of iron so maintenance of iron homeostasis depends on its absorption. Normally in men, children, and postmenopausal women iron is lost only in desquamated surface cells from gut and skin at an estimated rate of 1 mg/day or less.

Blood is by far the richest tissue in iron; 1 ml contains 0.5 mg so that a regular loss of only 2 ml/day—for example, from epistaxis or haemorrhoids—doubles the iron requirements. Women of reproductive age lose an average of 30 ml blood per period, corresponding to 0.5 mg iron per day over the month, so they need more iron than men. An important minority of women lose considerably more.

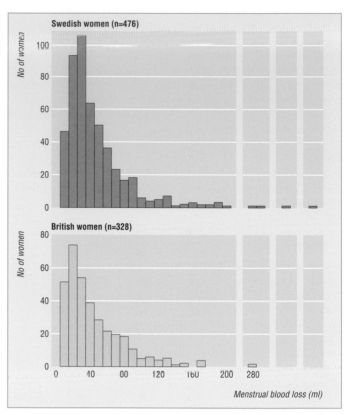

Menstrual blood loss per period in 476 Swedish and 328 British women[5]

### Iron content of some foods[6] (mg/100 g) (in descending order of total iron per usual serving)

| Food | Iron content |
| --- | --- |
| Cockles (boiled) | 26.0* |
| Black pudding (blood sausage) | 20.0* |
| Liver, cooked: ox – pig | 7.8-17.0* |
| Beef, rump steak, grilled, lean | 3.5* |
| Lamb, leg, roast, lean | 2.7* |
| Oatmeal | 3.8 |
| Legumes, cooked: baked beans – tofu | 1.4-3.5 |
| Green leafy vegetables: lettuce – watercress | 0.7-2.2 |
| Wines, white or red | 0.6-1.2* |
| Egg, boiled | 1.9 |
| Dried fruit: dates – figs | 1.1-4.2 |
| Fish: cod-anchovies | 0.4-4.1* |
| Chicken, roast, meat | 0.8* |
| Nuts: chestnuts – cashew | 0.9-6.2 |
| Chocolate, plain, dark | 2.4 |
| Potato, baked | 0.7 |
| Bread: white-wholemeal | 1.6-2.7 |
| Fresh fruit: apples – passion fruit | 0.1-1.3 |
| Milk, cows', whole | 0.05 |

\* Higher availability—haem and muscle iron or alcohol
Other foods with unusually high Fe content: curry powder (58 mg/100 g), All Bran (20 mg/100 g), wheat bran (13 mg/100 g), some other fortified breakfast cereals (13 mg/100 g), venison (8 mg/100 g), pigeon (15 mg/100 g), hare (11 mg/100 g), grouse (8 mg/100 g), hearts (5-8 mg/100 g), kidneys (5-8 mg/100 g)

These women, pregnant women, children growing fast, and anyone with chronic bleeding all need to absorb extra iron or they will use up what tissue stores they have.

Absorption of iron is inefficient. It averages roughly 10% from a mixed diet but is much less from many plant foods and from eggs and dairy foods. Haem iron is better absorbed than non-haem iron. Absorption of the latter is enhanced by animal flesh and by ascorbic and other organic acids (for example citric and lactic) and reduced by phytates and polyphenols (as in tea). Iron absorption is being studied by extrinsic labelling of foods with isotopes of iron (radio-iron was used earlier, but stable isotopes are now available and preferred). The different factors in foods combine algebraically to produce a high, medium, or low absorption from the meal. For example, tea reduces iron absorption from a meal but orange juice enhances it.

Iron is essential for haemoglobin formation. It is also part of myoglobin, of some enzymes required for neurotransmitter synthesis, and of an important enzyme in DNA synthesis. In deficiency, sometimes even before there is anaemia, adults have decreased capacity for heavy work, pregnant women have an increased risk of low birth weight or premature babies, and children do not concentrate or learn as well as they can after iron treatment.[7]

In people at risk of iron deficiency the haemoglobin (at least) should be checked, in:

- infants at the age of 1 year
- children and adolescents during phases of rapid growth
- through and after pregnancy
- after gastric surgery at least once a year
- women with heavy periods (direct questions may need to be asked)
- patients presenting with gastrointestinal symptoms or disease
- anyone with a history of recurrent bleeding, with a positive occult blood test, or a woman who is a frequent blood donor
- people (for example, with arthritis) taking aspirin or NSAIDs regularly.

Ferrous sulphate is standard **therapy** for iron deficiency. The traditional dose for anaemia has been three tablets per day ($3 \times 60$ mg Fe) but gastrointestinal side effects are common, related to the dose of iron and can lead to poor compliance. Absorption of iron is enhanced when there is deficiency and it may be practical to prescribe a more modest dose of 60 mg iron (one tablet) per day (given between meals). Iron is as well absorbed from ferrous fumarate (60 mg/tablet) or gluconate, but the latter only contains 35 mg per tablet. There is no advantage to more complex and expensive tablets containing iron. In developing countries trials are underway in which iron tablets are given only weekly for mild to moderate chronic iron deficiency.

### Prevention

A common cause of iron deficiency is that women, who require twice as much as men, consume only half as much. They often eat less liver, meat, and fish, the best sources of available iron. People who take no exercise or are on a weight reducing diet have such a low calorie intake that it is difficult for them to eat enough iron.[8] Iron absorption is increased in deficient individuals but this may not be enough to compensate for low intake or increased losses. Staple foods are fortified with iron in some countries (for example, many breakfast cereals in Britain) and old fashioned iron cooking pots add some iron to the food.

## Calcium and the bones

Calcium is the most obvious and persistent of the micronutrients, the fifth most abundant element (and the most

---

### Too much iron?

- There is no homeostatic mechanism for disposing of excess iron; if too much is absorbed it accumulates in liver, heart and other organs. Chronic iron overload occurs in three situations. In **hereditary haemochromatosis** absorption is enhanced on an ordinary diet. One in 300 men of North West European descent are affected and fewer women, who have a mutation of the HFE gene, discovered in 1996. Patients with intractable anaemias, (for example, thalassaemia) **and repeated blood transfusions** receive excess iron parenterally, and people who regularly imbibe **alcohol beverages with high iron content** receive excess absorbable iron by mouth (for example, Bantu siderosis).
- Free iron can damage tissues by catalysing the conversion of hydrogen peroxide to the destructive hydroxyl free radical (OH•). This is why in the body iron (and copper) are almost always bound to carrier proteins or locked away in storage proteins.

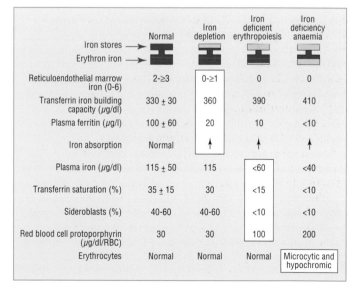

| | Normal | Iron depletion | Iron deficient erythropoiesis | Iron deficiency anaemia |
|---|---|---|---|---|
| Iron stores → | | | | |
| Erythron iron → | | | | |
| Reticuloendothelial marrow iron (0-6) | 2-≥3 | 0-≥1 | 0 | 0 |
| Transferrin iron building capacity (µg/dl) | 330 ± 30 | 360 | 390 | 410 |
| Plasma ferritin (µg/l) | 100 ± 60 | 20 | 10 | <10 |
| Iron absorption | Normal | ↑ | ↑ | ↑ |
| Plasma iron (µg/dl) | 115 ± 50 | 115 | <60 | <40 |
| Transferrin saturation (%) | 35 ± 15 | 30 | <15 | <10 |
| Sideroblasts (%) | 40-60 | 40-60 | <10 | <10 |
| Red blood cell protoporphyrin (µg/dl/RBC) | 30 | 30 | 100 | 200 |
| Erythrocytes | Normal | Normal | Normal | Microcytic and hypochromic |

Sequential changes in the development of iron deficiency[5]

abundant cation) in the body, yet it is more difficult to measure adequacy of intake for calcium than for other nutrients. There are two major questions about calcium.

(1) Will a generous intake during childhood and adolescence contribute to taller adult height or heavier bones, or both? If so how much is needed?
(2) Will a generous intake from about 45 years onwards delay the onset of osteoporosis, especially in women, who are more likely to be affected? If so how much is best and in what form?

Over 99% of body calcium is in the skeleton. Here it not only provides structural support but is a large reservoir for maintaining the plasma calcium concentration at very stable concentrations. Any reduction of absorbed calcium does not show in the plasma concentration, which is immediately reset by an increased parathyroid hormone concentration and the formation of active 1,25 dihydroxyvitamin D (in the kidney from 25 hydroxyvitamin D). Ionised calcium **in the plasma** has many vital functions—muscle contractility, neuromuscular irritability, blood coagulation, etc—which would be disturbed if its concentration fell. By different modulators the ionised calcium **inside cells** is also tightly controlled. An inadequate dietary calcium will therefore not normally be allowed to lower plasma or intracellular calcium concentrations and disturb their numerous important soft tissue functions; instead a little less will go into the bones in children or a little will be removed from the bones in adults.

Calcium in the bones amounts to 25 g at birth and builds up to about 1200 g in an adult. From the indices of growth and skeletal composition the amount of calcium which is being added to the bones each day in growing children can be calculated. It averages about 180 mg calcium per day but reaches 400 mg per day at the peak of adolescent linear growth. This amount is the required positive balance. Calcium absorption is inefficient—faecal calcium is about 70% of intake in adult calcium balances—and there is an obligatory loss of calcium in urine as well. The diet must therefore supply substantially more than the daily skeletal increment, and the recommended daily amount in Britain is 1000 mg in boys and 800 mg in girls aged 11-18 years. There is evidence that in some conditions a supplement of milk (the best source of calcium) has improved the growth rate of children. The great increase in the height of young Japanese adults from 1950 to 1970 coincided with a tripling of the national calcium intake from about the lowest in the world to 600 mg/day.

Yet it is hard to understand how poor children in developing countries on diets of cereals and vegetables and no milk obtain enough calcium to grow. Their final adult height is usually lower than in industrial countries, but osteoporosis in older people seems to be less of a problem. There are several possibilities to explain the more economical handling of calcium in people in countries where there is little or no milk.

- More skin synthesis of vitamin D from sunshine in the tropics.
- Regular weight-bearing exercise which promotes bone formation and muscle strength.
- Lower intake of animal protein (which is known to increase the obligatory urinary calcium).
- Lower intake of salt (which also increases urinary calcium loss).
- Genetic selection.

**Osteoporosis**
Osteoporosis is porosis of the bones. There are more holes in trabecular (inside) bone and thinning of cortical bone. The ratio of mineral (mostly $CaPO_4$) to organic matter (collagen

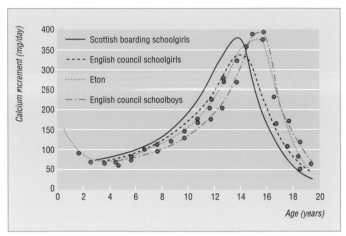

Estimated daily increment in skeletal calcium of children at various ages[9]

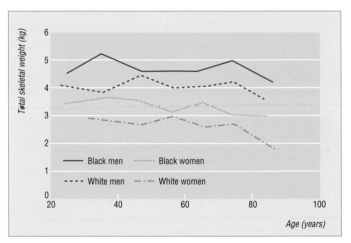

Age related changes in total skeletal weight of black and white people in the United States of America[10]

In 1927 a series of trials was carried out in Scotland in which about 1500 children in the ordinary elementary schools in the seven largest towns were given additional milk at school for a period of seven months. Periodic measurements of the children showed that the rate of growth in those getting the additional milk was about 20% greater than in those not getting additional milk. The increased rate of growth was accompanied by a noticeable improvement in health and vigour. This experiment was twice repeated by different observers who obtained substantially the same results on numbers up to 20 000 children.[11]

and cells) is normal but the amount of total bone is reduced. In other words osteoporosis is atrophy of bones. It causes no symptoms unless/until there is the only complication—a fracture associated with inadequate trauma.

The commonest sites of osteoporotic fracture are:

- neck of femur (hip) fracture, the most serious
- vertebral collapse fracture(s)
- arm fracture—Colles' wrist fracture.

Osteoporosis cannot be recognised by clinical examination. It can be diagnosed with DEXA (dual x-ray absorptiometry) of a femoral neck and/or lumbar spine and/or a distal forearm. WHO defines osteoporosis as a bone mineral density less than 2.5 standard deviations below the mean for young adults (separate standards for women and men; for Caucasians and African Americans).

Osteoporosis is thus analogous to atherosclerosis. They are both important pathological states because they are precursors of common and serious clinical diseases, but they can only be recognised by special techniques (special imaging for osteoporosis, invasive for atherosclerosis). There are two main types of **primary** osteoporosis: postmenopausal and senile. **Secondary** osteoporosis is due to conditions such as long-term corticosteroid treatment. Bone density is also reduced by vitamin D deficiency (disproportionate loss of mineral) or infiltration by different types of cancer.

# Dieting can be dangerous

Malnutrition can result from dietary regimens which happen to be very unbalanced nutritionally. Some of these were introduced by medical graduates, others are unscientific. The following are only a sample.

### "Liquid protein" combined with fasting
In the United States of America in the late 1970s this diet led to at least 60 deaths from cardiac arrhythmias in people with no history of heart disease. The product "Prolinn", an extract from beef hides, lacked several essential amino acids. It was withdrawn, but prolonged fasting with or without protein supplements (even those of good biological value) carries the risk of sudden fatal arrhythmias and has been criticised authoritatively.

### Zen macrobiotic diets
These diets consist of 10 levels. The highest level is 100% cereals and prescribes a very low fluid intake. These diets have led to scurvy and/or impaired renal function, anaemia, hypocalcaemia, and emaciation. In some cases these have been fatal. These diets have been condemned by the American Medical Association.

### Dr Atkins's diet revolution
This weight reducing diet in a popular paperback written in 1972 prescribed a minimal carbohydrate intake. Ketosis is inevitable; and the diet raises plasma lipid concentrations. It was condemned by the American Medical Association but the book can still be found on bookstalls, having sold millions of copies. It has been revived recently. This time it should be thoroughly tested for efficacy and safety.

### Strict vegan diets for infants
Plant foods contain no vitamins B-12 or D. The latter can be synthesised in the skin if a child is exposed to sunlight, but the most serious nutritional complication of strict vegetarian diets is vitamin B-12 deficiency in infants. The milk of vegan mothers

## Calcium and osteoporosis

- There have been several controlled trials of the effect in adolescent girls of extra milk or calcium tablets on bone density. Most reported small extra gains in the supplement group[12] but the trials were only of 1 or $1\frac{1}{2}$ year's duration and it is not known whether the effects persist.
- In postmenopausal women 20 trials have been reported with calcium tablets or extra milk (usually 1000 mg Ca for two years) added to usual diet. In most of the trials bone density increased 1-3% (not always significantly) in the treated group.[13] Presumably extra calcium has most benefit where the usual dietary calcium was low. The US Committee on Dietary Reference Intakes has set the dietary reference intake for people over 70 years at 1200 mg (30 mmol) Ca/day[14] but in the UK a COMA subcommittee's re-examination did not consider there was evidence for increase of the dietary reference value of 700 mg/day.[15]
- A good calcium intake is part of preventing (delaying) osteoporosis, along with regular weight bearing exercise and vitamin D from sun or diet. For treating osteoporosis calcium is less effective than hormone replacement but should be prescribed alongside the latter.

---

**Osteoporosis is only important because of these fractures. The most serious is hip fracture. Its pathogenesis is multifactorial. As well as low bone mineral density of the proximal femur, instability, muscle weakness and lack of adipose "padding" all contribute.[16]**

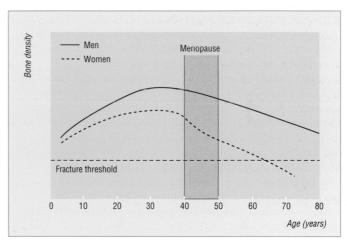

Average bone density with age and fracture threshold

---

## Articles which show the dangers of some diets
- *Liquid protein and fasting*—Isner JM *et al.* Circulation 1979; **60:** 1401-12.
- *Zen macrobiotic diets*—AMA Council on Foods and Nutrition. *JAMA* 1971; **218:** 397-8.
- *Dr Atkins's diet revolution*—AMA Council on Foods and Nutrition. *JAMA* 1973; **224:** 1415-19.
- *Vitamin B-12 deficiency in vegan infants*—Wighton MC *et al. Med J Aust* 1979; **ii:** 1-3 (see next box).
- *Beverly Hills diet*—Mirkin GB, Shore RN. *JAMA* 1981; **246:** 2235-7.

contains insufficient vitamin B-12 unless she takes a supplement. This vitamin is required for normal myelin formation, and infants' nervous systems are specially susceptible to deficiency. They can show impaired mental development, involuntary movements, and even coma responsive to vitamin B-12, as well as megaloblastic anaemia.

### The Beverley Hills diet

This weight reducing diet requires consumption of nothing but fruit (all in a certain order and only the designated fruits) for the first 10 days. Some bread, salad, and meat are added later. The theory behind this diet is unscientific, and it has been criticised in detail in the *Journal of the American Medical Association.*

## Eating disorders[17]

**Anorexia nervosa** is an illness of our time, although it was first described and named in 1874. Many teenage girls and young women say they are dieting to stay or become slim but most are not very successful. They do not stick to their diets. The young woman with anorexia nervosa is unusual: without talking about dieting she succeeds in losing a lot of the weight that the others say they would like to. But then she cannot stop. By rigid control of her eating she avoids foods that she understands to be fattening (appetite is usually there, but suppressed). She has a phobia of being fat and a distorted body image, seeing herself fatter than she really is. Amenorrhoea is characteristic.

Up to one in 100 middle class women aged 15 to 25 may be affected. Before this loss of weight the young woman with anorexia nervosa was often a model of good behaviour, conformism, and achievement though this probably concealed a sense of ineffectiveness and self doubt.

Some women not only abstain: they have learnt to induce vomiting or purging and may have eating binges between. When habitual this behaviour is **bulimia nervosa**.

The physical effects of a young woman starving herself to 45 kg and below are similar to those described for famine in chapter 8. But there are differences. The anorectic patient usually eats adequate protein and micronutrients and is restless and overactive. There is skinniness or emaciation, cold extremities, lanugo hair, bradycardia, low blood pressure, and normal pubic and axillary hair. Plasma potassium concentrations may be low if there has been vomiting or purging, and plasma cholesterol or carotene values are sometimes raised. The amenorrhoea is similar to that which occurs in starvation.

Early diagnosis is important because a long illness, and severe weight loss are all bad prognostic features. The young woman denies she is too thin or that she is dieting. Amenorrhoea may appear to have preceded the weight loss. Other organic diseases that can lead to emaciation and amenorrhoea have to be excluded—for example, thyrotoxicosis, malabsorption, and hypopituitarism. But the bigger challenge for the family doctor is to detect the characteristic features of anorexia nervosa and to convince the young woman that she needs treatment.

Treatment is usually best managed by a specialised team, most often a psychiatrist with special experience in anorexia nervosa working with a dietitian. Moderate cases are treated as out patients. Admission to a special anorexia unit is indicated if weight loss is severe (BMI 16.5) or there is some medical or psychological complication. The two lines of treatment are to persuade her to increase food intake and to get her weight up to a target figure (usually a compromise) and at the same time

---

**An exclusively breast fed infant of a vegan mother**

"Neurological deterioration commenced between 3 and 6 months of age and progressed to a comatose premoribund state by the age of 9 months. Investigations revealed a mild nutritional vitamin B-12 deficiency in the mother and a very severe nutritional B-12 deficiency in the infant with severe megaloblastic anaemia. Treatment of the infant with vitamin B-12 resulted in a rapid clinical and haematological improvement but neurological recovery was incomplete …"

By 17 months of age his general level of motor, social, and intellectual development was that of a child of 11 months.

Wighton *et al.,* 1979
(reference in previous box)

---

---

**Criteria for diagnosis**

*Anorexia nervosa*
1 Loss of weight to body mass index* under 17.5.
2 Disturbance of body image.
3 Refusal to maintain normal weight.
4 Intense fear of becoming fat.
5 Amenorrhoea.
6 No known medical illness leading to weight loss.

*Bulimia*
1 Recurrent episodes of binge eating, often secretive with rapid consumption of high caloric foods.
2 Binge followed by self-induced vomiting or purging.
3 Strict dieting between binges.
4 Body weight may be within the normal range.
5 Awareness of abnormal eating patterns and fear of not being able to stop voluntarily.
6 Not due to any physical disorder.

In practice intermediate and atypical forms are common
*Weight (kg)/height (m)$^2$

---

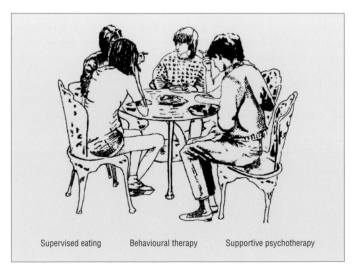

Supervised eating   Behavioural therapy   Supportive psychotherapy

Treatment in a special anorexia unit

to provide emotional support. Eating is tactfully supervised by nurses, and behavioural principles can be effective, more privileges for each step of weight gain, previously agreed by the patient. As she is refed and becomes physically stronger it becomes easier for the patient to tackle the changes needed so that she can adapt to society and develop a healthier body image.

> In a 5-year follow up study Ben Tovin *et al.* found that 3/95 anorexia patients died and 20 had persistent anorexia nervosa. Prognosis was better for bulimia: none died and only 8% still had bulimia. Many patients made a good recovery without accessing specialised treatments. Those with lengthy admissions did not necessarily have better long term outcome.[18]

## Interactions of food, nutrition, and drugs

**Particular drugs can affect the nutritional state**, changing the results of biochemical tests or even leading on occasions to clinical undernutrition, overnutrition, or malnutrition.

**Appetite may be decreased** by anorectic drugs, bulking agents, dexamphetamine, metformin, cardiac glycosides, glucagon, morphine, phenylbutazone, indometacin, cyclophosphamide, fluorouracil, methylphenidate, salbutamol, levodopa, etc, and by drugs that alter taste (griseofulvin, penicillamine, and lincomycin).

**Appetite may be increased** by sulphonylureas, oral contraceptives, cyproheptadine, chlorpromazine, androgens, anabolic steroids, corticosteroids, insulin, lithium, amitriptyline, pizotifen, clomipramine, benzodiazepines, and metoclopramide.

**Malabsorption** for more than one nutrient may be induced by neomycin, kanamycin, paromomycin, colchicine, phenindione, chlortetracycline, cholestyramine, colestipol, cyclophosphamide, indometacin, liquid paraffin (fat soluble vitamins), methotrexate, and methyldopa.

**Energy metabolism** may be stimulated by caffeine, smoking, and some sympathomimetic drugs.

**Carbohydrates**—Increased blood glucose concentrations may be produced by corticosteroids, thiazide diuretics, diazoxide, oral contraceptives, and phenytoin. Hypoglycaemia may be produced by propranolol and by alcohol (as well as by sulphonylureas, metformin and insulin).

**Lipids—Plasma total cholesterol** may be raised by thiazides (for example, chlorthalidone, hydrochlorothiazide), by phenobarbital, chlorpromazine, some oral contraceptives, and large intakes of boiled coffee. As well as specific cholesterol lowering drugs, aspirin, colchicine, prazosin, clonidine, neomycin, phenformin, and sulphinpyrazone may lower total cholesterol. **Plasma high density lipoprotein cholesterol** may be raised by phenytoin, ethanol, cimetidine, valproate, carbamazine, terbutaline, and prazosin. It may be lowered by danazol, propranolol, and oxprenolol.

**Plasma triglycerides** may be raised by propranolol, ethanol, and (oestrogenic) oral contraceptives. They may be lowered by norethisterone.

**Protein—Nitrogen balance** may be made negative by corticosteroids, vaccines, and tetracyclines. It may be made positive by insulin or anabolic steroids. **Plasma amino acids** may be increased by tranylcypromine and lowered by oral contraceptives. Plasma phenylalanine may be raised by trimethoprim and methotrexate.

**Thiamin** absorption can be reduced by ethanol.

**Riboflavin** status may be lowered by oral contraceptives and by chlorpromazine.

**Niacin** may be antagonised by isoniazid.

**Vitamin B-6** may be antagonised by isoniazid, hydralazine, cycloserine, penicillamine, oral contraceptives, oestrogens, hydrocortisone, imipramine, levodopa, piperazine, and pyrazinamide.

---

### Nutrients, foods, and drugs can interact in several ways

- **Foods can affect drugs**, for example, by affecting absorption, an acute effect of single meals. Grapefruit juice inhibits one of the cytochrome P450s that metabolises drugs such as calcium-channel blockers, statins, carbamazepine, and terfenadine.[19]
- **Nutrition can affect drugs.** The nutritional state can affect drug metabolism and hence dosage and toxicity, for example, in Kwashiorkor.
- **Particular drugs can affect the nutritional state.** Appetite, absorption, metabolism, and concentration of nutrients can be affected, positively or negatively, by different drugs (see Left).
- **Drugs can cause unpleasant reactions to minor components in some foods** whose metabolism we normally take for granted—for example, hypertension from tyramine in cheese in patients taking monoamine oxidase inhibitors.
- **A few drugs are used as drinks**, as part of the usual diet: alcoholic drinks, coffee, tea, and carbonated cola beverages.
- **Some nutrients are used as drugs.** The nutrients are all obtainable in pure form. They may, in doses above the nutrient requirement, sometimes have a useful pharmacological action—for example, nicotinic acid for hyperlipidaemia.

---

### Should I take the medicine before or after meals, doctor?

- Most drugs are best taken with or just after meals, because this is the easiest way to remember to take any drug and some are gastric irritants. Absorption of several drugs is a little delayed but this is unimportant and a few are better absorbed when taken with meals—for example, griseofulvin, metoprolol, and labetalol.
- Plenty of water should be taken with uricosurics (to prevent renal precipitation) and with cholestyramine and bulk formers like methyl cellulose.
- A few drugs should be taken **half an hour before meals**: antibiotics which are labile in acid—ampicillin, benzylpenicillin, cloxacillin, erythromycin, lincomycin, tetracycline, rifampicin, and isoniazid. So should one of the antidiabetic agents—glipizide—and, of course, appetite suppressant drugs.

**Folate** may be antagonised by ethanol, phenytoin, oral contraceptives (uncommonly), cycloserine, triamterine, and cholestyramine. In addition several drugs owe their antibacterial action to antagonism of folate metabolism—more in microbial than mammalian cells—pyrimethamine, trimethoprin, and pentamidine. Methotrexate is a potent folate antagonist which has more effect on rapidly dividing cells—for example, cancer cells.

**Vitamin B-12** absorption may be impaired by slow K, cimetidine, ranitidine, metformin, colchicine, trifluoperazine, and by high doses of vitamin C, cholestyramine, and methotrexate. Prolonged nitrous oxide anaesthesia oxidises vitamin B-12 *in vivo*. Smoking and oral contraceptives reduce the plasma concentration.

**Vitamin C**—Plasma concentrations are lowered by oral contraceptives, smoking, aspirin, and tetracycline. Ascorbate excretion is increased by corticosteroids, phenylbutazone and sulfinpyrazone.

**Vitamin A** plasma concentration is increased by oral contraceptives. Absorption may be reduced by liquid paraffin and cholestyramine.

**Vitamin D** status is lowered by anticonvulsants—for example, phenytoin, phenobarbitone, and when these are taken in high dose for long periods rickets can occur.

**Vitamin E** is antagonised by iron in premature newborns. Fish oils (refined) increase requirements.

**Vitamin K**—Coumarin drugs—for example warfarin—are antimetabolites. Purgatives and intestinal antibiotics, such as neomycin, tetracyclines, and sulphonamides, may remove the contribution from colonic bacteria. Salicylates and cholestyramine may reduce absorption, and some cephalosporin antibiotics antagonise the vitamin K-epoxide cycle.

**Potassium**—Drugs are important causes of potassium depletion: purgatives and laxatives increase faecal loss; thiazide diuretics and frusemide and ethacrynic acid increase renal loss. Other drugs that may increase urinary potassium are penicillin, glucocorticoids, liquorice, outdated tetracycline, gentamicin, and alcohol. Insulin can lower serum potassium. Drugs that raise serum potassium include ACE inhibitors, spironolactone, succinylcholine, triamterene, and potassium compounds.

**Calcium**—Absorption may be increased by aluminium hydroxide or by cholestyramine and decreased by phosphates and corticosteroids. Thiazide diuretics decrease urinary calcium excretion. Gentamicin, dactinomycin, frusemide, and ethacrynic acid increase it.

**Iron**—Gastrointestinal bleeding from aspirin and NSAIDS depletes the body's iron. Allopurinol, fructose, and ascorbic acid increase absorption. Antacids, phosphates, and tetracycline decrease it. Oral contraceptives tend to increase serum iron.

**Iodine**—Sulphonylureas, phenylbutazone, amiodorone, and lithium can cause goitre; they interfere with iodine uptake in the gland. Serum protein bound iodine is increased by oral contraceptives, x-ray contrast media, and potassium iodide, and decreased by phenytoin.

**Phosphate** absorption is decreased by aluminium or calcium compounds.

**Zinc** depletion from increased urinary excretion may be produced by thiazide diuretics and frusemide, by cisplatin, penicillamine, and alcohol.

**Magnesium** depletion from increased urinary loss may be produced by thiazides and frusemide, cisplatin, alcohol, aminoglycosides, amphotericin, ciclosporin, and gentamicin.

## References

1 United National Subcommittee on Nutrition, Focus on micronutrients. *SCN News* no 9: mid 1993; 1-34.
2 Bowden DK, Hill AVS, Higgs DR, Weatherall DJ, Clegg JB. Relative roles of genetic factors, dietary deficiency, and infection in anaemia in Vanuatu, south-west Pacific. *Lancet* 1985; ii: 1025-8.
3 Gregory J, Foster K, Tyler H, Wiseman M. *The dietary and nutritional survey of British adults.* London: HMSO, 1990.
4 Gregory J, Lowe S, Bates CT *et al.* National Diet and Nutrition Survey: young people aged 4 to 18 years. London: Stationery Office, 2000.
5 Bothwell TH, Charlton RW, Cook JD, Finch CA. *Iron metabolism in man.* Oxford: Blackwell, 1979, p 251.
6 Holland B, Welch AA, Unwin ID, Buss DA, Paul AA, Southgate DAT. *McCance & Widdowson's the composition of foods*, 5th edn. Cambridge: Royal Society of Chemistry, 1991.
7 Brunner AB, Joffe A, Duggan AK, Casella JF, Brandt J. Randomised study of cognitive effects of iron supplementation in iron-anaemic iron-deficient adolescent girls. *Lancet* 1996; **348**: 929-96.
8 Barber SA, Bull NL, Buss DH. Low iron intakes among young women in Britain. *BMJ* 1985; **290**: 743-4.
9 Leitch I, Aitken FC. The estimation of calcium requirements a re-examination. *Nutr Rev* 1959; **29**: 393-407.
10 Merz AL, Trotter M, Peterson RR. Estimation of skeletal weight in the living. *Am J Phys Anthropol* 1956; **14**: 589-610.
11 Orr JB. *Food, health and income. Report of a survey of adequacy of diet in relation to income.* London: Macmillan, 1936.
12 Cadogan J, Eastell R, Jones N, Barker ME. Milk intake and bone mineral acquisition in adolescent girls: randomised, controlled intervention trial. *BMJ* 1997; **317**: 1255-60.
13 Nordin BEC. Calcium and osteoporosis. *Nutrition (Elsevier)* 1997; **13**: 664-86.
14 Standing Committee on the Scientific Evaluation of Dietary Reference Intakes, Food and Nutrition Board, Institute of Medicine. *Dietary reference intakes for calcium, phosphorus, magnesium, vitamin D and fluoride.* Washington, DC: National Academy Press, 1997.
15 Report of the Subgroup on Bone Health, Working Group on the Nutritional Status of the Population of the Committee on Medical Aspects of Food and Nutrition Policy. *Nutrition and Bone Health: with particular reference to calcium and vitamin D.* London: Stationery Office, 1998.
16 Cummings SR, Melton LJ. Osteoporosis 1. Epidemiology and outcomes of osteoporotic fractures. *Lancet* 2002; **359**: 1761-7.
17 Fairburn CG, Harrison PJ. Eating disorders. *Lancet* 2003; **361**: 407–16.
18 Ben Tovin DI, Walker K, Gilchrist P, Freemen R, Kalucy R, Esterman A. Outcome in patients with eating disorders: a 5-year study. *Lancet* 2001; **357**: 1254-7.
19 Spence JD. Drug interactions with grapefruit: whose responsibility is it to warn the public? *Clin Pharm Therap* 1997; **61**: 395-400.

# 10 Vitamins and some minerals

No animal can live on a mixture of pure protein, fat and carbohydrate, and even when the necessary inorganic material is carefully supplied the animal still cannot flourish. The animal body is adjusted to live upon plant tissues or the tissues of other animals and these contain countless substances other than the proteins, carbohydrates and fats.

Sir Frederick Gowland Hopkins (1906)

Deficiencies of vitamins still occur in affluent countries: folate, thiamin, and vitamins D and C. Some of these deficiencies are induced by diseases or drugs. In developing countries deficiency diseases are more prevalent. Vitamin A deficiency (xerophthalmia), for example, is a major cause of blindness. Some vitamins may have useful actions above the dose that prevents classic deficiency disease—for example, vitamins A, C, and B-6; nicotinic acid has been used to treat hyperlipidaemia.

Vitamins have caught the popular imagination, and they are also big business. Many people take over the counter vitamins without medical advice and a few unorthodox practitioners prescribe "megavitamin therapy". Doctors therefore need to know the symptoms of overdosage.

## Definition

Vitamins are:

(a) Organic substances or groups of related substances
(b) found in some foods
(c) substances with specific biochemical functions in the human body
(d) not made in the body (or not in sufficient quantity)
(e) required in **very small** amounts.

Many people seem to have lost sight of point (e), but it appears in all dictionary definitions and can be seen in the table of requirements. The daily requirement of most vitamins is around 1 mg, the weight of one grain of raw sugar. There are no exceptions to points (a), (b), and (e). On point (c), the biochemical action of most vitamins can now be visualised, but those of vitamins A and C are not yet explained fully, and the active metabolite of vitamin D acts as a hormone. Exceptions to point (d) are that certain carotenoids can replace vitamin A; proteins (through the amino acid, tryptophan) can replace niacin; and exposure to sunlight can replace vitamin D.

## Vitamin A

Best understood of the actions of vitamin A is its role in night vision; 11-*cis* retinaldehyde is combined with a specific protein in the light-sensitive pigment, rhodopsin, in the rods of the retina. Night blindness occurs in children deficient in vitamin A in some developing countries, and in affluent countries it is seen rarely in patients with chronic biliary obstruction or malabsorption.

More recently discovered functions of vitamin A affect many different cell types. Retinol, carried in plasma on retinol binding protein, is taken up in cells by cellular retinol binding protein, oxidised to retinoic acid or 9-*cis* retinoic acid. These are transported to the nucleus where they are bound to specific receptors and initiate genetic transcription. In vitamin A deficiency there is metaplasia of conjunctival epithelium and

**Daily requirements for healthy adults***

| | |
|---|---|
| Vitamin A | 1 mg |
| Thiamin | 1 mg |
| Riboflavin | 1.5 mg |
| Niacin | 15-20 mg** |
| Vitamin B-6 | 1.5 mg |
| Pantothenic acid | 5 mg |
| Biotin | 30 μg |
| Folate | 200 μg[†] |
| Vitamin B-12 | 1.5 μg |
| Vitamin C | 40-60 mg |
| Vitamin D | 5 μg[‡] |
| Vitamin E | 10 mg |
| Vitamin K | 70 μg |

*Based on DHSS 1991[1] and rounded
**Part replaceable by tryptophan in proteins
†Double this in pregnancy
‡More for growth: no dietary requirement if adequate exposure to sunlight

**Recommended names for vitamins**

| Recommended name* | Alternative name | Usual pharmaceutical preparation |
|---|---|---|
| Vitamin A | Retinol | Retinol palmitate |
| Thiamin[†] | Vitamin B-1 | Thiamine hydrochloride |
| Riboflavin | Vitamin B-2 | Riboflavin |
| Niacin | Nicotinic acid and nicotinamide | Nicotinamide |
| Vitamin B-6 | Pyridoxine | Pyridoxine hydrochloride |
| Pantothenic acid | | Calcium pantothenate |
| Biotin | | Biotin |
| Folate | Folacin | Folic acid |
| Vitamin B-12 | Cobalamin | Hydroxocobalamin or Cyanocobalamin |
| Vitamin C | Ascorbic acid | Ascorbic acid |
| Vitamin D | Vitamins $D_2$ and $D_3$ | (Ergo) calciferol |
| Vitamin E | | α-Tocopheryl acetate |
| Vitamin K | | Vitamin $K_1$ |

* International Union of Nutritional Sciences
† Spelt 'thiamine' in the pharmaceutical literature

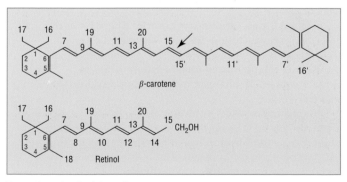

Formation of retinol from β-carotene

loss of mucus production, leading to xerophthalmia (chapter 8). Other epithelia, for example, respiratory, are similarly affected and their resistance to infection is lowered.

Preformed vitamin A (retinol) is found in animal foods: liver is the richest source, but about a quarter of vitamin A intake in Britain comes from carotenes, yellow and orange pigments in the leaves of vegetables and in some fruits, chiefly $\beta$-carotene. One molecule of $\beta$-carotene can be cleaved by a specific intestinal enzyme into two molecules of vitamin A. But this conversion is not very efficient, $6\,\mu g$ $\beta$-carotene is assumed to be equivalent to $1\,\mu g$ retinol. Vitamin A is stored in the liver; stores are enough for one to two years in most British adults (see chapter 8). Retinol is transported from the liver to the rest of the body on retinol binding protein, part of the pre-albumin complex. Its concentration is normally held constant and does not reflect vitamin A intake except when this is very low or high.

[International units of vitamin A can be confusing if used for $\beta$-carotene and are best avoided, but some pharmaceuticals continue to use them. For retinol $1\,IU = 0.3\,\mu g$ retinol, so the UK reference nutrient intake for men is either $700\,\mu g$ or $2333\,IU$.]

In supranutritional amounts vitamin A reduces both keratinisation of skin and sebum production. 13-*cis* retinoic acid (tretinoin) and its isomer isotretinoin, are used either topically in creams or orally in capsules, but oral retinoids are teratogenic and must not be prescribed for women in whom there is any possibility of pregnancy.

Because vitamin A is teratogenic there is no role for megadosage of this vitamin. Regular intakes should not exceed $3.3\,mg$ in early pregnancy (4.5 times the UK reference nutrient intake of $0.7\,mg$). Liver contains 13-40 mg vitamin A per $100\,g$ (depending on species), so women who are or might become pregnant are advised not to eat liver or products made from it. High doses of vitamin A are toxic to non-pregnant people and fatalities have occurred. Acute hypervitaminosis A causes raised intracranial pressure and skin desequamation. Chronic overdosage is more common and can occur after long term intakes of 10 times the nutritional requirement or more. Symptoms include headache, alopecia, dry itchy skin, hepatomegaly, bone and joint pains. A high plasma vitamin A confirms the diagnosis. High intakes of $\beta$-carotene, on the other hand, colour the plasma and skin (hypercarotenaemia) but are not dangerous.

## Thiamin (vitamin B-1)

Thiamin plays a part in the metabolism of carbohydrates, alcohol, and branched chain amino acids. The body contains only 30 mg—30 times the daily nutrient requirement—and deficiency starts after about a month, on a thiamin free diet sooner than for any other vitamin. The requirements are proportional to the non-fat energy intake. The two principal deficiency diseases are beriberi and Wernicke–Korsakoff syndrome.

**Beriberi** is now rare in the countries where it was originally described—Japan, Indonesia, and Malaysia. In Western countries occasional cases are seen in alcoholics: clinical features are a high output cardiac failure with few electrocardiograph changes and a prompt response to thiamin treatment alone.

**Wernicke–Korsakoff syndrome** is usually seen in alcoholics: it can also occur in people who fast (such as hunger strikers) or who have persistent vomiting (as in hyperemesis gravidarum). Early recognition is important. The ophthalmoplegia and lowered consciousness respond to thiamin (50 mg intramuscularly) in two days, but if treatment is delayed the

---

**Food sources of vitamin A**

**Preformed vitamin A (retinol)**
 Liver, fish, liver oils (very rich sources)
 kidney, dairy produce
 eggs, fortified margarine

**$\beta$-carotene**
 Carrots, red palm oil
 apricots, melon, pumpkin
 dark green leafy vegetables
 (spinach, broccoli, sprouts, etc)

In Britain the main sources in the diet are liver, margarine, butter and dairy products.

---

**Carotenoids**

**600 colours of flowers, autumn leaves and birds, yellow to red, have chemically similar structure to $\beta$-carotene, with variations usually at the end rings. Of the three carotenoids in higher concentration in human plasma (reflecting dietary intake) only $\beta$-carotene is pro-vitamin A. The other two are lycopene, the red colour of tomatoes, which has antioxidant properties, and lutein/zeaxanthin (stereoisomers) which give the yellow colour to the macula lutea in the retina.**

---

**Food sources of thiamin**

• whole wheat and wholemeal breads
• wheat germ (richest source) bran
• yeast, mycoprotein, nuts
• pork, bacon, Marmite
• fortified breakfast cereals
• oatmeal, potatoes, and peas

In Britain the main sources in the diet are bread and cereal products, potatoes, and meat.

memory may never recover. Red cell transketolase and the effect on it of thiamin pyrophosphate (TPP) *in vitro* are used to confirm thiamin deficiency, but fresh whole blood is needed and must, if it is to be meaningful, be taken before thiamin treatment is started. If thiamin deficiency is suspected treatment should be started without waiting for the laboratory result. Two days later there will either have been a clinical response and a positive laboratory report of high TPP effect (indicates deficiency) or the provisional diagnosis will not have been confirmed.

Patients on regular haemodialysis should routinely be given small supplements of thiamin and other water-soluble vitamins. Thiamin should also be given prophylactically to people with persistent vomiting or prolonged gastric aspiration and those who go on long fasts, as well as alcoholics. The toxicity of thiamin is very low, though occasional cases of anaphylaxis have been reported after intravenous injection.

# Riboflavin (vitamin B-2)

Riboflavin, a yellow substance with green fluorescence in the coenzymes flavin mononucleotide (FMN) and flavin adenine dinucleotide (FAD), has vital roles in cellular oxidation. Its biochemical functions do not easily explain the clinical manifestations that have been recorded in volunteers on a riboflavin deficient diet: angular stomatitis, cheilosis, atrophic papillae on the tongue, nasolabial dyssebacea, and anaemia. There are no real body stores of riboflavin, but the liver contains enough (in coenzyme form) to withstand depletion for about three months.

Most of the features of riboflavin deficiency have more than one cause. Angular stomatitis, for example, may occur with deficiencies of niacin, pyridoxine, or iron; after herpes febrilis; or with ill fitting dentures. Clinical riboflavin deficiency is very uncommon in milk drinking countries like Britain. Pregnant women, people with thyrotoxicosis, and those taking chlorpromazine, imipramine, and amitriptyline have increased requirements. Riboflavin has to be included in total diets: infant formulas, fluids for total parenteral nutrition, and supplements for patients on dialysis.

# Niacin

Niacin (nicotinamide and nicotinic acid) is the part of the coenzymes, nicotinamide adenine dinucleotide (NAD) and nicotinamide adenine dinulceotide phosphate (NADP), that has to be supplied by the diet. In addition the amino acid, tryptophan has a minor metabolic pathway via kynurenine to nicotinamide; about $\frac{1}{60}$ of ingested tryptophan goes this way. Tryptophan makes up about 1% of dietary proteins, so 70 g protein a day provides about 12 mg niacin equivalents towards the total niacin requirement of 15-18 mg a day (for adults).

**Pellagra**, caused by niacin deficiency, is now rare except in areas, such as parts of Africa, where people subsist on maize and little else. In maize the niacin is in a bound form, biologically unavailable (except when cooked after pre-treatment with calcium hydroxide water, the traditional Central American way), and tryptophan is its limiting amino acid (unlike other cereals). Secondary pellagra may occur in patients with chronic renal failure on low protein diets or dialysis, if niacin is not included in the regimen. Another rare cause is Hartnup disease, a recessive inborn error of tryptophan absorption.

Above the nutrient dose nicotinic acid (not the amide) produces cutaneous flushing from histamine release at doses of 100 mg/day or more; it has been used for chilblains.

---

**Wernicke–Korsakoff syndrome**

In 1880 Wernicke first described an encephalopathy. Characteristic features are:

- stupor or apathy
- ophthalmoplegia (lateral or vertical)
- nystagmus
- ataxia.

With treatment most patients pass through a phase in which they show the memory disorder, first described by Korsakoff (1887), which consists of inability to retain new memories and confabulation.

The pathological findings in Wernicke's encephalopathy and Korsakoff's psychosis are similar: capillary haemorrhages in the mamillary bodies and round the aqueduct in the mid brain.

Wernicke's encephalopathy responds rapidly to thiamin but Korsakoff's psychosis responds slowly or not at all.

---

**Food sources of riboflavin**

- liver, kidney (richest sources)
- milk, yoghurt
- cheese, Marmite
- fortified cereals
- eggs, beef
- wheat bran
- mushrooms, wheat germ

In Britain the main sources in the diet are milk, meat, fortified breakfast cereals, and vegetables.

---

**Food sources of niacin**

- liver, kidneys (richest source)
- meat, poultry
- fish
- brewer's yeast, Marmite
- peanuts
- bran, pulses
- wholemeal wheat
- coffee

The above are foods with useful amounts of niacin. Protein-rich foods also provide niacin equivalents via their tryptophan content.

---

At doses of 3 g/day or more it inhibits lipolysis in adipose tissue and lowers plasma cholesterol and triglyceride concentrations. It has been one of the treatments for combined hyperlipidaemia—hypercholesterolaemia plus hypertriglyceridaemia. Patients often develop tolerance to the flushing. Its other side effects (in high dosage) include gastric irritation, hyperuricaemia, impaired glucose tolerance and liver function tests, and occasionally cholestatic jaundice.

## Vitamin B-6

The term vitamin B-6 includes five closely related substances that all occur in foods and in the body: pyridoxal and pyridoxamine, their 5' phosphates, and pyridoxine, best known to doctors as the pharmaceutical form. Pyridoxal 5' phosphate is coenzyme for over 100 reactions in the body involving amino acids. Many foods contain moderate amounts. Primary dietary deficiency is rare. An outbreak of convulsions in infants in 1954 was traced to insufficient vitamin B-6 in milk formula because of a manufacturing error. Several drugs interfere with vitamin B-6: hydralazine, penicillamine, and possibly oestrogens. Peripheral neuropathy from high dose isoniazid is prevented with pyridoxine. There are several conditions for which pharmacological doses of 50 to 100 mg pyridoxine are probably beneficial. These include homocystinuria, hyperoxaluria, gyrate atrophy of the choroid, hypochromic sideroblastic anaemia, and radiation sickness. Some biochemical indices of vitamin B-6 state may be abnormal in women taking some oral contraceptives, but these are indirect indices. The more specific plasma pyridoxal phosphate concentration is usually normal. Premenstrual tension is a very variable condition: prescribed or self medication with pyridoxine has no physiological basis and has never been subjected to a convincing double-blind trial.

Above 100 mg/day pyridoxine in repeated dosage may cause severe sensory neuropathy.[2] All seven patients in the first report of this side effect were taking pyridoxine for an inadequate indication—mostly for premenstrual oedema—and most had increased the dosage on their own. Pyridoxine should not be available over the counter at tablet size above 50 mg (which is already 33 times the nutrient requirement).

**Food sources of vitamin B-6**
- wheat germ and bran
- potatoes
- nuts and seeds, peanut butter
- meat, fatty fish, and offal
- other fish
- fortified breakfast cereals
- banana, avocado, dried fruits
- vegetables (especially raw), baked beans
- milk

## Vitamin B-12

The red vitamin was the last to be isolated (1948). Humans eat it preformed in animal foods including fish and milk. It is synthesised by some micro-organisms—for example, in the rumen of cows and sheep (which require traces of cobalt in the pasture). No vegetable food has been shown to contain vitamin B-12 consistently unless it is contaminated—for example, by manure. Humans excrete in the faeces vitamin B-12 that has been synthesised by the colonic bacteria. Vitamin B-12 is the largest of the nutrients, with a molecular weight of about 1350. The physiological mechanism for its absorption requires intrinsic factor from the stomach, and the complex is absorbed only at a special site, in the terminal ileum. Deficiency occurs in several gastric, intestinal, and ileal diseases, including pernicious anaemia (gastric atrophy; no intrinsic factor), and in vegans (pure vegetarians). Adult body stores of vitamin B-12 in the liver last longer than those for any other vitamin, but deficiency occurs more quickly in infants. Vitamin B-12 cooperates with folate in DNA synthesis, so deficiency of either leads to megaloblastosis (anaemia and infertility). Vitamin B-12 has a separate biochemical role, unrelated to folate, in synthesising fatty acids in myelin,

**Food sources of vitamin B-12**
- liver (richest source)
- kidney
- sardines, oysters
- heart, rabbit
- other meats, fish
- eggs
- cheese
- milk
- some fortified breakfast cereals

so deficiency can present with neurological symptoms. Deficiency is diagnosed by measuring the serum vitamin B-12 and/or the concentration of methylmalonate which requires vitamin B-12 for its metabolism.

Supplementation with hydroxocobalamin is desirable for adult vegans and essential for their young children. Several drugs, such as colchicine and metformin, and prolonged anaesthesia with nitrous oxide, can interfere with absorption of vitamin B-12. Hydroxocobalamin can improve some cases of optic neuritis, possibly by detoxifying accumulated cyanide. Apart from rare hypersensitivity reactions there are no known toxic effects from vitamin B-12. It thus makes an ideal placebo, which may still be the commonest reason for its prescription!

# Folate

Folic acid (pteroylglutamic acid) is the primary vitamin from the chemical point of view, and this is the pharmaceutical form because of its stability. But it is rare in foods or in the body. Most folates are in the reduced form (tetrahydrofolate); they have one-carbon components attached to the pteroyl ring, and up to seven (instead of one) glutamic acid residues in a row at one end. Folate is the group name for all these compounds with vitamin activity. These folates have many essential roles in one-carbon transfers in the body, including one of the steps in DNA synthesis.

In folate deficiency there is first a reduction of serum folate below 3 ng/ml (7 nmol/l) and later megaloblastosis of blood cells and other cells with a rapid turnover because cells cannot double their DNA to enable nuclear division. As well as anaemia, diarrhoea is common when the deficiency results from antagonism (due to drugs) rather than dietary lack.

Folate deficiency may occur simply from a poor diet, but it is usually seen when there is malabsorption or increased requirements because of pregnancy (chapter 4) or increased cell proliferation (haemopoiesis, lymphoproliferative disorders) or antagonism from a number of drugs. Methotrexate, pyrimethamine, and co-trimoxazole act preferentially in cancer cells or micro-organisms by inhibiting the complete reduction of folate to the active form, tetrahydrofolate, preferentially in cancer cells or micro-organisms. Alcohol is the commonest antagonist.

Body stores of folate are not large and deficiency can develop quickly in patients on intensive therapy. In some cases this can be ascribed to intravenous alcohol or particular parenteral amino acid mixtures. Trauma, infection, uraemia, increased haemopoiesis, dialysis, vomiting, or diarrhoea may also be partly responsible. Folate deficiency appears to be the most common vitamin deficiency among adult hospital patients in countries such as Britain, so supplements should be prescribed whenever patients are fed intravenously for more than a few days.

The name comes from the Latin *folia* (= leaf), but liver, legumes, nuts, and even wholemeal bread are as good dietary sources as leafy vegetables. Prolonged boiling destroys much of the vitamin in hospital cabbage. No toxic effects are known from moderate doses up to 1000 μg/day; 200 μg folate/day is more than enough to prevent folate deficiency megaloblastic anaemia and had been accepted worldwide as the reference nutrient intake (or recommended dietary allowance). Two research developments in the late 1990s changed this concept. Firstly, maternal folate intakes at the start of pregnancy above this level have been shown to greatly reduce the risk of neural tube effects in the fetus (chapter 4). Secondly, extra folate can reduce raised plasma homocysteine levels which have been

## Food sources of folate

- liver (especially chicken)
- fortified breakfast cereals
- wheat germ, bran, soya flour
- blackeye beans (boiled)
- Brussels sprouts, peanuts
- kidney, other nuts and seeds
- broccoli, lettuce, peas, etc
- wholemeal bread, eggs
- citrus fruits, blackberries, potatoes
- cheese
- beef

In Britain the foods that provide most folate are potatoes, fortified breakfast cereals, bread, and fresh vegetables and some from beer

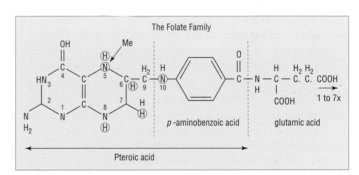

This is folic acid with extra hydrogens at 5, 6, 7 and 8. Tetrahydrofolate (pteroyl glutamic acid) monoglutamate.

Folic acid (pteroyl glutamic acid) is the primary vitamin from the chemical point of view, and it is the pharmaceutical form because of its stability. But it is rare in foods and in the body. Most folates are in the reduced form, tetrahydrofolate (THF); they also have 1-carbon components (methyl or formyl) attached to nitrogen atom 5 or 10, or bridging between them (5,10-methylene-tetrahydrofolate). In addition, they have up to 7 glutamic acid residues in a row (at the right in the figure)

shown to be an independent risk factor for cardiovascular disease (chapter 1).

In the USA fortification of cereal foods with folic acid was made mandatory in 1998 and the recommended intake has been increased to 400 μg per day for men and women (600 μg in pregnancy).

## Vitamin C

Ascorbic acid is the major dietary antioxidant in the aqueous phase of the body. The best established biochemical consequence of its deficiency is impaired reduction of the amino acid, proline to hydroxyproline. Hydroxyproline is an uncommon amino acid, except in collagen, of which it makes up an indispensable 12%. Impaired collagen formation is the biochemical basis of scurvy.

Small doses of vitamin C will cure scurvy. Lind achieved this with two oranges and a lemon in the first controlled trial on HMS *Salisbury* in 1747; 30 mg of vitamin C is more than enough to prevent scurvy. Desirable intakes of vitamin C can be thought of at three levels.

(1) The official reference nutrient intake for adults— 40 mg/day in Britain and 75 to 90 mg/day in the United States—is for healthy people. This is more than enough ascorbate to prevent scurvy.

(2) In hospital patients this is not enough. Absorption of the vitamin may be reduced or its catabolism increased by disease. Trauma and surgery increase the need for vitamin C for collagen synthesis. Several drugs antagonise vitamin C: adrenal corticosteroids, aspirin, indometacin, phenylbutazone, and tetracycline, together with smoking. Hence it is advisable to give a supplement of up to 250 mg ascorbic acid a day to cover major surgery.

(3) The third level is the great vitamin C debate: megadoses (up to 10 g/day) proposed by the late Linus Pauling for superhealth—or not? The best known claim for large intakes of vitamin C is that they prevent common colds. At least 31 controlled trials have been reported and in 23 of them (including the largest and best designed ones) there was no significant preventive effect. The eight supportive trials all had qualifications—for example, they were not double blind, had tiny groups, or showed an effect only in a subgroup.[4]

The present evolution of Pauling's hypothesis is that high intakes of ascorbate increase antioxidant capacity in the body and may help to prevent (or delay) degenerative diseases, such as cataract.[5] High intakes of fruits and vegetables appear epidemiologically to reduce the risk of stomach cancer. The active protective factor might be vitamin C.

At megadosage the law of diminishing returns comes in. The small intestine has limited capacity to absorb ascorbate (so it should be eaten, or taken as tablets, tds). When blood levels increase, the vitamin is excreted in the urine. Careful pharmacokinetic experiments show that little further increase of plasma ascorbate can be achieved above intakes of 250 mg/day.[6] At high intakes urinary excretion of oxalate (which is a metabolite of ascorbate) increases somewhat. Although oxalate is a common component of urinary tract stones, large epidemiological studies have not found more cases of stones in people who take vitamin C supplements.[7] People with a history of nephrolithiasis should nevertheless avoid these supplements, so should patients with chronic renal failure whose plasma ascorbate can rise to levels above the normal range.

Vitamin C enhances the absorption of non-haem iron taken at the same time. This works with mixtures of foods or juices and is a benefit from generous intakes for 299/300 people.

### Serum folate results 1994–1998 in a large clinical laboratory in California, USA

| Year | Number of tests | Rate of serum folate testing[*] | Test results < 2.7 μg/l | Test results ≥ 20 μg/l | Median serum folate value μg/l |
|---|---|---|---|---|---|
| 1994 | 14 493 | 7.3 | 183 (1.3) | 3709 (25.6) | 12.6 |
| 1995 | 14 750 | 6.7 | 186 (1.3) | 3652 (24.8) | 12.7 |
| 1996 | 17 642 | 7.5 | 223 (1.3) | 4130 (23.4) | 11,7 |
| 1997 | 22 805 | 8.9 | 134 (0.6) | 7185 (34.3) | 14.9 |
| 1998 | 26 662 | 10.2 | 89 (0.3) | 12 990 (45.3) | 18.7 |
| Total | 98 351 | 8.3 | 815 (0.8) | 31 666 (32.9) | 14.7 |

[*]Per 1000 members
Since mandatory fortification with folate in the USA (Jan 1998) and Canada (Nov 1998) serum folates have increased, homocysteines have declined and the incidence of neural tube defects is lower[3]

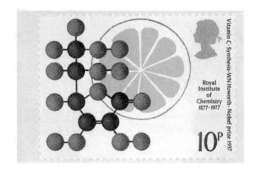

### Food sources of vitamin C

- blackcurrants, guavas
- rosehip syrup, green peppers
- oranges, other citrus fruit, strawberries
- cauliflower, broccoli
- sprouts, cabbage, watercress
- potatoes
- (liver and milk)

In Britain the main sources of vitamin C are fruit juices, potatoes, and other vegetables.

But for the 1/300 people with homozygous haemochromatosis genes vitamin C supplements are contraindicated.

Vitamin C is easily destroyed by cooking (aggravated by alkaline conditions, for example, sodium bicarbonate), so fresh fruit and juices and salads should be encouraged and vegetables cooked lightly and quickly.

## Vitamin D

Cholecalciferol is hydroxylated in the liver to 25-OHD$_3$, the plasma concentration of which is a good index of vitamin D status. In the kidney 25-OHD$_3$ is further hydroxylated either to $1,25(OH_2)D_3$ (calcitriol) or to an inactive metabolite. Calcitriol functions as a hormone whose best known action is to stimulate the synthesis of a calcium transport protein in the epithelium of the small intestines.

The natural substance cholecalciferol was originally called vitamin D$_3$. Vitamin D$_2$ is the artificially produced ergocalciferol. The natural and usual source of cholecalciferol is by the action of short wavelength ultraviolet light from the sun on a companion of cholesterol in the skin, 7-dehydrocholesterol. Cholecalciferol also occurs in a small minority of our foods. When people live in high latitudes, wear clothes, and spend nearly all the time indoors and the sky is polluted with smoke they have insufficient exposure in the winter to ultraviolet light to make the required amount of this substance; under these conditions dietary intake becomes critical and cholecalciferol assumes the role of a vitamin.

In rickets and osteomalacia there is reduced calcification of growing and mature bones respectively. These diseases have been more prevalent in Britain than in other Western countries. They tend to affect adolescents and the elderly, especially Asians in northern cities. In Britons with normal levels plasma 25-OHD$_3$ concentrations show annual fluctuations, with their trough in late winter and their peak after the summer holidays. It is not clear whether the lower prevalence of rickets in Canada and Sweden is because milk is fortified with vitamin D or because people receive more ultraviolet radiation of their skin over the year in these other northern countries.

The small dietary contribution of vitamin D is lost in malabsorption and chronic biliary obstruction. Long term anticonvulsants, phenobarbitone, and phenytoin, increase metabolic losses. Vitamin D is indicated in these conditions. In chronic renal failure and hypoparathyroidism 1 $\alpha$-hydroxylation to the active metabolite is impaired and renal bone disease responds only to $1,25(OH)_2D_3$ (calcitriol) or 1$\alpha$-OHD$_3$ (alfacalcidol), a synthetic derivative.

Irradiation of the skin may cause sunburn but does not lead to vitamin D toxicity. On the other hand, the margin of safety with oral vitamin D, between the nutrient requirements of up to 10 $\mu$g and toxic intakes, is narrow. Overdose with vitamin D causes hypercalcaemia, with thirst, anorexia, polyuria, and the risk of metastatic calcification. Some children have developed hypercalcaemia on vitamin D intakes only five times the recommended nutrient intake. More than this should not be taken except for rickets or osteomalacia. Here 25 to 100 $\mu$g vitamin D—for example, as ergocalciferol—is the usual therapeutic dose.

[One international unit (IU, obsolescent) of vitamin D = 0.025 $\mu$g of cholecalciferol or ergocalciferol—to convert IU to micrograms, divide by 40.]

## Vitamin E

$\alpha$-Tocopherol is the most active of eight very similar compounds with vitamin E activity. Being fat soluble, vitamin E

7-dehydrocholesterol

UV light (290–312 nm)

Cholecalciferol, vitamin D$_3$

(in the liver)

25-hydroxycholecalciferol

(in kidneys)

1,25-dihydroxycholecalciferol (calcitriol)

It may be difficult to remember which foods contain useful amounts of which vitamins but it's a good general rule that highly refined foods and drinks like fats, oils, sugar, cornflour, and alcoholic spirits contain little or no vitamins.

**Food sources of vitamin D**

- fish liver oils
- fatty fish (sardines, herring, mackerel, tuna, salmon, pilchards)
- margarine (fortified)
- infant milk formulas (fortified)
- eggs, liver

In Britain the main sources in the diet are margarines, fatty fish, dairy spreads, breakfast cereals, and eggs

is present in all cell membranes where, being an antioxidant, it is thought to reduce peroxidation of unsaturated fatty acids by free oxygen radicals.

The nutritional requirement for vitamin E is roughly proportional to the intake of polyunsaturated fat. Vitamin E is not easily transported across the placenta, and signs of deficiency, mild haemolytic anaemia, are sometimes found in premature infants.

The most severe cases of deficiency occur in patients with chronic fat malabsorption, especially fibrocystic disease of the pancreas and abetalipoproteinaemia. As well as mild anaemia, in these conditions ataxia, loss of tendon jerks, and pigmentary retinopathy have been reported, which respond to long term vitamin E treatment.

Many people take vitamin E supplements on their own initiative in large doses. Earlier it was rumoured to enhance virility (infertility had been the first reported effect of deficiency in rats) but double-blind trial did not confirm this. In the 1990s the focus is on whether vitamin E's antioxidant activity *in vitro* can reach sufficient concentrations inside the body to reduce atherogenesis. Two large cohort studies in the United States[8] suggest that vitamin E supplements may reduce the risk of coronary heart disease, but a large 5-year randomised trial in Finland[9] found no benefit from 50 mg $\alpha$-tocopherol/day (about five times average dietary intake). Two other large preventive trials in Italy and another in Canada have likewise found no benefit with even larger doses. Although it is a fat-soluble vitamin, tocopherol has a low toxicity. Few adverse effects have been reported from doses up to 3200 mg/day and none were observed consistently.[1]

# Vitamin K

The Koagulations vitamin (Dam, 1935) comes in two chemical forms. Vitamin $K_1$ (phytomenadione) is found mainly in vegetables. The $K_2$ vitamins (menaquinones) are a series produced by bacteria—for example, in the gut. Deficiency of vitamin K manifests itself as hypoprothrombinaemia and bleeding.

Cord blood levels of vitamin K are very low (evidently placental transfer is limited), and breast milk contains little of the vitamin unless the mother has been dosed with vitamin K. To prevent haemorrhagic disease of the newborn 1 mg of vitamin $K_1$ (by injection or by mouth) is given either to all infants or to those at increased risk (low birth weight or difficult delivery), depending on the hospital's policy. The single intramuscular injection of vitamin $K_1$ prevents both early and late vitamin K deficiency bleeding. In one British epidemiological study this injection at birth appeared to be associated with increased risk of childhood cancers. Subsequent studies in several countries have not confirmed this and in the United States there has been no increase of childhood cancer nationally since vitamin K injection at birth became common practice around 1961.[10] Oral vitamin K prevents early but not late haemorrhagic disease. Doubts still linger[11] and doctors should follow locally agreed policy.

In adults vitamin K deficiency is to be expected in obstructive jaundice and can occur in malabsorption syndromes. Vitamin $K_1$ must be given before surgery for these conditions. Anticoagulants of the warfarin group owe their therapeutic action to antagonism of vitamin K, and vitamin $K_1$ is the antidote for overdose.

Vitamin K promotes the synthesis of an unusual amino acid, $\gamma$-carboxyglutamic (gla) a component of coagulation proteins II, VII, IX, and X. Another protein that contains gla and

---

**Food sources of vitamin E**
- vegetable oils—wheat germ oil the richest
- margarines, mayonnaise
- nuts and seeds

Small amounts in wholegrain cereals, eggs, butter, some vegetables, and some fruits.

---

- Four members of the vitamin E family are $\alpha$-, $\beta$-, $\gamma$- and $\delta$-tocopherol. These differ chemically in the number and position of methyl groups on the double ring at one end of the molecule. Biologically $\alpha$-tocopherol is the most potent and $\beta$, $\gamma$, and $\delta$ are each in turn less active. The tocopherols are more active than the four *tocotrienols*, which have double bonds in the side chain; $\alpha$-tocotrienol is the most biopotent, next $\beta$-tocotrienol.
- The eight vitamin E compounds also show d- and l-stereoisomerism. Natural forms are d- (or RRR) and synthetic or dl- (or racemic). Both forms of $\alpha$-tocopherol are available commercially. The most biologically active compound is the natural d- (or RRR) $\alpha$-tocopherol, and vitamin E activity in foods or tissues is summed as d- (or RRR) $\alpha$-tocopherol equivalents.

---

**Food sources of vitamin K**
- turnip greens
- broccoli
- cabbage, lettuce
- liver

These are all good sources, though there is no systematic list.

requires vitamin K for its synthesis is osteocalcin, involved in bone formation.

# Vitamins that can usually be taken for granted (but are required in total parenteral nutrition)

**Biotin** is cofactor for several carboxylase enzymes concerned in fat synthesis and amino acid catabolism. It is widely distributed in foods, the requirement is small, and deficiency is rare. Deficiency has occurred in people who eat large amounts of raw eggs (which contain a protein that binds biotin and prevents its absorption) and in patients receiving total parenteral nutrition with biotin omitted. They suffer scaly dermatitis, loss of hair, hypercholesterolaemia, and a characteristic combination of organic acids in the urine. **Panthothenic acid** is a constituent of coenzyme A which has many functions and is widespread in the body and in foods. The name means "available everywhere". Spontaneous deficiency in man has never been proved. **Choline** is part of lecithin and of sphingomyelin, the two major phospholipids in the body, and it is also part of acetylcholine, the neurotransmitter. It is a dietary essential for the rat, but man seems to be able to synthesise it (partly from methionine) and does not have the active catabolising enzyme (choline oxidase) found in rat liver.

# Multivitamins

The sensible purpose of multivitamin preparations is an insurance policy for people whose diet may be restricted or unbalanced but neither they nor their adviser is sure which vitamin may be lacking. There is a case for multivitamin supplements for people with low calorie intake because of poor appetite or a weight reducing diet or frailty, also for food faddists, the emotionally disturbed and socially disadvantaged people.[12] The dose of each vitamin should be near the nutritional requirement so a multivitamin cannot do harm, even if it does not do good. A doctor prescribing multivitamins or talking to patients who choose to take them should sometimes check the small print—as one should with an insurance policy. How many vitamins of the maximum 13, or the 11 described above are in the ingredient list? Do they contain folic acid? Multivitamin preparations have no lucrative patents, so drug companies are not very interested in keeping them up to date; reformulating is expensive. They are also rather neglected by medicine committees and by dietitians.

# Some minerals

At least 13 inorganic elements *per se* are known to be essential for man (the same as the number of vitamins) while others are needed in compounds (P, S, Cl, Co). All must be provided for long term total parenteral nutrition and ensured in infant formulas. Of the nutritionally important inorganic elements, sodium and potassium are discussed in chapter 2, fluoride in chapter 3, iodine in chapter 8, calcium and iron in chapter 9. Zinc and selenium are sometimes taken as supplements and deserve mention here.

## Zinc
This metal is cofactor for over 100 enzymes (including superoxide dismutase) and "zinc fingers" are part of a number

## Not vitamins
The following compounds sold in "health food" shops and still included in some multivitamin pharmaceuticals are not vitamins. They are not required in infant formulas or in fluids for total parenteral nutrition:

- Bioflavonoids
- Inositol
- Orotic acid
- Aminobenzoic acid (PABA)
- Vitamin B-15 ("pangamic acid")
- Vitamin B-17 (laetrile)
- Vitamin P

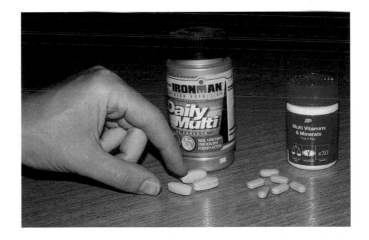

of important transcription factors for DNA. Tissue concentrations of zinc are highest in the choroid of the eye, the prostate and in semen.

The first recognised human deficiency disease (1963) was adolescent growth retardation and hypogonadism in rural Iran; absorption of the small zinc intake in their mainly vegetable diet was hindered by phytate in unleavened bread. The most florid clinical features of zinc deficiency—moist facial eczema, depression, hair loss and diarrhoea have been seen with total parenteral nutrition that omitted zinc and in acrodermatitis enteropathica, a rare inborn error of zinc absorption. Zinc is predominantly intracellular and serum zinc is not a reliable indicator of deficiency. Randomised controlled trials have demonstrated benefit from zinc supplements in children in developing countries with acute diarrhoea,[13] pneumonia, and stunting.[14] Universal zinc supplements will not, however, improve the growth of stunted children except where zinc is the primary growth-limiting nutrient. Reports of benefit in cases of the common cold in industrial countries were not confirmed. The best dietary sources of zinc are meat, fish, cheese, and whole grain cereals (though absorption is reduced by phytate).

## Selenium

Selenium compounds have long been known to be toxic. The content of this trace element in foods varies greatly, depending on the amount in the soil. Since the 1950s selenium deficiency in animals has been known to cause muscular dystrophy in sheep and liver necrosis in rats. Human deficiency has caused juvenile cardiomyopathy in Keshan, China (1979). In the body selenium replaces sulphur in selenomethionine and selenocysteine. It is part of glutathione peroxidase (antioxidant) and an enzyme that converts thyroxine to triiodothyronine. Blood selenium reflects intake and nutritional status and so does the Se content of toenails. Intakes have been moderately low in Finland and in South Island, New Zealand. Finland corrected this by fortifying fertilisers used for wheat fields with selenium from 1994. In New Zealand extensive research has been done at Otago University on selenium nutrition and metabolism. No clear human condition has been attributable to the local selenium level. Meanwhile intakes there are rising a little with more foods coming in from Australia. But in Britain selenium intakes have been declining[15] due to less wheat coming in from North America (high Se) and more from the continent of Europe (lower Se). Occasional cases of muscular disease have been reported in patients maintained long term on total parenteral nutrition if selenium was not included. A large randomised controlled trial with selenium in people with early skin cancer for five years, in low selenium areas in the south east United States of America showed an unexpected significantly reduced incidence of prostate cancer.[16]

## References

1 Department of Health. *Dietary reference values for food energy and nutrients for the United Kingdom.* Report on Health & Social Subjects no 41. London: HMSO, 1991.
2 Institute of Medicine. *Dietary Reference Intakes for Thiamin, Riboflavin, Niacin, Vitamin B-6, Folate, Vitamin B-12, Pantothenic Acid, Biotin and Choline.* Washington DC: National Academy Press, 1998.
3 Lawrence JM, Petitti DB, Watkins M, Umekubo MA. Trends in serum folate after food fortification. *Lancet* 1999; **354**: 915–6.
4 Truswell AS. Ascorbic acid and colds (letter). *N Engl J Med* 1986; **315**: 709.
5 Jacques PF, Taylor A, Hankinson SE *et al.* Long-term vitamin C supplement use and prevalence of early age-related lens opacities. *Am J Clin Nutr* 1997; **66**: 911-16.
6 Levine M, Corry-Cantilena C, Wang Y *et al.* Vitamin C pharmacokinetics in healthy volunteers: evidence for a recommended dietary allowance. *Proc Natl Acad Sci USA* 1996; **93**: 3704-9.
7 Gerster H. No contribution of ascorbic acid to renal calcium oxalate stones. *Ann Nutr Metab* 1997; **41**: 269-82.
8 Rimm EB, Stampfer MJ, Ascherio A, Giovannucci E, Colditz GA, Willett WC. Vitamin E consumption and the risk of coronary heart disease in men. *N Engl J Med* 1993; **328**: 1450-6.
9 Rapola JM, Virtamo J, Ripatti S *et al.* Randomised trial of α-tocopherol and β-carotene supplements on incidence of major coronary events in men with previous myocardial infarction. *Lancet* 1997; **349**: 1715-20.
10 American Academy of Pediatrics, Vitamin K ad hoc Task Force. Controversies concerning vitamin K and the newborn. *Pediatrics* 1993; **91**: 1001-3.
11 The 17 January 1998 issue of the BMJ contains an editorial, four research papers and a letter with a meta-analysis—a total of 24 pages—on neonatal vitamin K prophlaxis. *BMJ* 1998; **316**: 161, 173-93.
12 Truswell AS. Who should take vitamin supplements? *BMJ* 1990; **301**: 135-6.
13 Sazawal S, Black RB, Bhan MK, Bhandari N, Sinha A, Jalk S. Zinc supplementation in young children with acute diarrhoea in India. *N Engl J Med* 1995; **333**: 839-44.
14 Umeta M, West CE, Haidar J, Deurenberg P, Hautvast JGAJ. Zinc supplementation and stunted infants in Ethiopia: a randomised controlled trial. *Lancet* 2000; **355**: 2021-6.
15 Rayman MP. Dietary selenium: time to act. *BMJ* 1997; **314**: 387-8.
16 Clark LC, Combs GF, Turnbull BW *et al.* Effects of selenium supplementation for cancer prevention in patients with carcinoma of the skin. A randomised controlled trial. *JAMA* 1996; **276**: 1957-63.

# 11 Overweight and obesity

## Obesity is an increasing problem

Obesity is rising to alarming levels around the world.[1]
In England during the 15 years 1980 to 1995 some important
health statistics improved and life expectancy lengthened by
three years. But the numbers of obese men (16-64 years)
increased from 6% to 15% and obese women from 8% to
16.5%. Obesity is one of only four of the 25 targeted statistics in
the Health of the Nation strategy that has moved in the wrong
direction. Similar trends of increasing obesity have occurred in
almost all industrialised countries and in the prosperous class
in developing countries.

There have been recent advances in our understanding of
genetics, endocrinology and metabolism related to adiposity.
However treatment options have not kept pace; fenfluramine
and dexfenfluramine, sadly, in 1997 joined the list of
disappointing and/or potentially dangerous treatments for
obesity.[1] Resources for the management of obesity—dietetic,
pharmaceutical, and surgical—have been likened to treatment
options for hypertension 40 years ago.[3]

### Why is there an epidemic of increasing obesity?
Although the external influences and internal processes are
both very complex the ultimate causes of obesity are under-
exercising and/or over-eating: energy intake > energy
expenditure. But the development of obesity, via overweight is
usually so slow and insidious that people hardly notice it is
happening. The body's homeostatic energy regulation is better
able to defend against insufficient food than against a little
more food, a little less energy expenditure (see box opposite).

*Possible reasons for over-eating these days:*

- cheaper foods (relative to incomes)
- more varied foods; supermarkets
- advertising and promotion of foods
- more eating outside the home (pubs, ethnic restaurants, fast
  food chains, etc)
- more fatty food; more snack foods
- over-eating because of anxiety (for example, work stress) or
  depression (for example, unemployment)
- grazing and irregular meal times
- fewer people now smoke (smoking suppresses appetite)

*Possible reasons for under-exercising these days:*

- more labour-saving machinery at work and at home (fork-lift
  trucks, power tools, washing machines, even automatic doors
  and lifts)
- television (couch potatoes)
- personal computers ("mouse potatoes") and email
- more cars; less walking and cycling
- less open space for recreation
- fear of violence in the streets
- central heating might also reduce energy expenditure

Prentice and Jebb[4] considered the case for Britain. The
continuing series of food consumption data in households
shows a reduction in average total energy intake per head since
1980. But this is food disappearance data (not food actually
eaten) and does not include food eaten outside the home.
The National Food Surveys, year by year, also show that
consumption of fat (the most concentrated food energy) has

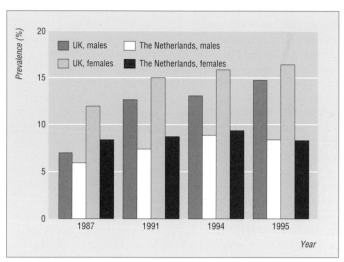

Prevalence of obesity in the UK and the Netherlands 1987-1995[2]

---

### Energy balance

1 kg body weight gained has energy of approx 7000 kcal

10 kg weight gain over 5 years $= \frac{70\,0000}{5 \times 365} = 38$ kcal/day

This is a daily error of energy balance of $+1.5\%$
OR 10 minutes' walk
OR one square (1/8) of a 2oz milk chocolate bar
OR half a digestive biscuit

---

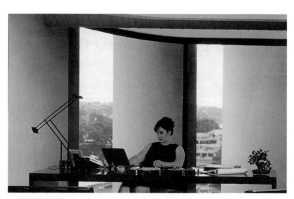

Email is more fattening than ice cream (Courtesy Roche with permission)

declined slightly since 1980. The evidence for reduced energy expenditure is more persuasive, though based on indirect indices. Car ownership and television viewing were strikingly related to the prevalence of obesity whether plotted against year or against socioeconomic status.

### Facing moderate obesity

It is easy to diagnose moderate and gross obesity before the patient undresses. The difficulty with these patients is to organise the time and summon up the enthusiasm to embark on management which will be lengthy and may be unsuccessful. While our profession can transplant a human heart, manage *in vitro* fertilisation, and eliminate smallpox, to manage obesity is a challenge for a conscientious practitioner. A health service, like the British NHS, which provides an annual fee per patient is a suitable framework.

Obesity is different from most other diseases. If the general practitioner feels they are not the best person to look after a patient's haemorrhoids or backache or poor vision there is usually a specialist at the nearest big hospital who has the skills and equipment and will be happy to manage this part of the patient. But there is unlikely to be a consultant with special skills or equipment for looking after obesity. Obesity is a continuum and all but the most complicated or severe cases would not be welcome in the district hospital.

Many obese patients are referred to dietitians but there are too many obese people for the number of dietitians in Britain, and hospital staff are not well placed for looking after obese "outpatients"—that is, people who live at home and have to go out to work each weekday.

To put in the hard work of treating the obese people on the practice's list reduces the likelihood of having to treat them later for complications of obesity. The best conditions for managing obesity are:

- regular visits, at least once a fortnight
- weighing the patient under the same conditions on the same scale
- about quarter of an hour's talk with the same practitioner each visit
- opportunity to bring wife, or husband
- the therapist is not obese.

### Complications of obesity

Most of the medical complications of obesity are well known. Risks of cardiovascular complications and diabetes are greater in people with abdominal obesity. This can be assessed clinically by measuring waist circumference. In men the normal measurement is up to 94 cm and metabolic complications are substantially increased at above 102 cm. The corresponding waist circumferences in women are: healthy <80 cm, increased risk 80-88 cm, substantially increased risk 88 cm.[5] Considerable weight gain in a short time carries greater risks than reaching the same weight slowly.[6]

The social complications are more immediate and may be very painful. Religious, racial, and gender prejudice are now unacceptable in mainstream Western societies, as is prejudice against the disabled. But prejudice against fat people is undisguised. It starts at school, affects the job opportunities and social status of obese people—and it is so pervasive that it probably colours many doctors' attitudes towards their obviously obese patients.

> Make less thy body hence, and more thy grace;
> Leave gormandising; know the grave doth gape
> For thee thrice wider than for other men.
> Shakespeare, *King Henry IV* Part II, V, v.

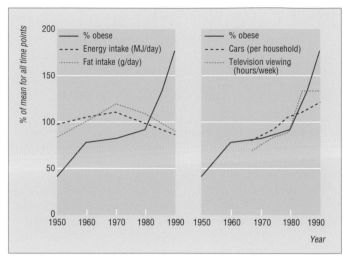

Secular trends in diet (left) and activity (right) in relation to obesity in Britain. (Adapted from Prentice and Jebb[4])

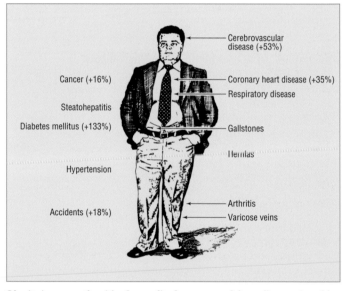

Obesity increases the risk of mortality from some of these diseases (notably diabetes) more than others

### Substances secreted by adipose tissue[7]

Adipose tissue liberates free fatty acids and glycerol under the stimulus of catecholamines on lipase. When it loses fat in this way some of the stored cholesterol and accumulated non-polar foreign substances, for example DDT, also go into the circulation.

Since the discovery (1994) of **leptin**—the chemical signal to the brain of the amount of adipose tissue—it is realised that adipocytes are more than simple fat stores. They also secrete:

- tumour necrosis factor α, TNF α
- interleukin 6, IL6
- resistin
- angiotensinogen
- adipsin (complement factor D)
- tissue factor (initiator of coagulation)
- adiponectin
- aromatase, etc

TNF α, IL6 and resistin appear to increase insulin resistance,[8] the extra angiotensinogen makes hypertension more likely and aromatase converts androstenedione to the oestrogen estrone.

### Recognising mild obesity/overweight

By contrast, for overweight or mild obesity diagnosis and recognition are where the management goes wrong. Yet there are several people with mild obesity for every case of obvious obesity in a practice. Mild obesity is much easier to treat, and prevention of gross obesity is much easier than cure.

People with mild obesity do not usually come to their practitioner complaining that they are too fat. The adiposity has been slowly creeping up on them and does not cause pain, distress, or fear. They come to the doctor with any other symptom and disease.

Patients may become mildly obese under their doctor's eyes, during the course of an illness which the practitioner is following and concentrating on: bed rest after myocardial infarction; giving up smoking; pregnancy and lactation; anxiety or depression from stress at work or at home. Recognition of overweight can be more difficult too in a patient in bed.

## Measuring obesity

It is part of good practice to have a system so that all patients on the list are weighed at regular intervals by the receptionist or nurse. The weight is entered on the record. Knowing the patient's height (without shoes) the doctor can then decide whether he or she is: underweight, in the normal range, overweight, or obese. Comparison with previous weights shows if the patient is putting on weight.

Weight measurements are objective. To show the patient his or her weight against the standards for his or her height is impressive and, if outside the normal range, the basis for action. Obesity is an excess of adipose tissue. There are two methods for deciding whether someone is too fat. One is **social** or according to fashion. The doctor's role here is to advise patients not to make themselves too thin, not to take unphysiological diets or drugs to lose weight unnecessarily, and not to start on the road to anorexia nervosa.

The other method for deciding whether someone is too fat (or too thin) is **actuarial**. Above (or below) a range of weights for a given height the risk of developing illness or of mortality increases. Weight/height$^2$ (in kg/m$^2$) is a convenient index of relative weight. It gives a single number and is almost independent of height. This is the body mass index (BMI) or Quetelet's index. Note that smoking carries a higher risk of mortality than overweight or the milder degrees of obesity.

The lower and upper ends of the acceptable range here are close to, respectively, the lowest weight for small frame and highest weight for large frame for men in the earlier "desirable weights" of the Metropolitan Life Insurance Company of New York (1959).

The unisex table on page 72 was introduced in the early 1980s. It is simpler than older standards. They had somewhat lower cut off points for women than men, but the numbers of women taking out life insurance were probably inadequate. Modern prospective data show no significant differences between men and women.

### BMI cut offs in different ethnic groups

**The range 18.5 to 24.9 may not be optimal for the whole world. Somewhat higher ranges probably suit Polynesians who tend to have more muscle, less fat. Somewhat lower ranges are probably optimal for south Asians who have insulin resistance at lower BMIs than Caucasians.[10]**

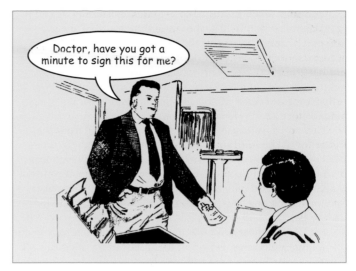

Have you got a minute doctor to sign this for me?

---

### Measuring the patient

- Beam and lever scales are more reliable but take more space and are slower to use.
- For screening it is a good idea to have a lever scale in the reception area and for the receptionist or nurse to weigh the patient with shoes and coat removed.
- Obese patients being treated can be weighed (ideally in their underclothes) at each visit by the doctor in his consulting room on the same platform scale with a quick reading dial.
- The patient's height can be measured with a rule or tape measure attached to a flat wall and recorded in the notes. Heights are lower in the evening than in the morning. If the patient has any weakness or deformity an assistant is needed to get them as straight as possible for the measurement.

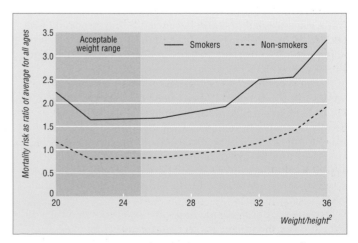

Variations in mortality by weight among 750 000 men and women.[9] Cut off for obesity starts at BMI of 30

Obesity is taken in this table as generally starting at a BMI of 30 kg/m$^2$, which is 20% above the upper end of the acceptable range of weights for height. Between the top of acceptable weight and start of obesity is "overweight", which is the BMI range 25-29.9. The column at the far right shows weights for BMI of 40 kg/m$^2$, the start of "gross obesity". Adiposity is thus graded; this grading is needed for deciding management, and reflects prognosis.

The cut off values in the table have to be read from the viewpoint of the individual patient, like normal ranges for laboratory tests. People with gracile bones should weigh less than heavy boned people. Unusual muscle development (as in weight lifters) and oedema increase body weight. The waist circumference or waist/hip ratio should also be included in the assessment.

In children there are no actuarial data on which to base cut off weights for obesity. However, the upper percentiles of BMI references for British boys and girls by Cole et al.[11] can be used. These are based on a total sample of 30 500 children and adolescents (also see chapter 6, page 24).

## Causes

Obesity **secondary** to hypothalamic conditions that increase appetite is rare, and to endocrine disorders uncommon.

Obesity may follow (*a*) enforced inactivity such as bed rest, arthritis, stroke, change to a less active job, sports injury, or (*b*) over-eating associated with psychological disturbances, for example, depression or anxiety, or some drugs that increase the appetite. Pregnancy and stopping smoking contribute to overweight.

---

**Drugs that can increase appetite and promote weight gain**

Corticosteroids, anabolic agents, some oral contraceptives, sulphonylureas, cyproheptidine, amitryptyline, clomipramine, lithium, pizotifen, metoclopramide, clozapine, olanzapine, some benzodiazepines

---

The genetic influence on obesity was clearly shown in a study using the Danish Adoption Register. A strong relation existed between the weight class of the adoptees (thin, acceptable, overweight, or obese) and the body mass index of their **biological**, but not their adoptive, parents. In twins body mass index is more strongly correlated between monozygotic than dizygotic twins, even when they are reared apart.[12]

Wide searches are going on to see if mutations of candidate genes for peptides and receptors involved in energy regulation are associated with obesity. Mutations of MC4R the melanocortin receptor, of $\beta_1$, $\beta_2$ and $\beta_3$ adrenoreceptors, of the leptin receptor and of leptin have been found associated with obesity. All are very rare except the MC4R mutation which is uncommon. In the great majority of obese people the weight gain is polygenic.

In most people obesity is **primary**. There is no obvious predisposing condition. If the patient says (s)he eats little: (1) the weight gain may have been in the past (2) some people undoubtedly need less food than others apparently comparable; they are efficient metabolisers with a low basal metabolic rate (but normal thyroid) and may feel the cold sooner than others, (3) repeated periods on low calorie diets, weight cycling, may lead to further adaptive lowering of the basal metabolic rate.

In surveys, obese people have often reported that they do not eat more than thin people. But the doubly labelled water technique (that measures rates of disappearance of the stable

---

### Guidelines for body weight in adults

| Height (without shoes) ft, in | (m) | Weight (kg) (minimal clothes) | | | |
|---|---|---|---|---|---|
| | | Normal BMI 18.5-25 | Overweight BMI 25-30 | Obese BMI 30+ | Grossly obese BMI 40+ |
| 4,9 | 1.45 | 39-53 | 53-64 | >64 | >85 |
| 4,10 | 1.48 | 40-55 | 55-65 | >65 | >88 |
| 4,11 | 1.50 | 42-55 | 55-68 | >68 | >90 |
| 5,0 | 1.52 | 43-58 | 58-69 | >69 | >93 |
| 5,1 | 1.54 | 44-59 | 59-71 | >71 | >95 |
| 5,1 | 1.56 | 45-61 | 61-73 | >73 | >97 |
| 5,2 | 1.58 | 46-63 | 63-75 | >75 | >100 |
| 5,3 | 1.60 | 47-64 | 64-78 | >78 | >103 |
| 5,4 | 1.62 | 48-66 | 66-79 | >79 | >105 |
| 5,5 | 1.64 | 50-67 | 67-81 | >81 | >108 |
| 5,5 | 1.66 | 51-69 | 69-83 | >83 | >111 |
| 5,6 | 1.68 | 52-71 | 71-85 | >85 | >113 |
| 5,7 | 1.70 | 53-73 | 73-87 | >87 | >116 |
| 5,8 | 1.72 | 55-74 | 74-89 | >89 | >119 |
| 5,9 | 1.74 | 56-76 | 76-91 | >91 | >121 |
| 5,9 | 1.76 | 57-78 | 78-93 | >93 | >124 |
| 5,10 | 1.78 | 59-79 | 79-95 | >95 | >127 |
| 5,11 | 1.80 | 60-81 | 81-97 | >97 | >130 |
| 6,0 | 1.82 | 61-83 | 83-99 | >99 | >133 |
| 6,0 | 1.84 | 63-85 | 85-102 | >102 | >136 |
| 6,1 | 1.86 | 64-87 | 87-104 | >104 | >139 |
| 6,2 | 1.88 | 65-88 | 88-106 | >106 | >141 |
| 6,3 | 1.90 | 67-90 | 90-108 | >108 | >145 |
| 6,4 | 1.92 | 68-92 | 92-111 | >111 | >148 |

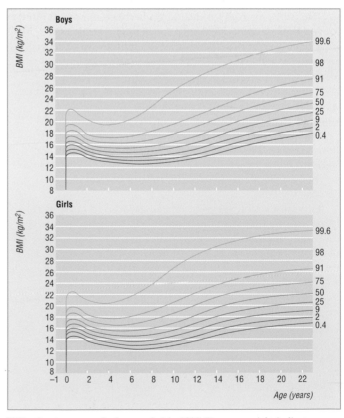

BMI reference curves for boys and girls: 1990. Figures on right indicate percentiles (Adapted from Cole et al.[11])

isotopes, $^2H$ and $^{18}O$) showed that the energy expenditure of a group of obese people was higher than their self-recorded food energy intakes. In other words, obese people tend to **under-report** their food intake.[13]

# Regulation of energy balance

Many outside influences and numerous complex biological mechanisms inside the body affect energy balance. No diagram or model can adequately describe how most people's energy metabolism and fat stores are unconsciously regulated with little or no cumulative error. The system can be visualised at four levels: cerebral cortex, satiety, control centres in the hypothalamus, and thermogenesis.

*Cerebral cortex*
Eating behaviour is initiated by cultural and psychological influences: meal times, habitual diet, olfactory and visual stimuli, perception of appetite, social norms, foods available, personal relationships, etc.

*Satiety*[14]
Signals to stop eating come from distension and from chemical stimuli in the stomach and upper small intestine. These send afferent impulses via the vagus and cause secretion of gut hormones, for example cholecystokinin (CCK) is the most potent. Satiety signals go to the tractus solitarus nucleus in the brain stem, which has connections to the hypothalamus. Serotonergic receptors are involved in the brain.

*Thermogenesis*[17]
Animals that hibernate or adapt to cold have brown fat in which (unlike white fat) noradrenaline stimulates uncoupling of energy flow in the mitochondria, with production of heat instead of ATP. After infancy humans possess little or no distinct area of brown fat but are capable of some thermogenesis (increased metabolic rate)—on exposure to cold and with overfeeding. There appear to be varying numbers of brown adipose cells dispersed in white fat depots. The agent that catalyses the proton leak in these cells is Uncoupling Protein 1 (UCP1) which is triggered by $\beta_3$ adrenergic receptors and influenced by thyroid hormone. Two other uncoupling proteins UCP2 and UCP3 have been recently discovered in humans.

> It is not possible to conjure a unifying theory which will explain why some people become fat while others remain lean. This is too much to expect; economists have no simple explanation for the commercial success or failure of businesses or nations, and the energy economy of a human being is subject to as many influences as any financial economic model.[18]

# Management

There are three phases in the management.

- First is for the obese patient to reach an agreement with the health professional about what they believe they can achieve.
- Second is the difficult phase of the patient modifying eating and exercise habits to lose this much weight.
- Third is the longer and sometimes more difficult phase of the patient maintaining the new lower weight.

**First: agreeing on the objective**
**To reduce weight to the acceptable range** is a reasonable aim that should be achievable for someone who is in the overweight category (BMI 25-30, or grade 1 obesity). With this grade of adiposity the weight loss required is only about 10 kg (22 lb).

---

**Control centres in the hypothalamus**[15]

Circulating leptin conveys information about the size and fluctuation of the adipose tissue stores to receptors in the hypothalamus. There are also receptors there for insulin. If leptin or insulin is injected directly into the brain it reduces food intake: deficiency of either hormone increases intake. Decreased leptin (reduced energy stores) activates neurones in the arcuate nucleus that express two neuropeptides that increase appetite: **neuropeptide Y** (NPY) and **agouti-related protein** (AGRP). Increased leptin inhibits these neurones and instead activates neurones that express **melanocortin**, which suppresses appetite. These different neuropeptides act on specific receptors in the paraventricular nucleus, notably Y1 and Y5 for NPY and MC4 for melanocortin. (Drugs that could block NPY receptors are already being studied.)

**Ghrelin** is a newly discovered peptide secreted by the stomach during fasting.[16] It acts on the hypothalamus to stimulate the neurones that express NPY and AGRP.

---

"Obesity cannot be prevented or managed solely at the individual level. Communities, governments, the media and the food industry need to work together to modify the environment so that it is less conducive to weight gain. Such partnerships are required to ensure that effective and sustainable changes in diet and everyday levels of physical activity can be achieved throughout the community."[19]

---

**Three phases in management of obesity**

- Agreement on what can be achieved
- Modification of eating and exercise habits
- Maintenance of new lower weight

---

But for someone considerably obese, BMI 35 or more, we know that most people cannot manage, with present resources, to reduce their food intake and increase their exercise sufficiently for long enough to bring their weight down all the way to the acceptable range. For someone with a BMI of 35 and a height of 175 cm this means taking off 31 kg (68 lb). It is better to set a **more realistic, intermediate goal** (which could always be extended later). A weight loss of 10 kg brings with it real health benefits.

For any overweight or obese patient the medical adviser can at least hope to help them to **hold their weight stable** and not let it creep up further. To achieve this may involve discovering why the patient has been putting on weight and discussing how these conditions can be modified.

Because there are now so many people in any general practice with overweight and obesity and these increase risks for many degenerative diseases, it is important work for the doctor (1) to recognise overweight and give early warning, and (2) in patients with obesity to take a structured therapeutic role.[20] For patients with type 2 diabetes (especially), hypertension, coronary disease, hernias, etc, action to reduce weight is not just preventive medicine, it is a central part of the treatment. The Nutrition Task Force and the Physical Activity Task Force of the UK Health of the Nation strategy proposed that prevention of obesity rather than its treatment should be a national priority.

### Second: reducing weight

Two main treatments are indispensable: eating less dietary energy and increasing energy expenditure. Both are needed; they are synergistic. The cupboard of drugs for obesity is rather bare at present, and surgery—perhaps gastric stapling—should only be considered for the very fat minority.

> You can lose weight only by achieving a cumulative negative energy balance. Calories in must be less than calories expended. An average loss of 2000 kJ (500 kcal) per day—14 000 kJ (3500 kcal) over a week—is equivalent to a loss of about 0.5 kg (1 lb) per week or more at the start, when water is lost.

### The new way of eating

- Try to avoid the word "diet" that has discouraging overtones and suggests temporary hardship rather than a lifestyle that can last. Habits are more important than diets.
- It does not matter what you eat as long as it is less. This may sound irresponsible and obviously could not be taken to extremes (but there is sometimes too much technical detail in weight-loss programmes and malnutrition is a very rare complication).
- Eat smaller portions of what you usually eat, no second helpings, no snacks between meals.
- Have three regular meals each day. It is more difficult to control one's weight when meal occasions are irregular.
- Eat more low energy (calorie) foods—salads, fruits, vegetables, low fat milk, and yoghurt (left side of "energy values of foods" table on page 75).
- Avoid or ration energy (calorie)-dense foods with a high fat content—and fats in some foods are invisible; cakes, biscuits, cheese, chocolate, nuts, potato crisps, standard meats, chicken skin, and of course fried foods.
- The household should be involved and supportive. Husband and wife or partners should share in discussions with the doctor and dietitian.

---

### Likely benefits of 10 kg weight loss[20]

- *Blood pressure*
  Fall of 10 mmHg systolic     Fall of 20 mmHg diastolic
- *Diabetes*
  Fall of 50% in fasting blood glucose
- *Plasma lipids*
  Fall of 10% total cholesterol     Fall of 15% LDL
  Fall of 30% triglycerides     Rise of 8% HDL
- *Mortality*
  Fall of >20% total mortality

---

### Starting measurements

If an agreement has been reached between patient and doctor that they will start a weight-loss programme this is a good time to make baseline measurements that are likely to improve. As well as accurate height and unclothed weight, hence BMI, waist circumference should be measured and fasting blood taken for plasma lipids (including triglycerides) and glucose.
Risks of metabolic complications are greater in people with abdominal obesity[21]

- For women: increased risk above 80 cm waist circumference (32 inches) substantial risk above 88 cm (35 inches)
- For men: increased risk above 94 cm waist circumference (37 inches) substantial risk above 102 cm (40 inches)

---

### Successes

Klem *et al.*[22] collected records of 629 women and 155 men in the United States who successfully lost at least 30 lb (13.6 kg) and maintained the weight loss for at least one year. Their average starting BMI was 35, they lost an average of 30 kg and their new BMI was 24.5 kg/m$^2$.

A little over half of this sample lost weight through formal programmes; the rest lost weight on their own. All of them used diet **and** exercise. Three-quarters of them reported that a triggering event had preceded their successful weight loss. Some limited classes of foods, some limited quantities of foods, some counted calories. They said that their weight loss led to improvements in energy, physical mobility, mood, self-confidence, and physical health.

---

### Satiety

Satiety is a function that has been neglected in weight reduction programmes. People stop eating because of internal feelings of satiety, "I've had enough, thank you". But this feeling of having eaten enough is not directly related to the energy (calories) of a meal or food. Some foods give stronger satiety per MJ than others. High fat foods have weak satiety for their energy values compared to predominantly carbohydrate foods.[23] Short-term studies indicate for example that boiled potatoes have twice the satiety effects of chips for the same calories and fruits have greater satiety effect than biscuits or confectionery.[24]

**Representative energy values of (stated) typical servings of some common foods**

| | kJ | kcal | | kJ | kcal | | kJ | kcal |
|---|---|---|---|---|---|---|---|---|
| Lettuce (30 g) | 17 | 4 | Bread (1 slice, 30 g) | 280 | 67 | Biscuits (2 digestive) | 670 | 160 |
| Cucumber (45 g) | 21 | 5 | Egg (1 boiled) | 305 | 73 | Peanuts (30 g) | 711 | 170 |
| Carrot (50 g) | 42 | 10 | Banana (1 fruit) | 334 | 80 | Avocado (1/2 fruit) | 711 | 170 |
| Cauliflower (90 g, raw) | 50 | 12 | Beer (1/2 pint) | 360 | 86 | Chicken roast, meat only, 120 g) | 744 | 178 |
| Tomato (90 g) | 54 | 13 | Wine (125 g) | 393 | 94 | Cheese (Cheddar, 45 g) | 752 | 180 |
| Grapefruit (1/2, no sugar) | 75 | 18 | Yoghurt (carton, low fat) | 418 | 100 | Chocolate biscuits (2) | 794 | 190 |
| Milk (full cream, 30 g, in tea) | 84 | 20 | Cornflakes (30 g) | 460 | 110 | Beef steak (grilled, 150 g) | 1003 | 240 |
| Sugar (1 level teaspoon) | 84 | 20 | Butter (15 g) | 460 | 110 | Potato crisps (50 g) | 1108 | 265 |
| Crispbread (10 g) | 134 | 32 | Fish (cod, grilled, 120 g) | 481 | 115 | Rice (75 g, raw) | 1129 | 270 |
| Jam (15 g) | 168 | 40 | Potatoes (boiled, 150 g) | 481 | 115 | Macaroni (75 g, raw) | 1170 | 280 |
| Orange juice (120 g) | 192 | 46 | Carbonated soft drink (323 ml) | 543 | 130 | Sponge cake (65 g) | 1212 | 290 |
| Apple (100 g) | 192 | 46 | Dates (60 g) | 585 | 140 | Fish (fried in batter, 120 g) | 1338 | 320 |
| Peas (90 g) | 209 | 50 | Baked beans (240 g) | 606 | 145 | Chips (fried, 180 g) | 1902 | 455 |
| Whisky (25 g) | 234 | 56 | Milk chocolate (30 g) | 648 | 155 | Pork chops (fried, including fat, 210 g with bone) | 2257 | 540 |

- Simple food tables can help in planning lifestyle, shopping, meals, and menus. But note that they give kilojoules (kilocalories) and fat per 100 g. Typical servings of some foods are less, of other foods more than this (see "energy values of foods" table).
- A dietitian, preferably nearby and linked with the practice, can help with detailed suggestions.

Crash diets do not work.

**A weight loss of 1 kg (2 lbs) per week is the most that can be expected but half this is useful (and all that some can manage).**

A valuable technique for managing obesity is modification of eating behaviour. Its introduction by RB Stuart in 1967 changed the expectation of treatment from poor to fair and refinements are improving prospects further.

Firstly the patient makes notes of everything he or she eats for a week and where they were at the time, what they were doing, and how they felt. The calories can be worked out later. The therapist guides and encourages the patient to fill in the form. In the process the patient discovers in what circumstances he or she eats most. The doctor or dietitian discusses the completed form with the patient and suggests behaviour modifications. Obese people do not eat so much because they are hungry, but more in response to external cues—boredom, anger, delicious taste, other people eating, food that would be wasted, etc. The patient can make arrangements to minimise these cues.

| Time | Food | Taste rating | Amount | kcal | Where? | Who with? | Mood | Hunger | Associated activity | Why eaten? |
|---|---|---|---|---|---|---|---|---|---|---|
| 4.45pm | Chocolate Cake | My weakness V.Good | 3 slices | 510 | Kitchen | Children | Fed up | No | Giving children their tea | Irritated |
| 5.00pm | Egg Sandwich | Nothing special | 1½ sandwiches | 200 | Kitchen | Alone | OK | No | Clearing | Leftovers |

Record of what is eaten, where and when

*Rules for modifying eating behaviour*

- Buy non-fattening foods. Do not buy foods that specially tempt you. Use a shopping list and stick to it. Do not shop when you are hungry.
- Always eat in one room, in only one place in that room—for example, seated at the dining table—and avoid other activities (except conversation). Make eating a pure experience.
- Look for times when you are most likely to eat unnecessarily—for example, when giving children their tea, or because you cannot bear to throw food away—and take steps to change your routine.
- Always have nearby a variety of low calorie foods to use as snacks—like raw vegetables.
- Recruit others to help you curb your eating—spouse, coworkers, friends—they can help most by praising when you do not over-eat.

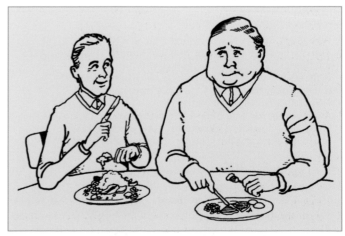

Fatty and thinny eating side by side

- Build in rewards for sticking to the programme—something you would like to do, or a present. Family and friends are usually happy to cooperate. Of course, the reward cannot be a meal or food.
- Make small portions of food appear to be large (small plate, food cut up and spread all over it). Make second helpings hard to get; do not keep serving dishes on the table. Leave the table as soon as you have eaten.
- Slow down the rate at which you eat. Chew each mouthful for longer. Always use a knife and fork or a spoon and put them down between mouthfuls. Swallow one mouthful before the next.
- Take steps to minimise hunger, loneliness, depression, boredom, anger, and fatigue, each of which can set off a bout of overeating. This needs discussion and planning. Hunger is minimised by three regular meals daily.
- Increase the exercise you take each day.
- Keep a record of how much you eat and exercise, and of your weight.

*Exercise*

During an hour's walk at ordinary speed, mostly on the level, 21 kJ/min × 60 = 1260 kJ (or 5 × 60 = 300 kcal) of energy are used up. But at rest about 4.2 × 60 = 252 kJ (1 × 60 = 60 kcal) would be spent per hour. The energy used by going for an hour's walk is therefore the difference between 1260 and 252 = 1008 kJ (300 and 60 = 240 kcal). This is equivalent to about two slices of bread and butter (60 g bread + 15 g butter, see "energy value of foods" table). People can be discouraged by the small amount of food which is directly equivalent to the use of quite a lot of precious time taking exercise.

There are, however, additional benefits from increased regular exercise.

(1) Obese people, with a heavier body to move, use more energy than in the table for the same amount of work.
(2) Exercise can be valuable as a diversion from sitting indoors and being tempted to eat.
(3) Exercise is more likely to reduce than increase appetite.
(4) After exercise, the resting metabolic rate may increase for some hours (though the effect is evidently small, and some experimenters have not been able to measure it).
(5) When exercise is taken after meals the thermic effect of the meal may be increased.

Exercise also limits the proportion of lean tissues lost in slimming programmes and helps in weight maintenance. Fat people cannot usually manage vigorous sports and may be embarrassed to dress in sports gear. Walking in all its varieties is the most important exercise.

---

**Exercise advice could include[20]:**

- Walking is the key to controlling your weight
- Travel whenever possible by foot and aim for 30 minutes' brisk walking per day
- Walk all or part of your journey to work or the shops
- If you usually travel by bus get off a stop earlier
- Use the stairs instead of a lift
- Avoid sitting for long periods; be active during TV adverts
- If you have a garden, spend more time working in it
- If you have a dog, take it for more frequent or longer walks

---

### Third: maintaining the lower body weight

After a weight-loss programme with the new eating plan, and increased exercise and behaviour modification for 12-20 weeks, the motivated and well-supported patient should have lost near to 10 kg. Now starts the longer phase of keeping the weight off. This is where temptations and disappointment lie in wait.

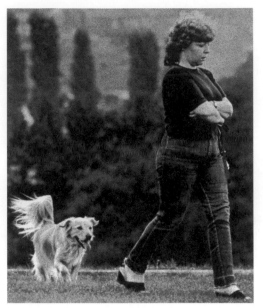

Walking the dog

---

**Energy/minute used in activities**
(rounded approximate figures)

| At rest | kJ | kcal |
| --- | --- | --- |
| (Men +10%, women −10%) | 4 | 1 |
| **Moderate exercise** | | |
| For example, walking, gardening, golf | 21 | 5 |
| **Intermediate** | | |
| For example, cycling, swimming, tennis | 29 | 7 |
| **Strenuous** | | |
| For example, squash, jogging, hill climbing, heavy work | 42 | 10 |

In SI units: 1 kcal/min = 4.2 kJ/min = 70 watts

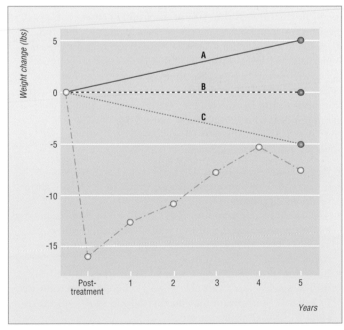

Mean weight loss of behavioral programmes post-treatment and at 1, 2, 3, 4, and 5 years follow up. Lines A, B, and C represent hypothetical groups of people against which to compare the results of behavioral programmes. Line A, natural history of obese persons receiving no treatment as gradually weight is gained; line B, stable weight; line C, gradual loss. (Adapted from Brownell and Kramer[25])

The graph on page 76 shows combined average results of several behavioural programmes.

Weight loss was satisfactory but gradually the subjects' weight slowly crept up so that after five years about half the weight lost had been put back on. The same slow regain of weight has been reported whatever treatment was used for the weight loss phase (very low calorie diet, appetite suppressant drugs, etc). The challenge, therefore, is for therapist and subject to be aware of this tendency to re-gain and work to minimise it.

If the weight-loss diet was drastic and incompatible with a normal lifestyle, food habits will rebound. Some restriction of diet has to continue in the maintenance phase. An *ad lib* low fat (high carbohydrate) diet has been shown to be more effective for weight maintenance than a fixed energy intake.[26] An active lifestyle with regular adequate exercise seems to be essential to keep body weight down.[27]

## Other treatments

*Drug therapy*

It is futile to prescribe drugs unless the patient is committed to eating less calories and/or exercising more. Only a limited range of drugs are available at present, though pharmaceutical companies are researching hard to find safe additional types.

**Orlistat** ("Xenical") is an inhibitor of pancreatic lipase. It reduces digestion of fat (triglycerides) and increases faecal fat. Oily spotting and faecal urgency can be controlled by eating a low fat (so lower energy) diet.

**Sibutramine** inhibits the reuptake of serotonin and noradrenaline in the central nervous system. It decreases appetite and may increase thermogenesis (metabolic rate). Blood pressure can rise.

The serotonergic appetite suppressants fenfluramine and dexfenfluramine have been withdrawn because of rare but severe cardiac valve disease and pulmonary hypertension. Of the catecholaminergic drugs, amphetamines cannot be used because of their potential for abuse. Only phentermine is in the *British National Formulary*. It should only be used to support someone with moderate to severe obesity who is restricted to a 12-week prescription.

Commercial organisations, for example, Weight Watchers or similar organisations, use group therapy and can help some people with mild to moderate obesity. The Scottish Obesity guidelines[20] have a set of useful criteria for evaluating the local organisation of this type. Other patients prefer a more individual approach.

More radical treatments sometimes used are **very low calorie diets** and **gastric stapling**. They are in the specialist's domain. Ideally patients with a BMI over $35 \, kg/m^2$ should be referred to a specialist centre,[20] but these are not well developed in all areas.

## References

1 McLellan F. Obesity rising to alarming levels round the world. *Lancet* 2002; **359**: 1412.
2 Caterson I. Obesity 1998 – has anything changed? *Modern Med* 1998; **41**: 52-66.
3 Bray G. Drug treatment of obesity: don't throw the baby out with the bath water. *Am J Clin Nutr* 1998; **67**: 1-4.
4 Prentice A, Jebb SA. Obesity in Britain: gluttony or sloth? *BMJ* 1995; **311**: 437-9.
5 Report of a WHO Consultation. *Obesity: Preventing and managing the Global Epidemic.* Geneva: WHO, 2000.
6 Wannamethee G, Shaper AG. Weight change in middle-aged British men: implications for health. *Eur J Clin Nutr* 1990; **44**: 133-42.
7 Trayhurn P, Beattie JH. Physiological role of adipose tissue: white adipose tissue as an endocrine and secretory organ. *Proc Nutr Soc* 2001; **60**: 329-39.
8 Flier JS. The missing link with obesity. *Nature* 2001; **409**: 292-3.
9 Lew EA, Garfinkel L. Variations in mortality by weight among 750 000 men and women. *J Chron Dis* 1979; **32**: 563-76.
10 Whincup PH, Gilg JA, Papacosta O *et al.* Early evidence of ethnic differences in cardiovascular risk: cross sectional comparison of British South Asian and white children. *BMJ* 2002; **324**: 635-8.
11 Cole TJ, Freeman JV, Preece MA. Body mass index reference curves for the UK, 1990. *Arch Dis Childhood* 1995; **73**: 25-9.
12 Stunkard A, Harris JR, Pedersen NL, McClearn GE. The body mass index of twins who have been reared apart. *N Engl J Med* 1990; **332**: 1483-7.
13 Prentice AM, Black AE, Coward WA. High levels of energy expenditure in obese women. *BMJ* 1986; **292**: 483-7.
14 Blundell JE, Goodson S, Halford JCG. Regulation of appetite: role of leptin in signalling systems for drive and satiety. *Int J Obesity* 2001; **25** (Suppl 1): S29-34.
15 Schwartz MW, Woods SC, Porte D, Seeley RJ, Baskin DG. Central nervous system control of food intake. *Nature* 2000; **404**: 661-71.
16 Pinkney J, Williams G. Ghrelin gets hungry. *Lancet* 2002; **359**: 1360-1.
17 Lowell BB, Spiegelman BM. Towards a molecular understanding of adaptive thermogenesis. *Nature* 2001; **404**: 652-9.
18 Garrow J. Luxuskonsumption, brown fat, and human obesity. *BMJ* 1983; **286**: 1684-6.
19 Report of a WHO Consultation. *Obesity: Preventing and Managing the Global Epidemic.* Geneva: WHO, 2000: p241.
20 Obesity in Scotland. *Integrating prevention with weight management. A National Clinical Guideline recommended for use in Scotland.* Edinburgh: Scottish Intercollegiate Guidelines Network (SIGN), 1996.
21 Després J-P, Lemieux I, Prud'homme D. Treatment of obesity: need to focus on high risk abdominally obese patients. *BMJ* 2001; **322**: 16-20.
22 Klem ML, Wing RR, McGuire MT, Seagle HM, Hill JO. A descriptive study of individuals successful at long-term maintenance of substantial weight loss. *Am J Clin Nutr* 1997; **66**: 236-46.
23 Blundell JE, MacDiarmid JI. Fat as a risk factor for overconsumption: satiation, satiety and patterns of eating. *J Am Dietetic Assoc* 1997; **97** (Suppl): S63-9.
24 Holt SHA, Brand Miller JC, Petocz P, Farmakalides E. A satiety index of common foods. *Eur J Clin Nutr* 1995; **49**: 675-90.
25 Brownell KD, Kramer FM. Behavioural management of obesity. In: Blackburn GL, Kander BS (eds). *Obesity: pathophysiology, psychology and treatment.* New York: Chapman & Hall, 1994.
26 Toubro S, Astrup A. Randomised comparison of diets for maintaining subjects' weight after major weight loss: ad lib, low fat, high carbohydrate diet v. fixed energy intake. *BMJ* 1997; **314**: 29-34.
27 Anderson JW, Konz EC, Frederick RC, Wood CL. Long-term weight-loss maintenance: a meta-analysis of US studies. *Am J Clin Nutr* 2001; **74**: 579-84.

# 12  Measuring nutrition

## Energy (calories)

Methods of measuring calories (food energy) are different from those for the other essential nutrients.

### Energy expenditure

Measurement of energy balance is technically difficult. *Energy expenditure* can be measured in one of five ways.

(1) By measuring a subject's heat output in a special insulated room. This is **direct calorimetry**, a costly and complicated experiment. There are very few direct calorimeter rooms anywhere in the world. The method has been replaced by (2).

(2) **Indirect calorimetry** measures oxygen consumption and the production of $CO_2$ and urinary nitrogen. From these the mixture of carbohydrate, fat (exogenous or endogenous), and protein metabolised can be calculated. Urinary N indicates protein catabolism and $CO_2/O_2$ (the respiratory quotient) indicates the ratio of carbohydrate to fat metabolised. Energy production per gramme differs with the metabolic fuel (greater when fat is oxidised). These measurements can be made for up to 24 hours in a *respiration chamber*, in which a subject can live and carry out various somewhat restricted activities.[1]

The energy produced per litre of oxygen consumed happens to be much the same whichever of the three macronutrients is oxidised. Oxygen consumption alone gives an adequate quantification of energy expenditure *over short periods*. It can be measured with different types of apparatus: Douglas bag, or a portable electronic respirometer carried on the back, a ventilated hood or a bedside metabolic monitor. The former are used to estimate the energy cost of different activities. The latter apparatus is used clinically to measure resting or **basal metabolic rate**, which can be increased in patients—for example, after burns or trauma or with infections.

(3) The **doubly labelled water** method measures the decay of body water concentrations of the stable isotopes $^2H$ and $^{18}O$. It is an ingenious method, developed for human work in the 1980s, suitable for measuring total energy expenditure over 7-10 days. It depends on the principle that labelled oxygen is lost partly as carbon dioxide and partly as water while the rate of water loss is given by the decay of labelled hydrogen.[2] The isotopes are given as a very accurately weighed dose of water. Disappearance is measured (by dedicated mass spectrometer) in repeat timed urine specimens. From $CO_2$ production (knowing the average respiratory quotient from the diet record and estimate of any changes in body fat) energy expenditure can be calculated as for indirect calorimetry. Unfortunately the heavy oxygen is very expensive.

(4) It ought to be possible to assess energy expenditure from an estimate of basal metabolic rate (from the patient's age, sex, and weight) and from recording all his activities (lying, sitting, walking upstairs, etc) throughout the day. Energy values for the different activities have to be assumed from reported values. The method is tedious and inaccurate.

(5) The possibilities for estimating energy expenditure are better by counting the heart rate for a day or more with a small portable cardiac monitor. (Practical details for this and the other methods are reviewed by Murgatroyd *et al*.[2])

> **1 kcal = 4.184 kJ**
> **kilojoules and megajoules are the SI units**

**The nutritional state** for energy, or for any essential nutrient, depends on the balance (B) between intake (I) (dietary or parenteral) and output (O) or expenditure: $B = I - O$.

When the balance is negative the nutritional state tends to go down towards depletion, but there may be an adaptive reduction in output (losses). When the balance is positive the nutritional state tends to go up: the nutrient may be stored somewhere in the body but some nutrients can start to become toxic. "You can have too much of a good thing."

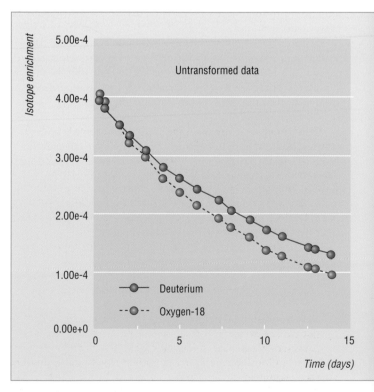

Doubly labelled water measurement of energy expenditure over 14 days. Isotope disappearances from a typical adult subject[2]

### Energy intake

For *energy intake* the energy (calorie) contents of foods eaten should ideally be analysed chemically by measuring the protein, available carbohydrate, fat, and alcohol contents and multiplying each of these by their metabolisable energy values. Energy values in food tables are only estimated averages.

The usual way of estimating *energy balance* is, of course, from the resultant **changes in body weight**. A gain or loss of energy by the body of about 25-29 MJ (6000-7000 kcal) should, respectively, increase or reduce the weight by 1 kg. Most of this weight change is in fat, with a variable amount of water and a minority of muscle. Gain or loss of tissue needs to be over 1 kg to be detectable, because, even with accurate weighing and on a constant regimen, healthy people's weights fluctuate within the day and from day to day. Furthermore, many scales and weighing techniques are not accurate.[4]

Reference standards for body weights at different heights based on body mass index (BMI) are given for adults in chapters 8 and 11 and for children in chapter 6.

It is difficult to weigh deformed or paralysed people. Very sick bedfast people cannot be weighed unless they are in a specially designed weighing bed. It is nearly always easy to weigh an ambulant patient—it just takes a little time and trouble. But in hospital patients confined to bed—for example, those with fluid lines or splints—some idea of loss of tissue can be obtained by measuring the arm circumference with or without one or more skinfold thicknesses.

**Measuring arm circumference** needs only a tape measure, put round the arm (preferably left) midway between the tip of the acromion and the olecranon. The enclosed area is made up of muscles and subcutaneous fat over the constant humerus.

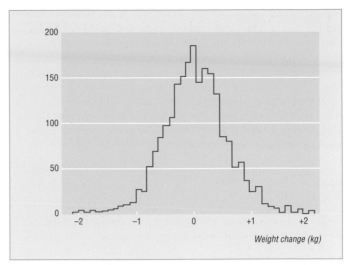

Distribution of day to day weight change (kg) on 2078 occasions on consecutive days in healthy young men[3]

### Weight measurement

Beam or lever balances are most reliable, not the usual bathroom scales. The best scales are not easily portable: they are heavy and the knife edge balancing part can be damaged. The patient should if possible be brought to the scale. It should be serviced regularly (as recommended by the manufacturer) and checked frequently against known weights, such as a heavy weight kept nearby. Subjects should be weighed in light underclothing and no shoes and with any heavy jewellery removed. A meal or full bladder increases the reading and a bowel action reduces it.

Adults and older children should stand straight on both feet on the centre of the scale's platform without touching anything else.

Pictures of how to weigh young children are shown in Valman B, Thomas R. *ABC of the First Year*, 5th edn. London: BMJ Books, 2001.

### Reference standards for mid-upperarm circumference (mm)[5,6]

| | Men | | | Women | | |
| | | Centiles | | | Centiles | |
| Age | 50th | 10th | 5th | 50th | 10th | 5th |
|---|---|---|---|---|---|---|
| 19-24 | 308 | 272 | 262 | 265 | 230 | 221 |
| 25-34 | 319 | 282 | 271 | 277 | 240 | 233 |
| 35-44 | 326 | 287 | 278 | 290 | 251 | 241 |
| 45-54 | 322 | 281 | 267 | 299 | 256 | 242 |
| 55-64 | 317 | 273 | 258 | 303 | 254 | 243 |
| 65-74 | 307 | 263 | 248 | 299 | 252 | 240 |

### Reference standards for triceps skinfold thickness (mm)[5,6]

| | Men | | | Women | | |
| | | Centiles | | | Centiles | |
| Age | 50th | 10th | 5th | 50th | 10th | 5th |
|---|---|---|---|---|---|---|
| 18-24 | 9.5 | 5 | 4 | 18 | 11.5 | 10 |
| 25-34 | 12 | 6 | 4.5 | 21 | 12 | 10 |
| 35-44 | 12 | 6 | 5 | 23 | 14 | 12 |
| 45-54 | 12 | 6 | 6 | 25 | 16 | 12 |
| 55-64 | 11 | 6 | 5 | 25 | 16 | 12 |
| 65-74 | 11 | 6 | 4 | 24 | 14 | 12 |

*Figures based on a large sample of healthy US citizens from Frisancho[5] and Bishop *et al.*[6]

**Measuring skinfold thickness** requires special calipers. The best are obtainable from Holtain Ltd, Crymych, Dyfed SA41 3UF. Cheap plastic ones are unreliable. The most common sites for measuring skinfold thickness are over the *mid-triceps*, halfway between the acromion and the olecranon, and the *subscapular* skinfold, 1 cm below the inferior angle of the scapula. Reference standards are available for skinfolds at these sites (see table opposite).

The triceps skinfold measurement can be used to calculate the mid-upperarm muscle circumference, AMC.

$$\text{AMC} = \text{arm circumference} - \pi \times \text{triceps skinfold (mm)}$$

Before substantial weight changes are detectable, or if weight cannot be measured, a rough idea of energy balance can be obtained by calculating the energy per day in recent food intake from food tables and comparing this with the estimated average requirements for energy published by the DoH.[7]

These reference values for energy intake are estimates and averages. They differ with gender, age, body weight, and

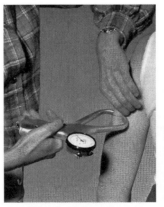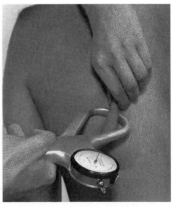

Measuring skinfold thickness with Holtain calipers: left—triceps site; right—subscapular site

especially with activity level.[7] About half of any group of similar people can be expected to need more, and half to need less, than these values. Individual requirements might well range from 50% to 150% of these averages. Furthermore, on any single day an individual might consume considerably less or more than their average daily intake.

There are no biochemical tests that reliably indicate energy balance. Acetone appears on the breath in people who fast for longer than 12 hours and $\beta$ hydroxybutyrate concentrations increase in body fluids but these cannot be used to show the extent of energy deficit.

# Protein

Tests for protein status estimate two variables: total body protein and visceral protein.

## Total body protein

This is predominantly muscle and can be estimated in several ways. At the clinical level:

- Body weight for height —that is, BMI, partly reflects body protein. Though the usual cause of a high BMI is excess fat, a less common cause is unusually well developed muscles in body builders and weight lifters.
- Total protein may also be estimated approximately from the mid-upperarm muscle circumference (mid-upperarm circumference $- \pi \times$ triceps skinfold).
- Twenty-four-hour urinary creatinine gives a biochemical measure of muscle mass because creatinine is a metabolite from the turnover of muscle creatine. One gram of creatinine/day comes from about 20 kg of muscle but urinary creatinine shows quite large day to day fluctuations even if collection is complete, and it is spuriously increased by eating meat and by exercise.

Three research procedures are potentially available to give the most reliable estimates of lean body mass.

- Total body nitrogen may be measured by *in vivo* neutron activation with simultaneous counting of the 10.8 MeV gamma rays produced from the protein nitrogen[9]; then $N \times 6.25$ = total body protein.
- Potassium is predominantly intracellular and normally proportional to body protein. Total body potassium can be measured non-invasively by placing a subject in a heavily screened whole-body counter and counting the natural weak gamma-ray emissions from the subject's own $^{40}K$ which is mixed as 0.012% with the stable $^{39}K$ throughout our bodies.
- Body density can be measured by underwater weighing in a special bath (a harmless procedure but only available in research centres). As the density of body fat is 0.9 and of lean body mass 1.1, the proportions of fat and lean can be calculated.

Other methods are available which are more accessible investigations but tend to be less precise.

- Use of bioelectrical impedance depends on the greater electrical conductivity of lean body mass than fat. A weak current is passed from ankle to hand. The equipment is portable and relatively inexpensive.
- Imaging methods such as dual x-ray absorptiometry can also provide estimates of body fat and lean.
- From total body water, by dilution of deuterium, lean body mass can be estimated because body water is in the lean not the fat.
- Total body fat can be estimated approximately by applying a formula to the sum of four skinfolds.[10]

## Estimated average requirements of food energy for people in the United Kingdom[7]

| Age | Males MJ/d (kcal/d) | Females MJ/d (kcal/d) |
|---|---|---|
| 0-3 months | 2.28 (545) | 2.16 (515) |
| 4-6 months | 2.89 (690) | 2.69 (645) |
| 7-9 months | 3.44 (825) | 3.20 (765) |
| 10-12 months | 3.85 (920) | 3.61 (865) |
| 1-3 years | 5.15 (1230) | 4.86 (1165) |
| 4-6 years | 7.16 (1715) | 6.46 (1545) |
| 7-10 years | 8.24 (1970) | 7.28 (1740) |
| 11-14 years | 9.27 (2220) | 7.92 (1845) |
| 15-18 years | 11.51 (2755) | 8.83 (2110) |
| **19-59 years** | **10.60 (2550)** | **8.05 (1920)** |
| 60-74 years | 9.82 (2355) | 7.98 (1900) |
| 75+ years | 8.77 (2100) | 7.61 (1810) |

Values from 0 to 18 years are based on average energy intakes. From 19 years on, however, they are based on measured energy expenditure, assuming low physical activity levels at work and leisure (physical activity level = 1.4 × BMR (basal metabolic rate)). More active people need to consume more than the figures here. In the light of recent measurements, the figures for children under 5 years may be too high by about 10%[8]

## Reference nutrient intake for protein*, based on British dietary reference values[7]

| Age and sex | Body weight (kg) | Protein (g/kg body weight) | Reference nutrient intake (RNI) (g/day) |
|---|---|---|---|
| 0-3 months | 5.9 | — | 13 |
| 4-6 months | 7.7 | 1.7 | 13 |
| 7-9 months | 8.8 | 1.6 | 14 |
| 10-12 months | 9.7 | 1.55 | 15 |
| 1-3 years | 12.5 | 1.2 | 15 |
| 4-6 years | 17.8 | 1.1 | 20 |
| 7-10 years | 28.3 | 1.0 | 28 |
| **Males** | | | |
| 11-14 years | 43.0 | 1.0 | 42 |
| 15-18 years | 64.5 | 0.85 | 55 |
| 19-50 years | 74.0 | 0.76 | 56 |
| 50+ years | 71.0 | 0.75 | 53 |
| **Females** | | | |
| 11-14 years | 43.8 | 0.94 | 41 |
| 15-18 years | 55.5 | 0.81 | 45 |
| 19-50 years | 60.0 | 0.75 | 45 |
| 50+ years | 62.0 | 0.76 | 47 |
| Pregnancy | | | +6 |
| Lactation | | | +11 |

British dietary reference values are based on FAO/WHO (1984) safe levels of protein intake.
*These recommended intakes assume that the protein comes from a mixed diet, as in the average British diet. Requirements may be higher if digestibility of the protein is incomplete or if one (or more) of the indispensable amino acids is poorly represented

### Visceral protein

*Visceral protein* is sometimes disproportionately reduced in protein deficiency, as seen most strikingly in kwashiorkor. There is fatty liver, intestinal mucosal and pancreatic atrophy, and impaired lymphocyte function. The usual tests measure concentrations of plasma albumin or transferrin, proteins synthesised in the liver. These are disproportionately reduced when there is visceral protein depletion and often within normal limits in total body protein depletion. Plasma albumin concentrations are also moderately reduced in the metabolic response to severe injury or infection as well as in liver cirrhosis and nephrotic syndrome. Transferrin concentrations are increased in iron deficiency.

## Other nutrients

Other nutrients do not affect anthropometric measurements directly. Inadequate intake can be suspected from the dietary intake or shown by specific biochemical tests.

### Assessment of dietary intake

The sequence of assessing nutrient intake is to:

- estimate **food intake** as g/day of different foods
- use **food tables** to convert g/day of each individual food to g, mg, or μg/day of various nutrients. These calculations can, and always used to be done manually but computers are generally used
- compare this patient's intake of one or several nutrients likely to be inadequate with the dietary reference values[7] of food energy and nutrients. Note: the reference nutrient intake[7] covers the individual nutrient requirements of the great majority of normal people, which means that an intake somewhat below the recommended daily amount would be adequate for most people (see page 85). The other consideration is whether the day(s) on which food intake was measured were typical.

### Food intake measurements

Food intake data may be obtained at the national, household or individual level. **National figures** come from food production plus imports minus exports, divided by the estimated national population. They report **apparent consumption** because some of the food is wasted, fed to tourists or pets, used in industry, etc. All developed countries publish annual figures for average consumption. **Household food consumption** has been measured in large samples across England, Wales and Scotland every year since 1940 and the National Food Survey provides a unique continuous series of national consumption of different foods.[11] The survey cannot show average individual intakes because until recently food and drink consumed outside the home was not estimated, and distribution of foods and nutrients within families varies between its members.

Although these macrofigures provide a background of trends in food consumption for clinical work and analytical epidemiology, we want to know what an **individual** has been eating and drinking. There are four types of method used to estimate individual food intake.

- **Dietary history**—"What do you eat on a typical day?" This is a good method in the hands of a skilled and patient interviewer. Food models, cups, plates, and spoons are used to estimate portion sizes.
- **24-hour recall**—"Tell me everything you've had to eat and drink in the last 24 hours." This is less subject to wishful thinking about what the person ought to have eaten. The weakness is that yesterday may have been atypical; 24-hour recalls can, however, be repeated.

---

**Checklist on patient's diet**

In a busy practice a short checklist about the patient's eating habits is a useful screening method.

- What is your appetite like?
- Do you eat more or less than other comparable people?
- Has what you eat changed—type of food or amount?
- Are you on a special diet?
- Is there any food you can't eat because it doesn't agree with you?
- Are you losing or gaining body weight?
- What do you usually have for the main meal of the day?
- Do you eat meat/fruit/fat on meat/salt/etc?
- What sort of bread do you eat?
- What sort of alcohol do you drink, how many drinks per week or per day?
- What do you have for breakfast and lunch?
- Do you take vitamin or mineral tablets?

---

**Individual food intake**

There are four types of method used to estimate individual food intake, and these are:

- Dietary history
- 24-hour recall
- Food dietary or record
- Food frequency questionnaire

---

3. (CONTINUED) PLEASE FILL IN YOUR **AVERAGE** USE, **DURING THE PAST YEAR**, OF EACH SPECIFIED FOOD

| FOODS AND AMOUNTS | NEVER, OR LESS THAN ONCE A MONTH | 1–3 PER MO. | 1 PER WEEK | 2–4 PER WEEK | 5–6 PER WEEK | 1 PER DAY | 2–3 PER DAY | 4–5 PER DAY | 6+ PER DAY |
|---|---|---|---|---|---|---|---|---|---|
| YOGHURT (1 CUP) | ○ | ○ | W | ○ | ○ | D | ○ | ○ | ○ |
| COTTAGE OR RICOTTA CHEESE (1/2 CUP) | ○ | ○ | W | ○ | ○ | D | ○ | ○ | ○ |
| CREAM CHEESE (1oz) | ○ | ○ | W | ○ | ○ | D | ○ | ○ | ○ |
| OTHER CHEESE, eg AMERICAN, CHEDDAR, etc, PLAIN OR AS A PART OF A DISH (1 SLICE OR 1 oz SERVING) | ○ | ○ | W | ○ | ○ | D | ○ | ○ | ○ |
| MARGARINE (PAT), ADDED TO FOOD OR BREAD; EXCLUDE USE IN COOKING | ○ | ○ | W | ○ | ○ | D | ○ | ○ | ○ |
| BUTTER (PAT), ADDED TO FOOD OR BREAD; EXCLUDE USE IN COOKING | ○ | ○ | W | ○ | ○ | D | ○ | ○ | ○ |

**FRUITS**

PLEASE TRY TO AVERAGE YOUR SEASONAL USE OF FOODS OVER THE ENTIRE YEAR. FOR EXAMPLE, IF A FOOD SUCH AS CANTALOUPE IS EATEN 4 TIMES A WEEK DURING THE APPROXIMATE 3 MONTHS THAT IT IS IN SEASON, THEN THE **AVERAGE** USE WOULD BE ONCE PER WEEK.

| | NEVER | 1–3/M | 1/W | 2–4/W | 5–6/W | 1/D | 2–3/D | 4–5/D | 6+/D |
|---|---|---|---|---|---|---|---|---|---|
| RAISINS (1oz OR SMALL PACK) OR GRAPES | ○ | ○ | W | ○ | ○ | D | ○ | ○ | ○ |
| PRUNES (1/2 CUP) | ○ | ○ | W | ○ | ○ | D | ○ | ○ | ○ |
| BANANAS (1) | ○ | ○ | W | ○ | ○ | D | ○ | ○ | ○ |
| PEACHES, APRICOTS OR PLUMS (1 FRESH, OR 1/2 CUP CANNED) | ○ | ○ | W | ○ | ○ | D | ○ | ○ | ○ |
| FRESH APPLES OR PEARS (1) | ○ | ○ | W | ○ | ○ | D | ○ | ○ | ○ |
| APPLE JUICE OR CIDER (SMALL GLASS) | ○ | ○ | W | ○ | ○ | D | ○ | ○ | ○ |
| ORANGES (1) | ○ | ○ | W | ○ | ○ | D | ○ | ○ | ○ |
| ORANGE JUICE (SMALL GLASS) | ○ | ○ | W | ○ | ○ | D | ○ | ○ | ○ |
| GRAPEFRUIT (1/2) | ○ | ○ | W | ○ | ○ | D | ○ | ○ | ○ |
| GRAPEFRUIT JUICE (SMALL GLASS) | ○ | ○ | W | ○ | ○ | D | ○ | ○ | ○ |
| OTHER FRUIT JUICES (SMALL GLASS) | ○ | ○ | W | ○ | ○ | D | ○ | ○ | ○ |
| STRAWBERRIES, FRESH, FROZEN OR CANNED (1/2 CUP) | ○ | ○ | W | ○ | ○ | D | ○ | ○ | ○ |
| BLUEBERRIES, FRESH, FROZEN OR CANNED (1/2 CUP) | ○ | ○ | W | ○ | ○ | D | ○ | ○ | ○ |
| CANTALOUPE (1/4 MELON) | ○ | ○ | W | ○ | ○ | D | ○ | ○ | ○ |
| WATERMELON (1 SLICE) | ○ | ○ | W | ○ | ○ | D | ○ | ○ | ○ |

**VEGETABLES**

| | | | | | | | | | |
|---|---|---|---|---|---|---|---|---|---|
| BROCCOLI (1/2 CUP) | ○ | ○ | W | ○ | ○ | D | ○ | ○ | ○ |
| CABBAGE OR COLESLAW (1/2 CUP) | ○ | ○ | W | ○ | ○ | D | ○ | ○ | ○ |
| CAULIFLOWER (1/2 CUP) | ○ | ○ | W | ○ | ○ | D | ○ | ○ | ○ |
| BRUSSELS SPROUTS (1/2 CUP) | ○ | ○ | W | ○ | ○ | D | ○ | ○ | ○ |
| CARROTS (1 WHOLE OR 1/2 CUP COOKED) | ○ | ○ | W | ○ | ○ | D | ○ | ○ | ○ |

Example of a page from a food frequency questionnaire

- **Food diary or record**—"Please write down (and describe) **everything** you eat and drink (and estimate the amount) for the next 3 (4 or 7) days." Amounts are usually recorded in household measures but for more accuracy subjects can be provided with quick reading scales to weigh food before it goes on the plate (and any leftovers).
- **Food frequency questionnaire**—"Do you eat meat/fish/bread/milk … on average: more than once a day/2 or 3 times a week/once a week/once a month etc?" (see example above).

The self-administered food frequency questionnaire is the newest of the four methods. It is much more economical of investigator's time and suitable for computer analysis. This method has made possible cohort studies with thousands of subjects' food intakes related to disease outcome.[12] It asks for usual, typical intake.

Estimating food intake quantitatively is labour intensive (and so expensive). It depends on adequate memory and the honesty and interest of the subject. Some people's food habits are very irregular and most people eat differently on Saturday and Sunday from during weekdays and on holiday.

There is no "gold standard" method for food intake. Methods that ask subjects to record or remember the food/drinks they really consumed are better for national nutrition surveys of samples of the population. Items may be forgotten (or not listed because of embarrassment) but the exact types of food, product or dish are actually captured, including unusual ones. For large epidemiological surveys food frequency questionnaires have enabled tens of thousands to be included. What these lose in precision they gain in numbers of subjects. Usually quintiles (fifths) of intake of food components

---

**Two pages from The *Composition of Foods*.**[14] **Each set of foods has four pages of nutrients. Pages 3 and 4 (not shown here) report vitamins and minerals**

**Cereals and cereal products** *continued*

|  |  |  | | Composition of food per 100 g | | | | | |
|---|---|---|---|---|---|---|---|---|---|
| No. | Food | Description and main data sources | Edible proportion | Water g | Protein g | Fat g | Carbo-hydrate g | Energy value kcal | kJ |
| *Rice* | | | | | | | | | |
| 18 | Brown rice, *raw* | 5 assorted samples | 1.00 | 13.9 | 6.7 | 2.8 | 81.3 | 357 | 1518 |
| 19 | *boiled* | Water content weighed, other nutrients calculated from raw | 1.00 | 66.0 | 2.6 | 1.1 | 32.1 | 141 | 597 |
| 20 | Savoury rice, *raw* | 10 samples, 5 varieties, meat and vegetable | 1.00 | 7.0 | 8.4 | 10.3 | 77.4 | 415 | 1755 |
| 21 | *cooked* | Calculation from raw, boiled in water | 1.00 | 68.7 | 2.9 | 3.5[a] | 26.3 | 142 | 599 |
| 22 | White rice, easy cook, | 10 samples, 9 different brands, parboiled | 1.00 | 11.4 | 7.3 | 3.6 | 85.8 | 383 | 1630 |
| 23 | *raw* easy cook, *boiled* | Calculation from raw | 1.00 | 68.0 | 2.6 | 1.3 | 30.9 | 138 | 587 |
| 24 | fried in lard/dripping | Recipe | 1.00 | 70.3 | 2.2 | 3.2 | 25.0 | 131 | 554 |
| *Pasta* | | | | | | | | | |
| 25 | Macaroni, *raw* | 10 samples, 7 brands; literature sources | 1.00 | 9.7 | 12.0 | 1.8 | 75.8 | 348 | 1483 |
| 26 | *boiled* | 10 samples, 7 brands boiled in water | 1.00 | 78.1 | 3.0 | 0.5 | 18.5 | 86 | 365 |
| 27 | Noodles, egg, *raw* | 10 samples, 8 brands | 1.00 | 9.1 | 12.1 | 8.2 | 71.7 | 391 | 1656 |
| 28 | egg, *boiled* | 10 samples, 8 brands boiled in water | 1.00 | 84.3 | 2.2 | 0.5 | 13.0 | 62 | 264 |
| 29 | Spaghetti, white, *raw* | 10 samples, 7 brands | 1.00 | 9.8 | 12.0 | 1.8 | 74.1 | 342 | 1456 |
| 30 | white, *boiled* | 10 samples, 7 brands boiled in water | 1.00 | 73.8 | 3.6 | 0.7 | 22.2 | 104 | 442 |
| 31 | wholemeal, *raw* | 10 samples, 5 brands | 1.00 | 10.5 | 13.4 | 2.5 | 66.2 | 324 | 1379 |
| 32 | wholemeal, *boiled* | Water content weighed, other nutrients calculated from raw | 1.00 | 69.1 | 4.7 | 0.9 | 23.2 | 113 | 485 |

|  |  |  | Fatty acids | | | |  |  | Dietary fibre | |
|---|---|---|---|---|---|---|---|---|---|---|
|  |  | Total nitrogen g | Satd g | Mono unsatd g | Poly Unsatd g | Cholesterol mg | Starch g | Total sugars g | Southgate method g | Englyst method g |
| *Rice* | | | | | | | | | | |
| 18 | Brown rice, *raw* | 1.10 | 0.7 | 0.7 | 1.0 | 0 | 80.0 | 1.3 | 3.8 | 1.9 |
| 19 | *boiled* | 0.43 | 0.3 | 0.3 | 0.4 | 0 | 31.6 | 0.5 | 1.5 | 0.8 |
| 20 | Savoury rice, *raw* | 1.41 | 3.2 | 3.7 | 1.8 | 1 | 73.8 | 3.6 | 4.0 | N |
| 21 | *cooked* | 0.48 | 1.1 | 1.3 | 0.6 | Tr | 25.1 | 1.2 | 1.3 | 1.4 |
| 22 | White rice, easy cook, | 1.23 | 0.9 | 0.9 | 1.3 | 0 | 85.8 | Tr | 2.7 | 0.4 |
| 23 | *raw* easy cook, *boiled* | 0.44 | 0.3 | 0.3 | 0.5 | 0 | 30.9 | Tr | 1.0 | 0.1 |
| 24 | fried in lard/dripping | 0.37 | 1.4 | 1.2 | 0.5 | 3 | 23.1 | 1.9 | 1.2 | 0.6 |
| *Pasta* | | | | | | | | | | |
| 25 | Macaroni, *raw* | 2.11 | 0.3 | 0.1 | 0.8 | 0 | 73.6 | 2.2 | 5.0 | 3.1[b] |
| 26 | *boiled* | 0.52 | 0.1 | Tr | 0.2 | 0 | 18.2 | 0.3 | 1.5 | 0.9[b] |
| 27 | Noodles, egg, *raw* | 2.12 | 2.3 | 3.5 | 0.9 | 30 | 69.8 | 1.9 | 5.0 | (2.9) |
| 28 | egg, *boiled* | 0.40 | 0.1 | 0.2 | 0.1 | 6 | 12.8 | 0.2 | 1.0 | (0.6) |
| 29 | Spaghetti, white, *raw* | 2.11 | 0.2 | 0.2 | 0.8 | 0 | 70.8 | 3.3 | 5.1 | 2.9 |
| 30 | white, *boiled* | 0.63 | 0.1 | 0.1 | 0.3 | 0 | 21.7 | 0.5 | 1.8 | 1.2 |
| 31 | wholemeal, *raw* | 2.30 | 0.4 | 0.3 | 1.1 | 0 | 62.5 | 3.7 | 11.5 | 8.4 |
| 32 | wholemeal, *boiled* | 0.81 | 0.1 | 0.1 | 0.4 | 0 | 21.9 | 1.3 | 4.0 | 3.5 |

[a] Calculated assuming water only was added; savoury rice cooked with fat contains approximately 8.8 g fat per 100 g
[b] Wholemeal macaroni contains 8.3 g (raw) and 2.8 g (boiled) Englyst fibre per 100 g. Reproduced by permission of the Royal Society of Chemistry

are related to disease outcomes. Relative consumption across the population is the aim here, rather than precise and specific quantitative results (examples are in chapter 1).

## Biomarkers of dietary intake

All estimates of food intake are subjective. Some subjects forget, some did not notice what food they ate, some do not report because they would be ashamed to admit having that food, drink, or amount. The search is on for biomarkers, which are objective biochemical indices of dietary intake. For some food components there are useful biomarkers; for others there is nothing available. Protein intake is reflected by 24-hour urinary nitrogen. Intake of non-endogenous fatty acids (18:2, 18:3, 20:4 and *trans* unsaturated) are reflected well in serum or adipose tissue fatty acid pattern but there is no biomarker for total fat or carbohydrate intake. Intake of individual carotenoids can be seen in the plasma. Plasma lycopene, for example, reflects tomato intake. Of the inorganic nutrients 24-hour urinary sodium is a much better indicator of salt intake than dietary history because the salt content of foods and dishes varies greatly and without the subject's knowledge. Vitamin A and calcium are nutrients whose plasma concentrations cannot serve here; they are held constant across the range of usual intakes. Toenail selenium has been used to reflect selenium intake.

## Food tables and nutrient databases

The British food tables are among the best in the world thanks to the original work of McCance and Widdowson,[13] their continuation by Paul and Southgate and colleagues, and the support of the Medical Research Council; Ministry of Agriculture, Fisheries, and Food; the Agriculture and Food Research Council; and the Royal Society of Chemistry. The 5th edition of *McCance & Widdowson's the composition of foods* was published in 1991,[14] and there is a growing list of supplements.

In the main volume 1188 foods and drinks arranged in 14 groups are given code numbers (which can be used for computer input—software packages are also available). The total publications, including supplements, cover around 2000 foods. Figures are given (per 100 g edible portion) for over 40 constituents.

The two example pages from the *Composition of foods* show the proximate constituents or macronutrients printed in the main tables.[14] Where relevant, alcohol content is also included. The other two pages for each food show inorganic nutrients—Na, K, Ca, Mg, P, Fe, Cu, Zn, Cl, Mn, Se, I—and all the vitamins—retinol, carotene, vitamins D and E, thiamin, riboflavin, niacin, tryptophan/60, vitamins B-6 and B-12, folate, pantothenate, biotin, vitamin C.

Individual amino acids and fatty acids are in the (1978) 4th edition of *McCance & Widdowson*[14] and a 1980 supplement. For any large scale work the nutrient data bank behind *McCance & Widdowson* is used in computer software, from the Royal Society of Chemistry, Letchworth, Herts., SG6 1HN or MAFF or a specialist software company. This software should contain the latest updates, revisions and additions to the database.

### Variability of nutrient content

The British tables give a single value for each nutrient in each food—an estimated average. The American tables,[16] which are published in loose leaf sections as analyses are completed, give an indication of variability to be expected round each average figure. There is no legal guarantee that any food contains what the food tables say it should. For some constituents—for example, fat—the food could easily contain 25% less or 25% more.

## Food composition tables[15]

Food composition analysis is work that is never finished. It is a bottomless pit. No country has food composition tables which have kept up with all the concepts of modern nutritional science, the proliferation of foods and dishes eaten in a country and the ever-growing list of substances in foods that may or could have biological functions.

The numbers in existing food tables are derived in three ways:

- By direct analysis in the country where the food tables are produced. These may be based on multiple samples and a modern, specific analytical method or they may be antique figures based on a single sample.
- From literature. Figures may be a subjective decision (even if experienced) of the best representative one from an array of original results, or they may be "borrowed" from another country's food tables.
- Imputed figures, estimates from similar foods or from the known composition of most of the ingredients of mixed dishes.

As a rule food tables do not say where each number comes from.

Food components/nutrients are not the same if analysed by different methods. Carbohydrate can be obtained by subtracting per cent water, fat, protein and ash from 100—"by difference" or by direct chemical analysis adding up the different classes of carbohydrate. There is still no agreement on which of some four different methods should be the standard one for dietary fibre. Cholesterol may be obtained by an older colorimetric method or by more specific gas-liquid chromatography.

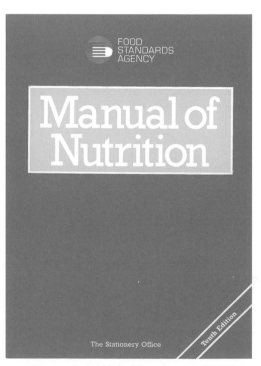

The *Manual of Nutrition* has a useful simplified food table, which gives calories and 11 nutrients for 150 common foods[17]

## Dietary reference values and requirements

For nutrient intakes to have any meaning they have to be compared against some number representing physiological requirements for each nutrient. The major number for this is the estimated upper end of the range of individual requirements. In Britain, the name for this was changed in 1991 to *reference nutrient intake* (RNI)[7] from recommended daily amount (RDA). The latter had the same abbreviation as the American term, recommended dietary allowance.

The North American dietary reference intakes are being revised in sections.[18] These new reference values have similar terminology to the British and also have numbers for a **tolerable upper intake level** (above which adverse effects might occur).

Ten of the new North American dietary reference intakes (DRIs) are similar to the 1991 UK set but five are different. A DRI has been added for selenium on which there has been interesting research since 1991 (see chapter 10) and daily requirements for vitamin D are provided. The folate requirement has been increased because prevention of neural tube defects and hyperhomocystinaemia have emerged in the 1990s. The North American committee set higher recommendations for vitamin C by using an optimal blood level of ascorbate rather than prevention of scurvy and maintenance of measurable ascorbate in plasma. The calcium recommendation is also higher, based more on balance data than the British recommendations, based more on epidemiology.

The RNI/RDA values differ for the two sexes and several age groups and are published in tables. They are for intakes averaged over several days. Since the RNI/RDA is estimated to meet the requirements of practically all healthy people, most people's requirements are less than this upper or prescriptive reference value. For assessment of people's intakes a lower, diagnostic, reference should be used, such as the **estimated average requirement** for groups of people and the **lower reference nutrient intake** for individuals.[7] An intake below this does not necessarily mean inadequacy but the lower it is the greater that probability. As elsewhere in medicine, for complete nutritional diagnosis, findings on examination (clinical, anthropometric, and biochemical) must be considered together with the food intake history.

Sick people have requirements not covered by the reference values. For example with bed rest, energy requirements are reduced; with fever they are increased. Losses of several nutrients are increased in different ways by illness, such as protein loss in nephrotic syndrome, potassium loss in diarrhoea, iron loss with bleeding. The allowances apply to oral feeding of conventional foods. For total parenteral nutrition the requirements are different; absorption is 100%, but minor vitamins like pantothenate and biotin and trace elements like molybdenum, manganese, chromium, etc, which can usually be ignored because there is enough in the diet, cannot be taken for granted and have to be provided in the infusion solution(s).

## Biochemical methods for nutritional status

Biochemical tests are an integral part of modern medical diagnosis. Plasma sodium and potassium concentrations, for example, are essential for diagnosing and treating difficult electrolyte disorders, and plasma or red cell folate and plasma vitamin B-12 should be measured before treating a patient with megaloblastic anaemia.

With most of the other nutrients also, biochemical tests have been developed which can be used (a) to confirm the diagnosis of a deficiency disease in places where it is uncommonly seen or where the clinical picture is complicated,

### British dietary reference values[7]: estimated average requirement for food energy (calories) and reference nutrient intakes (RNIs) for the other nutrients

| Nutrient | Men 19-50 years | Infants 4-6 months |
|---|---|---|
| Energy, kcal (MJ) | 2550 (10.6) | 670 (2.8) |
| Protein (g) | 56 | 13 |
| Vitamin A (RE, μg) | 700 | 350 |
| Thiamin (mg) | 1.0 | 0.2 |
| Riboflavin (mg) | 1.3 | 0.4 |
| Niacin (NE, mg) | 17 | 3 |
| Vitamin B−6 (mg) | 1.4 | 0.2 |
| Folate (total, μg) | 200 | 50 |
| Vitamin B−12 (μg) | 1.5 | 0.3 |
| Vitamin C (mg) | 40 | 25 |
| Vitamin D (μg) | — | 8.5 |
| Vitamin E (mg) | 7 | 0.4/g PUF |
| Calcium (mg) | 700 | 525 |
| Iron (mg) | 8.7 | 4.3 |
| Magnesium (mg) | 300 | 60 |
| Iodine (μg) | 140 | 60 |
| Potassium (mmol) | 90 | 22 |
| Sodium (mmol) | 70 | 12 |
| Zinc (mg) | 9.5 | 4 |

Some figures are slightly rounded. Figures for women are generally about 75% of those for men, except iron (higher until the menopause) and in pregnancy and lactation. Figures for children are interpolated between infants and adults.
RE = retinol equivalents; NE = niacin equivalents; PUF = polyunsaturated fat

### Biochemical methods for diagnosing nutritional deficiencies

| Nutrient | Indicating reduced intake | Indicating impaired function (IF) or cell depletion (CD) | Supplementary method |
|---|---|---|---|
| Protein | Urinary nitrogen | Plasma albumin (IF) | Fasting plasma amino acid pattern |
| Vitamin A | Plasma β-carotene | Plasma retinol | Relative dose response |
| Thiamin | Urinary thiamin | Red cell transketolase and TPP effect (IF) | |
| Riboflavin | Urinary riboflavin | Red cell glutathione reductase and FAD effect (IF) | |
| Niacin | Urinary N' methyl nicotinamide or 2-pyridone, or both | Red cell NAD/NADP ratio | Fasting plasma tryptophan |
| Vitamin B-6 | Urinary 4-pyridoxic acid | Plasma pyridoxal 5' phosphate | Urinary xanthurenic acid after tryptophan load |
| Folate | Plasma folate | Red cell folate (CD) | Urinary FIGLU after histidine load |
| Vitamin B-12 | Plasma holo-transcobalamin II | Plasma vitamin B-12 | Schilling test |
| Vitamin C | Plasma ascorbate | Leucocyte ascorbate (CD) | Urinary ascorbate |
| Vitamin D | Plasma 25-hydroxy-vitamin D | Raised plasma alkaline phosphatase (bone isoenzyme) (IF) | Plasma 1,25 dihydroxy-vitamin D |
| Vitamin E | Ratio of plasma tocopherol to cholesterol + triglyceride | Red cell haemolysis with $H_2O_2$ *in vitro* (IF) | |
| Vitamin K | Plasma phylloquinone | Plasma prothrombin (IF) | Plasma des-γ-carboxy-prothrombin |
| Sodium | Urinary sodium | Plasma sodium | |
| Potassium | Urinary potassium | Plasma potassium | Total body potassium by counting [40]K |
| Iron | Plasma iron and transferrin | Plasma ferritin (CD) | Free erythrocyte protoporphyrin |
| Magnesium | Plasma magnesium | Red cell magnesium (CD) | |
| Iodine | Urinary (stable) iodine | Plasma thyroxine (IF) | Plasma TSH |
| Zinc | Plasma zinc | Red cell zinc | |

TPP = thiamine pyrophosphate; FAD = flavin adenine dinucleotide;
NAD = nicotinamide-adenine-dinucleotide; NADP = NAD phosphate;
FIGLU = formiminoglutamic acid; [40]K = natural radioactive potassium;
TSH = thyroid stimulating hormone
There are no reliable simple methods for assessing *calcium* status (total body calcium can be measured by *in vivo* neutron activation analysis)

or (b) in community surveys and general practice to find individuals with subclinical nutrient deficiencies.

Tests which can be used for the major nutrients are listed in the table on page 85. As with other tests in chemical pathology, there may be false positive and false negative results. For example plasma vitamin B-12 concentrations are increased in acute hepatitis, and alkaline phosphatase may not be raised if rickets is accompanied by protein-energy deficiency.

When the intake of a nutrient is inadequate (less than obligatory losses) an individual generally goes through **three stages**. The first is adaptation to the low intake: urinary excretion of the nutrient or its metabolites typically falls but there is no evidence of abnormal function or of depletion of the cells.

In the second stage there are also biochemical changes indicating either impaired function or cellular depletion, but clinical manifestations of deficiency are absent or non-specific. A good example of a test showing impaired function is red cell transketolase activity. For each blood sample this enzyme is assayed in two test tubes, one with extra thiamin pyrophosphate (TPP), the other without. If the activity is more than 25% higher in the supplemented tube (TPP effect + 25%) this indicates functional thiamin deficiency. The third stage of depletion is that of clinical deficiency disease.

Most clinical biochemistry laboratories provide only some of the methods in the table as a routine but others could be set up in special circumstances or, alternatively, a laboratory specialising in nutrition research could be asked to help.

## References

1 de Boer JO, van Es AJH, van Raaij JMA *et al.* Energy requirements and energy expenditure of lean and overweight women, measured by indirect calorimetry. *Am J Clin Nutr* 1987; **46**: 13-21.
2 Murgatroyd PR, Shetty PS, Prentice AM. Techniques for the measurement of human energy expenditure: a practical guide. *Int J Obesity* 1993; **17**: 549-68.
3 Edholm OG, Adam JM, Best TW. Day to day weight changes in young men. *Ann Hum Biol* 1974; **1**: 3-12.
4 McKay K, Fozdan-Faroudi S, Bowman CE. How heavy the patient? *BMJ* 1991; **303**: 1608.
5 Frisancho AR. New norms of upper limb fat and muscle areas for assessment of nutritional status. *Am J Clin Nutr* 1981; **34**: 2540-5.
6 Bishop CW, Bowen PE, Ritchey SJ. Norms for nutritional assessment of American adults by upper arm anthropometry. *Am J Clin Nutr* 1981; **34**: 2530-9.
7 Department of Health. *Dietary reference values for food energy and nutrients for the United Kingdom. (Report on Health & Social Subjects no 41.)* London: HMSO, 1991.
8 Scrimshaw NS, Waterlow JC, Schürch B. Energy and protein requirements. Proceedings of an IDECG workshop. *Eur J Clin Nutr* 1996; **50** (Suppl 1): S11-S81.
9 Allman MA, Allen BJ, Stewart PM *et al.* Body protein of patients undergoing haemodialysis. *Eur J Clin Nutr* 1990; **44**: 123-31.
10 Durnin JVGA, Womersley J. Body fat assessed from total body density and its estimation from skinfold thickness: measurements on 481 men and women aged from 16 to 72 years. *Br J Nutr* 1974; **32**: 77-97.
11 Slater JM (ed) (Ministry of Agriculture, Fisheries & Food). *Fifty years of the National Food Survey 1940-1990.* London: HMSO, 1991.
12 Willett W. *Nutritional epidemiology* 2nd edn. New York: Oxford University Press, 1998.
13 Ashwell M. *McCance and Widdowson, A Scientific Partnership of 60 Years.* London: British Nutrition Foundation.
14 Holland B, Welch AA, Unwin ID, Buss DA, Paul AA, Southgate DAT. *McCance & Widdowson's the composition of foods*, 5th edn. Cambridge: Royal Society of Chemistry, 1991.
15 Greenfield H, Southgate DAT. *Food composition data. Production, management and use.* London: Elsevier Applied Science, 1992.
16 Human Nutrition Information Service, US Department of Agriculture. *Composition of foods: raw, processed, prepared.* Washington DC: US Government Printing Office. (This is a growing set of 23 volumes for different food groups, each with looseleaf supplements, providing nutrient analyses for over 3600 foods. Handbook 8-1 is for dairy and egg products, 8-2 for spices and herbs, 8-3 for baby foods … 8-22 for mixed dishes and 8-23 for miscellaneous foods.)
17 Ministry of Agriculture, Fisheries & Food. *Manual of nutrition*, 10th edn. London: HMSO, 1995.
18 The most recent is: Institute of Medicine. *Dietary Reference Intakes for vitamin A, vitamin K, arsenic, boron, chromium, copper, iodine, iron, manganese, molybdenum, nickel, silicon, vanadium and zinc.* Washington DC: National Academy Press, 2002.

# 13   Therapeutic diets

A person may be advised to change his or her diet to help treat or prevent disease.

- For essential or lifesaving treatment—for example, in coeliac disease, phenylketonuria, galactosaemia, hepatic encephalopathy.
- To replenish patients who are malnourished because of diseases such as cancer, intestinal diseases, and anorexia nervosa.
- To produce a negative energy balance in obese people.
- As helpful treatment, alternative or complementary to drugs, as in diabetes mellitus, mild hypertension, dyspepsia.
- To deal with the side effects of some drugs—for example, diets with increased potassium for patients taking long term diuretics or diets with restricted tyramine for patients taking monoamine oxidase inhibiting antidepressants.
- To provide standard conditions for diagnostic tests—for example, for measuring faecal fat. Also, an elimination diet is the mainstay in diagnosis of food sensitivity.
- Prophylactic diets like those described in chapter 7 on nutrition for adults (dietary goals or guidelines for the general public) often combine mild restriction of energy, saturated fat, and sodium with a moderate increase of dietary fibre.

Therapeutic diets ask patients to make one or more of the following changes: reduce or (virtually) eliminate one or more components, increase one or more food components, change the consistency of the diet, or change the feeding pattern. These are all changes to the patient's usual diet (which, of course, varies somewhat from day to day) or in comparison with a hypothetical "normal" or average diet for the country, culture, age, and sex.

The prescription for a diet should state:

- the nature of the modification(s)
- the degree of each modification
- the planned duration of these
- any compensation for essential nutrients compromised by the modifications.

The degree of the modification is as important as the dose in pharmacotherapy. People talk loosely about a "low salt" diet but its sodium intake can range from 25 to 100 mmol/day compared with a normal British sodium intake of around 150 mmol/day. Likewise with protein, a protein restricted diet may vary from 20 to 50 g/day compared with the standard of about 75 g/day (1 g/kg).

The dietary prescription has to be adjusted for the individual patient:

- for the foods disliked and liked
- for any sensitivity or intolerance to food
- for any religious food prohibition (including Ramadan for Moslems, the month when all eating has to be after dark)
- for vegetarians
- to include foods eaten away from home
- for income, occupation, and level of education
- for cooking facilities and the patient's domestic situation
- for the need for variety in foods (some insist on variety; others like the same foods from day to day)
- for the patient's motivation and degree of obsessionality
- for calorie (energy) expenditure and needs

For the purposes of describing therapeutic alternatives to diets a "normal" or average diet provides for a hypothetical healthy 70 kg Western man something like:

- **Energy** 10.5 MJ (2500 kcal)
- **Protein** 14% of energy or 85 g
- **Fat** 35% of energy or about 100 g
- **Carbohydrates** 48% of energy or 300 g
- **Alcohol** 3% of energy or 1 drink/day.

If the percentages of energy for macronutrients omit alcohol (as some do) carbohydrates here go up to 50% of energy and fat to 36%.

A "normal" diet provides around 75% of these absolute figures for the hypothetical woman (not pregnant or lactating), but the same percentages of energy for the macronutrients.

## The naming of diets

Diets are sometimes described eponymously (Giovanetti diet) or as belonging to a specific disease (renal failure diet). But neither type of name is recommended. Diets named after their (supposed) originator give no clue about their composition and particular diets do not necessarily relate to specific diseases. A "renal failure diet" may also be used for hepatic encephalopathy or rare inborn errors of the ornithine cycle. There have been many "diabetic" and "renal failure" diets.

"Cholesterol lowering diet" is ambiguous (and "low cholesterol diet" is worse). Several diets may lower the plasma concentration of cholesterol—low fat, vegetarian, or increased seed oil ($\omega$-6 polyunsaturated fatty acids)—and it is not necessary to lower the **dietary** cholesterol.

The most reliable way of naming diets is by the major change (from an average diet) in its composition.

## Degree of modification
### Sodium

- 100 mmol Na (2.3 g) is a mild low sodium diet
- 50 mmol Na (1.2 g) is a moderate low sodium diet
- 25 mmol Na (0.6 g) is a strict low sodium diet

### Protein

- 50 g/day (0.75 g/kg) is a mild protein restricted diet
- 30 g/day (0.5 g/kg) is a moderate protein restricted diet
- 20 g/day (0.33 g/kg) is a severe protein restricted diet

- for the duration of the diet. If a diet is necessary for only a week or two then it is not serious if it provides less than the recommended daily amount of (say) calcium or magnesium, but if the diet is continued these elements must be provided, by supplements if necessary
- for the patient's prognosis. A strict diet may not be justifiable for someone with a short life expectancy
- when two or more dietary prescriptions are combined. Sometimes these are more or less incompatible—for example, a low calorie plus high potassium diet or a high calcium plus lactose free diet (supplements would have to be used for these).

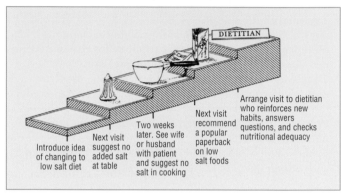

## Strategy

Essential, or lifesaving, diets should be looked after in collaboration with a dietitian. For some diseases—for example, gout, mild hypertension, and hyperlipidaemia—drugs or diet are alternative or complementary treatment options. Drugs appear to act more quickly, are easier to administer and more reliable, and take less of the doctor's time, but they may cause more side effects. Diet appears more natural and safer but it will take longer to explain. Sometimes the best choice is a synergistic combination so the dose of drug can be low (hence fewer side effects) and the diet not too irksome.

We know from results with obese people who are on weight reducing diets, and from studies in diabetics, that most people do not follow the diet prescribed. It is difficult and time consuming to explain what is intended and how it may be done. It is difficult too for a patient to make major changes to his or her food habits. Minor changes are much easier to incorporate and some places in the day's food sequence are easier to change than others. Each family and each individual has different feelings and ideas about foods. Some foods are given up more readily than others.

Outside hospital a therapeutic diet ("I'm on a low salt diet") is a strange association of an occasional talk by the doctor or dietitian with daily action by the patient and his or her family in the supermarket, kitchen, dining room, works canteen, and pub. The reality is different from what is on paper.

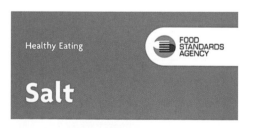

Building up therapeutic diet at successive visits

## Techniques

Essentially the doctor or dietitian has a list of foods rich in the component to be changed and of foods with medium and

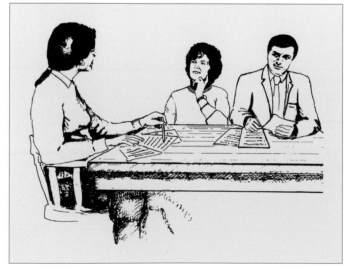

Three at the table

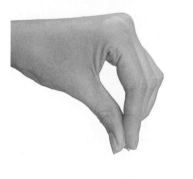

'Salt'—Food Standards Agency leaflet

low amounts of it. The trouble with scientific food tables, such as *McCance & Widdowson's The Composition of Foods*,[1] is that they give the content of nutrients per 100 g whereas what matters is the content per usual serving or portion (see box: typical serving sizes).

The patient, with his or her spouse, can produce a list of what the family usually eats and how it is cooked. Ideally the next series of steps is for the doctor or dietitian and these two to work out the most comfortable way for them to incorporate the dietary prescription into the family's food patterns. This cannot be completed at one session. It requires trial and error, questions and compromises.

There are two fairly easy ways of changing the diet. First, a food that tastes and functions like the original but has a different composition may be substituted. Examples are: polyunsaturated margarine for butter; sunflower (etc) oil for dripping; skimmed or 2% fat milk for whole milk; salt free bread for ordinary bread; wholemeal bread for white bread; high fibre breakfast cereal for low fibre brand.

Second, a simple addition may be made to less important parts of the day's diet. Examples are: a sprinkling of bran on the breakfast cereal to increase fibre; casein powder (such as Casilan) sprinkled on to food three times a day to increase protein; spoonful(s) of fish oil (such as Maxepa) to increase long chain highly polyunsaturated fatty acids.

Diets are more likely to be followed and persisted with by patients who are well motivated, have stable mood, normal intelligence, good home support, and lead a well organised life. Indeed, in some obsessional patients there can be the opposite problem of overdoing a diet suggested long ago on thin scientific evidence or for a condition that has since disappeared.

### Checking compliance and effectiveness

From an authoritarian viewpoint patients often do not properly **comply** with the doctor's instructions. This can be checked by asking revealing questions, by calling into the home at meal times, or by objective tests (for example biomarkers).

But for an intelligent patient who thinks that dieting is his or her own responsibility and that of his or her partner, with the doctor or dietitian one of their sources of information, what needs to be checked is the **effectiveness** of what they are doing.

Whatever the viewpoint or words used the same objective tests are available:

- change of body weight for reduced or increased energy diets
- increase of faecal weight for high (wheat) fibre diets
- 24-hour urinary sodium and potassium for dietary changes of sodium or potassium
- 24-hour urinary nitrogen for high or low protein diets, and also as general check on food intake (on average protein intake is 10-15% of energy intake)
- plasma fasting triglyceride fatty acid pattern to indicate consumption of polyunsaturated fat
- blood urea, urate, glucose, cholesterol, haemoglobin for respective diets prescribed to moderate these.

A Royal Pharmaceutical Society report urges clinicians to take a more egalitarian view of the relationship between prescribing and medicine taking, between patient and prescriber.[3] This is even more needed for dietary management.

## Diets for treating diabetes

Diabetic diets changed greatly throughout the 20th century. They have undergone further change since about 1970, as several facts emerged:

(1) Oral hypoglycaemic drugs may predispose to heart disease.
(2) There is no evidence that eating sugar **causes** diabetes.

### Typical serving sizes, approximate weight in grams

Bread (1 slice) 30 g
Crispbread (1 slice) 10 g
Biscuits about 12 g each
Breakfast cereal 30 g
Butter or margarine (for 1 slice bread) 7 g
Oil (1 tablespoonful) 20 g
Cake (portion) 40-50 g
Jam (for 1 slice bread) 15 g
Marmite (for 1 slice bread) 2 g
Milk (for 1 cup tea) 30 g
Milk (6 oz glass) 200 g
Cream (1 tablespoonful) 20 g
Sugar (1 level teaspoon) 5 g
Yoghurt (1 carton) 125-150 g
Cheese (1 portion) 30 g
Egg (1 edible portion) 50 g
Meat (chicken or beef) little or no bone 90-120 g
Meat (with bone, for example, chop) 160-200 g
Bacon (1 strip, raw) 30-40 g
Liver 80 g
Sausage (one) 50 g (approx)
Fish (fresh and canned) 110-120 g
1 fish finger 28 g
Macaroni and other pasta (for main course) 100 g (before cooking)
Vegetables (for example, peas, cauliflower) 60-100 g (before cooking)
Potato (1 medium, raw) 90 g
Lettuce 30 g
Parsley (chopped) 3 g
Fruit (1 apple, 1 banana peeled, raw) 100 g (approx)
1 grape 5 g
Nuts 30 g
Pepper 0.2 g
Wine (glass) 110-125 g
Spirits 25 g
Beer (1/2 pint) 285 g
Carbonated soft drink 240-330 g
Coffee powder 2 g

For more detail on individual British foods, see Crawley's handbook.[2]

### History of diets for diabetics 1900-80

| | |
|---|---|
| 1900-25 | Fasting (Naunyn, Allen); 5% *carbohydrate*, 85% fat (Newburgh 1923) |
| 1922 | Insulin discovered (but not generally available for a few years) |
| 1930 | 15% *carbohydrate* and 70% fat |
| 1940 | All *carbohydrate low*, for example, 40% and fat 50% |
| 1950 | Lawrence's lines in UK |
| 1970 | *Carbohydrate round* 40%; sugar prohibited. Emphasis on oral drugs or insulin rather than diet |
| 1980 | *Carbohydrates* 50% or more; emphasise "complex" $CH_2O$, fibre and legumes; restrict sugar |
| 2000 | Emphasis on lower glycaemic index foods |

(3) Asian people with diabetes on high starch diets have fewer complications (especially atherosclerotic) than their counterparts in Western Europe and North America.

(4) Westerners with diabetes are dying of excess atherosclerotic disease, have higher plasma cholesterol values, and have been eating higher saturated fat diets than people with no diabetes.

(5) Viscous dietary fibres such as that in guar, pectin, and legumes (though carbohydrates) improve diabetic control.

(6) Increased dietary carbohydrate improves the response to a glucose tolerance test. Increasing the (complex) carbohydrate of diabetic diets is not usually followed by deteriorating control.

(7) Individual foods containing carbohydrate do not give the same glucose and other metabolic responses at a standard intake. When put to the test, in human subjects some foods give much higher blood glucose curves than others. They have a higher or lower **glycaemic index** (area under the 2-hour blood glucose curve after eating a food containing 50 g carbohydrate as percentage of the corresponding area after the same weight of glucose). This means that carbohydrate exchange lists can no longer be relied on. (It was always hard to believe that 2 oz of grapes had the same effect in the body as 7 oz of whole milk.) The main cause of a low glycaemic index is that the starch in some foods is digested slowly by pancreatic amylase.

(8) Diabetics also have an increased chance of developing hypertension. The sodium content of their diets has been largely ignored.

## Principles of dietary treatment for diabetes[6,7]
*Type 1: insulin dependent diabetes (IDD)*

(1) **Integrate and synchronise meals (that is, the metabolic load) with the time(s) of action of the insulin treatment** to minimise high peaks of blood glucose as well as episodes of hypoglycaemia. The American Diabetes Association, for example, recommended that the individual's usual food intake is used as a basis for integrating insulin therapy into the eating and exercise patterns. Patients on insulin therapy should eat at consistent times synchronised with the time-action of the insulin preparation used.

(2) **Reduce saturated fat to 10% of total energy or less.** People with diabetes have an increased risk of coronary heart disease and this dietary change may reduce it.

(3) **Keep salt intake low**, because people with diabetes have an increased risk of hypertension.

(4) **Be very moderate with alcohol.** Large intakes carry the risk of hypoglycaemia; irregular drinking can disturb glycaemic control. But regular 1 to 2 glasses with a meal are acceptable and might be beneficial (except in pregnancy).

(5) **If still growing** make sure intakes of essential nutrients are adequate.

*Type 2: non-insulin dependent diabetes (NIDD)*
Dietary change has a greater potential to improve type 2 diabetes.

(1) **Reduce body weight by eating fewer kilojoules and taking regular exercise, and keep at it!** Even modest losses of weight improve metabolic control.[8] About three-quarters of type 2 diabetics are overweight or obese, and weight reduction is the first line of dietary management. To help patients lose weight and keep it off is a challenge for the physician and dietitian (cf chapter 11). Diabetics have a stronger incentive to lose weight because this improves their disease as well as their figure, but sulphonylureas or insulin (not metformin) tend to stimulate appetite. Some

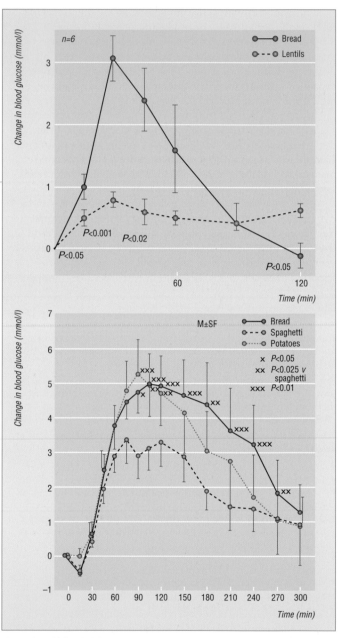

**Measurement of glycaemic index**

Mean rise of blood glucose after 50 g carbohydrate from four different foods. In the top graph the six subjects were not diabetic: lentils gave very low rise of blood glucose but at 2 hours lentil levels were higher than bread (now below fasting level).[4] In the lower graph the seven subjects had type 2 diabetes (two on insulin, two on glibenclamide). Blood glucose rises were higher than in the subjects with no diabetes and more sustained but over five hours area under the blood glucose curve for spaghetti was 60% that of bread[5]

who succeed in losing weight may be able to go off medications or go off insulin.

(2) **Reduce saturated fat**. Increased LDL-cholesterol may be more pathogenic in type 2 diabetes than non diabetic people.[10]

(3) Emphasise **low glycaemic index** foods.[9]

(4) Increase intake of **vegetables, fruit, legumes, and whole grain cereals** (which increase fibre intake and mostly have low glycaemic indices).

(5) Keep **salt intake low**.

(6) **Avoid excess alcohol** but 1-2 drinks per day with meals are acceptable.

(7) Forget carbohydrate exchanges

(8) There is no need to be obsessional about reducing sucrose. The glycaemic effect of sucrose is about the same as that of most starchy foods.[7]

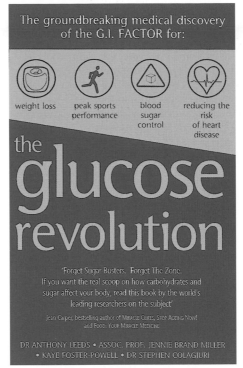

An up-to-date book written for the interested diabetic patient[9]

---

### Complex carbohydrates

The term "complex carbohydrates" has been used since 1977 for carbohydrates other than sugars (designated "simple carbohydrates")—that is, for polysaccharides, or for carbohydrates in whole grains, vegetables, and fruits. Diabetic patients have been advised to eat foods containing complex carbohydrates rather than simple carbohydrates. But the carbohydrates in fruits and many vegetables are predominantly sugars and food starches vary in rate of digestion so that some give higher rises of blood glucose than sucrose. The term has become confusing.[11] It is better to discuss carbohydrate components by using their chemical names or the names of the foods that contain them and in general to choose those with lower glycaemic index.

---

**Foods that have been shown to have low glycaemic indices (55 or less) compared to glucose = 100[12]**

| | | |
|---|---|---|
| Soya beans (18) | Pearl barley (28) | Bananas (53) |
| Lentils (29) | All pastas (40-45) | Apples (36) |
| Dried peas (31) | Rolled oats (55) | Apple juice (36) |
| Canned baked beans (40) | Oat bran (50) | Grapefruit (25) |
| Frozen peas (boiled) (48) | All Bran (40) | Oranges (43) |
| Other dried legumes, (around 30) | Pumpernickel (rye) bread (41) | Orange juice (57) |
| | | Plums (24) |
| | | Peaches (28) |
| | | Milk (full cream or low fat) and yoghurt (25-35) |

The glycaemic index of glucose is 100, of fructose 20, of sucrose (half way between) 60, of lactose 45.
High fat foods may also give a low glycaemic index, because of delayed gastric emptying, but are not recommended and are not on this list.

---

These dietary prescriptions look very similar to the general dietary guidelines in chapter 7. Indeed it can be said that a modern diabetic diet is the dietary guidelines for the general population pursued with more seriousness. At Birmingham General Hospital "Rather than tell the patients that this is a diabetic diet, we emphasise that it is a normal, healthy diet that everyone should be adhering to".[13]

## Diets for renal failure

A strict therapeutic diet is needed for patients with renal failure during the few days between diagnosis and dialysis and for the minority for whom dialysis will not be used. The diet should be low in protein (40 g/day) or very low in high biological value protein (25 g/day) with low potassium and a controlled sodium and water intake.

Most patients with chronic renal failure in Western countries however, are nowadays treated with regular dialysis while awaiting a transplant. For them the outpatient diet is not very different from a normal one. Protein should be about 1.2 g/kg body weight, a little more than the recommended daily intake for healthy people. Rather more protein is lost, and so is needed, on continuous ambulatory peritoneal dialysis than on haemodialysis. Potassium is carefully monitored but usually needs to be only a little restricted, sometimes not at all. It is controlled by adjusting the concentration in the dialysing fluid; 50 mmol/day is an average amount for the diet. This is achieved by eating fruits which have a low potassium content (apples, pears, and canned fruits) and boiled leafy vegetable and avoiding higher potassium vegetables (legumes), nuts, dried fruits, chocolate, and potato chips and crisps.

Patients can usually take an ordinary amount of sodium (about 110 mmol/day) or need only mild restriction. Fluid intake is restricted to about 1000 ml/day. Supplements of water soluble vitamins should not be given above nutrient requirement dosage.[14] Fat soluble vitamin supplements are not required; they tend to accumulate.

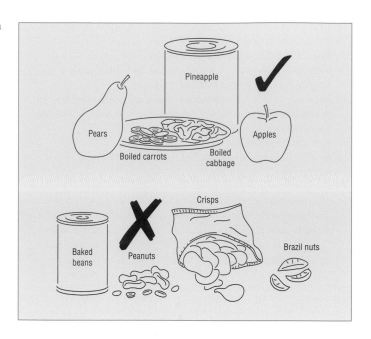

## Other conditions

### Diets for phenylketonuria

Phenylketonuria is one of the better known examples of an inborn error of amino acid metabolism. It leads to mental retardation and other abnormalities if patients are not started on a low phenylalanine diet in the first few weeks of life. Diagnosis is by routine screening of blood phenylalanine after adequate intakes of milk, on about the seventh day of life. Bottle feeding is essential in infancy and a special low phenylalanine formula has to be used, such as Lofenalac or Minafen. When the child is weaned, the diet has to be very different from that of other children: a combination of low protein foods (controlled by phenylalanine content) and a phenylalanine free mixture of other essential amino acids—for example, Aminogran—with sugars and fats and vitamin and mineral supplements. The relative amounts of the first two are adjusted to maintain plasma phenylalanine neither too high (toxicity) nor too low (inadequate growth). The diet has to be strictly maintained and monitored until the child is about 8 years old, after which it can usually be relaxed. But it is required again in women during pregnancy.

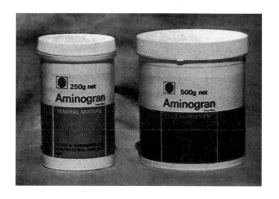

### Diets for gluten-sensitive enteropathy

Patients with gluten-sensitive enteropathy, coeliac disease, and dermatitis herpetiformis have to modify their diets to eliminate all wheat gluten, rye and barley gluten, and possibly oats. Fresh milk, fresh meat, fish and eggs, fresh vegetables and fruit, rice and maize, tea, coffee, sugar, wine, and spirits are all safe but many processed foods have wheat flour or gluten added. With many of these foods some brands contain gluten, others do not. The only thing to do is to check ingredients on the label or check brands against an up-to-date copy of Coeliac UK's list of gluten free manufactured products (PO Box 220, High Wycombe, Bucks HP11 2HY, http://www.coeliac.co.uk). Gluten free breads and pasta and other products, even communion wafers, are available, some on prescription. Unlike many other diets, even a small lapse and inclusion of the harmful component can lead to prompt return of symptoms.

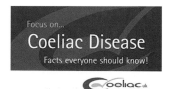

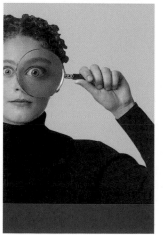

Coeliac booklet (produced with permission from Coeliac UK)

### Diets for dyspepsia

These diets present a contrast to the two preceding essential diets. Classic diets for peptic ulcer have not been found to accelerate healing in controlled barium meal studies. Modern drug treatment, especially with $H_2$ receptor antagonists and antibacterial treatment for *Helicobacter pylori* is usually effective. Diet is therefore much less emphasised than before for gastroduodenal diseases. Nevertheless, some foods are known to cause gastric irritation or stimulate acid secretion, including chilli powder, coffee, tea, peppers, alcohol, and cola beverages. Other foods commonly cause heartburn by lowering the tone of the lower oesophageal sphincter: peppermint, garlic, onion, fatty meals. Frequent, small volume feeds are beneficial in oesophageal reflux. Traditional bland foods such as milk, chicken, mashed potatoes, bananas, apples, and ice cream usually relieve symptoms in patients with dyspepsia, though individuals vary.

### Diets for diagnostic tests

For several days before a **glucose tolerance test** patients should be standardised on enough carbohydrate—that is, about 300 g or at least 50% of calories, the amount of carbohydrate in ordinary Western diets. Before a **faecal fat** test for malabsorption, patients should be on a known, controlled, and adequate fat intake, 70 to 100 g/day. Before **urinary screening for hypercalciuria** patients should be on a high normal calcium intake of about 1000 mg/day. Before urine is collected for **5-hydroxyindoleacetic acid (5-HIAA)** measurement dietary sources of it or of serotonin should be excluded: bananas, plantains, tomatoes, plums, avocadoes, pineapples, passion fruit, and walnuts. For urinary **4-hydroxy-3-methoxy-mandelic acid** (VMA) specific laboratory methods are now used, and dietary preparation should be unnecessary. Even urinary **creatinine** is affected (increased) by meat consumption.

### Diet for patients taking monoamine oxidase inhibitors

The diet for depressed patients taking these antidepressants is the most striking example of dietary adjustment to prevent side effects from drugs. Monoamine oxidase inhibitors interfere with the normal breakdown of tyramine, dopamine, and other amines that occur naturally in foods in which flavour is enhanced by protein breakdown. Dangerous increases of blood pressure may follow ingestion of cheese, but other foods contain these amines and should be excluded too: wines, bananas, aged game, salami, pickled herrings, broad beans, and yeast and meat extracts, and any stale foods. The drugs which require this dietary modification include tranylcypromine, phenelzine, and isocarboxazid.

In practice the most commonly needed diet is one with reduced energy and the second most needed is a regimen with reduced alcohol intake. Both are prescribed much more often than they are successfully followed. This discrepancy remains a challenge for medical practice and research.

Elsewhere in this book, diets are described which are low in saturated fat, with increased polyunsaturated fat (chapter 1); low in sodium (chapter 2); low in oxalate (chapter 3); low in energy (calories) (chapter 11); and elimination diets (chapter 15).

### Further reading

Thomas B (ed). *Manual of dietetic practice*, 3rd edn. Oxford: Blackwell Science, 2001

### References

1 Holland B, Welch AA, Unwin ID, Buss DH, Paul AA, Southgate DAT. *McCance & Widdowson's the composition of foods*, 5th edn. Cambridge: Royal Society of Chemistry, 1991.

2 Crawley H. (Ministry of Agriculture, Fisheries and Food.) *Food portion sizes*. London: HMSO, 1988.

3 Mullen PD. Compliance becomes concordance. Making a change in terminology produces a change in behaviour. *BMJ* 1997; **314**: 691-2.

4 Jenkins DJA, Wolever TMS, Taylor RH *et al*. Rate of digestion of foods and postprandial glycaemia in normal and diabetic subjects. *BMJ* 1980; **2**: 14-17.

5 Parillo M, Giacco R, Riccardi G, Pacioni D, Rivellese A. Different glycaemic responses to pasta, bread and potatoes in diabetic patients. *Diabet Med* 1985; **2**: 374-7.

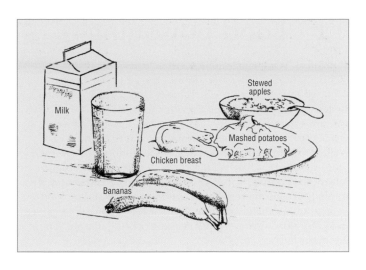

### Diagnostic tests

- Glucose tolerance tests
- Faecal fat test for steatorrhoea
- Urinary screening for hypercalciuria
- 5-hydroxyindoleacetic acid (5-HIAA) for carcinoid tumours
- 4-hydroxy-3-methoxy-mandelic acid (VMA) for phaeochromocytoma
- Creatinine

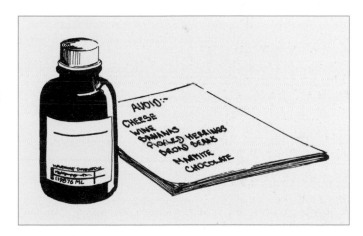

6 Ha TKK, Lean MEJ. Technical review. Recommendations for the nutritional management of patients with diabetes mellitus. *Eur J Clin Nutr* 1998; **52**: 467-81.

7 Franz MJ, Bantle JP, Beebe CA *et al*. Technical review. Evidence-based nutrition principles and recommendations for the treatment and prevention of diabetes and related complications. *Diabetes Care* 2002; **25**: 148-98.

8 Jung R. Obesity as a disease. *Br Med Bull* 1997; **53**: 307-21.

9 Leeds A, Brand Miller J, Foster-Powell K, Colagiuri S. *The Glucose Revolution*. London: Hodder and Stoughton, 1998.

10 Turner RC, Millins H, Neil HAW *et al*. Risk factors for coronary artery disease in non-insulin dependent diabetes mellitus: UK prospective diabetes study (UKPDS:23) *BMJ* 1998; **316**: 823-8.

11 Report of a Joint FAO/WHO Expert Consultation (Rome 14-18 April 1987). *Carbohydrates in human nutrition*. Rome: FAO, 1998.

12 Foster-Powell K, Miller JB. International tables of glycaemic index. *Am J Clin Nutr* 1995; **62**: 871S-93S.

13 Baxter A, Wright AD. Diabetic dietary prescriptions (letter). *BMJ* 1989; **299**: 124.

14 Allman MA, Truswell AS, Stewart PM *et al*. Vitamin supplementation of patients receiving haemodialysis. *Med J Aust* 1989; **150**: 130-3.

# 14    Food poisoning

Patrick G Wall, Ciara E O'Reilly

Bovine spongiform encephalopathy/new variant Creutzfeldt–Jakob disease (CJD), foot and mouth disease, *E. coli* O157:H7, salmonella in poultry and eggs, antibiotic-resistant strains of bacteria and residues in food, listeria in paté and cheeses, have all damaged the public's confidence in our food supply. Coupled with this, consumers' confidence in the ability of the regulatory agencies to protect the food supply, and in the commitment of the food industry to protecting consumers' health, has also been damaged. There are many factors contributing to consumers' concerns regarding food safety as outlined in the box opposite.

Changes in consumer behaviour including more eating out, bulk shopping, and a desire for more convenience foods have contributed to the increasing incidence of foodborne infectious disease. Busy lifestyles, two parents working outside the home and a decreasing knowledge of cooking are contributing to an increasing demand for convenience "ready to cook" and "ready to eat" food, and more and more food is being prepared outside the home. This is increasing the length of the food chain, providing more opportunities for things to go wrong. Microbes do not respect national frontiers and the increasing global distribution and mass processing of food products has given microbes the opportunity to disseminate widely.[2] In the poorer non-industrialised countries other factors that contribute to an unsafe food supply are expanding urbanisation, the increased dependence on stored foods, insufficient access to safe water and essential facilities for safe food preparation. For example an increased volume of street foods prepared under poor sanitary conditions increases the risk of foodborne illness.

Producing safe food involves a chain of responsibility including primary producers, processors, distributors, wholesalers, retailers, commercial caterers and consumers. Everyone in the chain from "plough to plate" has a role to play. See box on page 100 for details. There is no room for complacency with foodborne diseases, as what may be a mild dose of diarrhoea for a robust young adult can be a life-threatening illness for an infant, a frail elderly person or an individual suffering from some concurrent morbidity. Globally hundreds of millions of people are affected by illnesses caused by contaminated food. The toll in terms of human life and suffering is enormous, particularly among infants and young children, the elderly and other vulnerable groups. Over the next few decades the number of elderly people in the world is predicted to increase rapidly. By the year 2025 more than 1000 million of the global population will be over 60 years old and more than two-thirds will live in developing countries.[3] There are several key factors which relate to an increased risk of foodborne disease among the elderly: (a) the increase in the proportion and number of elderly people,[3] (b) physiological factors, such as changes in the functions of the gastrointestinal tract and immune systems, that predispose an elderly person to infections, (c) pathological factors associated with ageing, such as disability and losses in sensory functions, and (d) social changes in health care of the elderly.[1]

Animals and poultry are the reservoir for many foodborne infections (salmonella, campylobacter, *E. coli* O157:H7, cryptosporidia, and yersinia). Intensive farming of livestock to produce more and cheaper food has brought with it inherent dangers. It is possible to control the food, water, air and environment in these units and produce virtually disease-free

**Factors contributing to food safety concerns[1]**

- New food preparation
- New storage methods
- Changing lifestyles—convenience foods
- Globalisation in food trade
- Changes in food production on the farm
- New systems of food processing
- Longer distribution chains
- Increasing number of vulnerable groups (the elderly, immunocompromised individuals, etc)

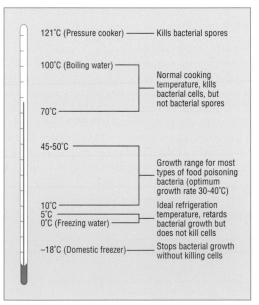

Summary of the effects of temperature on bacterial growth

animals. Husbandry practices are not always ideal, however, and the high stocking density facilitates the transmission of microbes, which can result in large amounts of contaminated material entering the food chain. Farms and abattoirs are not operating theatres and even with the best operational procedures a proportion of raw meat and poultry may contain harmful microbes. Care must be taken, therefore, to avoid transferring microbes from raw product to other foods that will not be heat-treated before consumption. Raw meat and poultry should be sufficiently cooked to kill all harmful microbes and refrigerated prior to cooking to prevent multiplication of harmful microbes. Bacteria such as *Listeria monocytogenes* (found in soil and silage as well as animals) and *Bacillus* species (soil, dust, etc) are widely distributed in the environment and may thus be found in plant (for example, coleslaw, rice) as well as animal (for example, soft cheeses, unpasteurised milk) products.

## Protozoal pathogens

| Causative agent | Incubation period | Usual duration of symptoms | Common clinical features* | Mode of transmission* |
|---|---|---|---|---|
| *Cryptosporidium* sp | 2-5 days | <3 weeks | D | W, An, X |
| *Entamoeba histolytica* | 2-4 weeks | Variable | D, B | X |
| *Giardia intestinalis* | 5-25 days | Variable | D, P | X, F, W |

\* See key in table on page 97
Adapted from Department of Health[4]

## Bacterial pathogens

| Causative agent | Usual incubation period | Duration of symptoms | Common clinical features | Mode of transmission |
|---|---|---|---|---|
| *Aeromonas* sp | Unknown | Varied | V, D | W, F |
| *Bacillus* sp | | <36 h | | F |
| B. cereus | | | | |
|   Emetic syndrome | 1-5 h | | N, V, D, P | |
|   Diarrhoeal syndrome | 8-16 h | | D, V, N, P | |
| B. subtilis | 1-4 h | | N, V, D | |
| B. licheniformis | 2-14 h | | D, P | |
| *Campylobacter* sp | 2-5 days | 2 days to 1 week | D, P, Fe | F, W |
| *Clostridium perfringens* | 12-18 h | 24 h | D, P | F |
| *Clostridium botulinum* | 12-36 h | Can be several months | Neurological signs | F, wound contamination |
| *Escherichia coli* | | | | |
|   Attaching and effacing (AEEC) | Unknown | Unknown | D | F |
|   Enteroaggregative (EAggEC) | 20-48 h | Unknown | D, B | F |
|   Enteroinvasive (EIEC) | 12-72 h | 5-7 days | D, B | F, W |
|   Enteropathogenic (EPEC) | 12-72 h | <2 weeks | D | X, F, W |
|   Enterotoxigenic (ETEC) | 12-72 h | 3-5 days | D | F, W |
|   Verocytotoxin-producing (VTEC) | 1-6 days | 4-6 days (not HUS) | D, B, HUS | F, X, W |
| *Listeria monocytogenes* | 1-10 weeks | Variable | Flu, meningitis, abortion | F, congenital, DC |
| Salmonellas (non-enteric fever) | 12-72 h | <3 weeks | V, D, Fe | F, X |
| *Salmonella typhi/paratyphi* | 1-3 weeks | 10-14 days | N, Fe | F, X, W |
| *Shigella* sp | 1-7 days | <2 weeks | D, B | X, F, W |
| *Staphylococcus aureus* | 2-4 h | <12-48 h | V, P, Fe | F |
| *Vibrio cholerae* (O1, O139) | 2-3 days | <7 days | D | W, F |
| *Vibrio parahaemolyticus* | 12-18 h | <7 days | D | F |
| *Vibrio vulnificus* | 12 h to 3 days | High mortality if concurrent liver disease or immunosuppression | Septicaemia, shock | F, DC |
| *Yersinia* sp. | 3-7 days | 1-3 weeks | D, P, Fe | F |

Adapted from Department of Health (2000)[5]
*Key to tables:* Bacterial pathogens, protozoal pathogens, viral pathogens and food poisoning biological toxins associated with seafood

**Clinical features:**
B   Blood in stool
D   Diarrhoea
Fe   Fever
HUS  Haemolytic uraemic syndrome
N   Nausea
P   Abdominal pain
J   Jaundice
V   Vomiting

**Mode of transmission:**
Aer  Aerosol
An  Animal contact
F   Food
W   Water
X   Person to person (faecal-oral)
DC  Direct contact with infected material

# ABC of Nutrition

Food poisoning is defined by WHO as: "Any disease of an infectious or toxic nature caused by or thought to be caused by the consumption of food and water".[5] This definition includes all food and waterborne illness regardless of the presenting symptoms and signs. Thus it includes not only acute illnesses characterised by diarrhoea and/or vomiting, but also illnesses presenting with manifestations not related to the gastrointestinal tract. Heavy metals, pesticides, and other chemicals can also cause food poisoning.

Most food poisoning whether caused by bacteria, viruses, protozoa or toxins usually results in symptoms which include diarrhoea, vomiting, nausea, abdominal pain, and occasionally fever. However, there are other agents that result in food poisoning but do not usually result in gastrointestinal symptoms. These include *Clostridium botulinum*, *Listeria monocytogenes*, hepatitis A virus, and poliovirus. Laboratory tests are required to identify the aetiological agent but the symptoms, incubation period, and duration of illness may suggest the likely cause.

National figures on the incidence of food poisoning in most countries arise from a combination of notifications of clinical disease, reports of laboratory-confirmed infections, and details on outbreaks. In the United Kingdom all clinicians have a statutory duty to notify to the proper officer of the local authority, cases, or suspected cases, of food poisoning. The meaning of the term "food poisoning" is not defined in the relevant UK legislation, the Public Health (Control of Diseases) Act 1984, and this has previously led to confusion as to which cases should be notified, but in 1992 the WHO definition was adopted. Notification is not contingent on laboratory confirmation of infection, and delaying notification until laboratory confirmation is available defeats the purpose of a rapid notification system designed to enable effective timely intervention at local level. An outbreak is defined as an incident in which two or more people, thought to have a common exposure, experience a similar illness or proven infection.[5] A general outbreak is defined as one that affects members of more than one household or residents of an institution, distinguishing it from an outbreak affecting one family.[5]

Notifications of food poisoning based on clinical diagnosis are a very crude estimation of the true extent of the burden of ill health due to food poisoning. The symptoms can occur unrelated to food poisoning and only a proportion of cases are actually notified (clinicians being unaware of the need to notify or omitting to do so). Gross under-notification of food poisoning occurs as is well documented for more serious infections.[6] Furthermore, many cases do not seek medical attention.[6]

Similarly the reports of laboratory-confirmed gastrointestinal pathogens represent just a fraction of the true incidence of these pathogens, as only a proportion of cases seek medical attention and only a subset of these have a sample submitted for analysis.[7] Not all of these will have a pathogen

## Viral pathogens

| Virus | Incubation period | Duration of symptoms | Common clinical features* | Mode of transmission* |
|---|---|---|---|---|
| Adenovirus | 7-8 days | 9-12 days | D, V | X |
| Astrovirus | 3-4 days | 2-3 days | V, D, Fe | X, F, Aer |
| Calicivirus | 1-3 days | 1-2 days | V, D, Fe | X, F, Aer |
| Hepatitis A | 15-50 days | Variable | J | F, W, X |
| Rotavirus | 1-2 days | 4-6 days | D, V | X, F |
| SRSV | 1-3 days | 1-3 days | V, D, Fe | X, F, Aer |

* See key in table on page 97
Adapted from Department of Health[4]

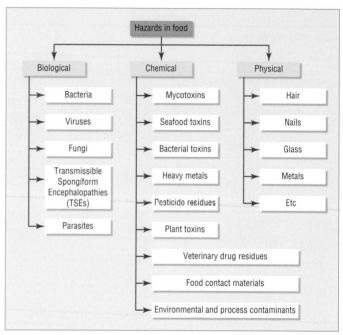

The biological, chemical, and physical hazards in food (adapted from[1])

## Food poisoning biological toxins associated with seafood

| Agent | Incubation period | Duration of symptoms | Common clinical features* | Mode of transmission |
|---|---|---|---|---|
| Paralytic shellfish poisoning | Minutes to hours | Several days | Tingling, numbness, incoordination, respiratory distress | F |
| Scombrotoxin | Minutes to hours | <12 hours | Allergic type; facial flushing V, N | F |
| Ciguatera fish poisoning | 1-24 hours | Weeks | V, D + neurological | F |

*See key in table on page 97

identified (particularly if the agent is a virus) and not all pathogens identified are reported centrally. The exact proportion in each category is unclear and may vary for different organisms. The National Infectious Intestinal Diseases Study attempts to estimate the true prevalence of the different pathogens and the degree of under-diagnosis and under-reporting.[4] Laboratory reports most likely represent patients at the severe end of the spectrum of diarrhoeal disease and are therefore a biased sample. In addition, laboratory reports of potentially foodborne microbes may not all have arisen by this route, with animal contact and person-to-person transmission accounting for a proportion. It is often only when cases are investigated epidemiologically that the exact route of transmission is identified. In England and Wales reports of laboratory confirmed infections are collated and published by the Communicable Disease Surveillance Centre (CDSC), the Epidemiology Unit of the Public Health Laboratory Service (PHLS). Similar national surveillance centres exist in most countries. Campylobacter and salmonella are by far the most commonly reported enteric pathogens and the most likely aetiological agents in a lot of the food poisoning notifications.

Food poisoning notifications and laboratory reports of campylobacter and salmonella: England and Wales 1992-2000 (Source: PHLS CDSC)

## Diagnosis

A microbiological diagnosis is often not necessary for successful treatment of an individual suffering from food-related gastroenteritis (see box opposite for details when it is necessary).

Faecal culture remains the gold standard for the identification of most foodborne pathogens. Electron microscopy is used for the identification of Norwalk and other viruses. Newer more rapid molecular methods are coming on stream. Clinicians should consult their local laboratory for information on the exact diagnostic tests on offer so that they can take the appropriate specimens and request the optimum investigations.

## Treatment

In uncomplicated cases of acute gastroenteritis, symptomatic therapy alone is recommended; that is oral rehydration combined with antipyretics. Antimotility drugs are not advised for acute attacks as they have a very limited role as adjuncts to fluid and electrolyte replacement. Antibiotic therapy is only recommended in high-risk groups, for example, patients with underlying disease such as sickle cell anaemia, immunocompromised patients, cases who are more likely to develop complications, and those with prolonged fever and extraintestinal infections. Metronidazole is indicated if symptoms are caused by giardia.

## Economic consequences of foodborne illness

As well as morbidity and mortality associated with foodborne diseases, there are direct economic costs to society in treating sick people. There are also economic losses due to food being rejected in export markets, and loss of consumer confidence in brand names on the domestic market. The US government has estimated the cost of human illnesses of seven foodborne pathogens to be between US$ 5.6 to 9.4 billion annually. The cost of salmonellosis in England and Wales in 1992 was estimated at between US$ 560 and 800 million.

---

**Microbiological diagnosis and food-related gastroenteritis**

Microbiological diagnosis is necessary for individuals suffering from food-related gastroenteritis:

- in severely ill, septicaemic or immunosuppressed patients;
- if clusters of similar cases are to be recognised and outbreaks controlled early;
- if the priority pathogens are to be identified to permit tailored public health interventions;
- to monitor ongoing trends and evaluate interventions;
- in nursery children, special needs children and the elderly in institutions where personal hygiene may be poor and there is a risk of secondary spread;
- for food handlers and healthcare workers to exclude excretors of typhoid and verocytotoxic *E. coli* (VTEC);
- when a patient wishes to take legal action against a restaurant or food retailer.

---

**Economic consequences contributing to food safety concerns[1]**

- Economic costs to society in treating sick people
- Economic losses due to rejection of food in export markets
- Loss of consumer confidence in brand names

---

Over 70% of costs were directly associated with treatment and investigation of cases, and costs to the economy of sickness related to absence from work. Estimates in 1999 showed that foodborne diseases annually cause approximately 76 million illnesses, 325 000 hospitalisations and 5000 deaths in the United States each year.[8] The BSE crisis in Britain is predicted to cost over US$ 5.5 billion. These costs are associated with the loss of export sales, compensating farmers, paying slaughterhouses and renderers, and research and control measures. The dioxin crisis in Belgium in 1999 saw the fall of the national government and economic costs in excess of US$ 2 billion to the Belgium economy.[1]

The true estimates of foodborne disease and the likely economic costs are unknown. In industrialised countries only a small proportion of cases of foodborne diseases come to the notice of health services and even fewer are investigated. Very few non-industrialised countries have established foodborne disease reporting systems, and in those that have, only a small fraction of cases are reported. The incidence of foodborne disease is likely to be far higher than in industrialised countries because of such factors as poor nutritional status, inadequate sanitation, low standards of hygiene and reduced likelihood of immediate medical attention. There are many hidden costs associated with foodborne illnesses. Tourists will shun regions with a high incidence of foodborne illness as will multinational firms choosing the location of foreign investment. Repeated bouts of diarrhoea damage children's mental and physical development and play havoc with their schooling.[1]

# Principal foodborne pathogens

**Bacteria**

*Campylobacter*

The importance of campylobacter as a human pathogen was recognised in the 1970s and it is the commonest gastrointestinal pathogen isolated from humans in the United Kingdom.[9] These bacteria do not usually multiply on food as they will not grow at temperatures below 28°C and grow best at 42°C. Infection in humans usually causes an acute self-limiting enterocolitis. Bacteraemia and reactive arthritis are rare complications and an association with Guillain–Barré syndrome has been observed.[10] Large outbreaks are rarely recognised and reported to the Communicable Disease Surveillance Centre in England and Wales: only 240 (0.2%) of 122 250 cases of campylobacter infections reported between 1992 and 1994 were associated with general outbreaks.[11] There are two principal species, *C. jejuni* and *C. coli*, although most cases are reported without a species. *C. jejuni* is the most common cause of bacterial food poisoning in many industrialised countries. These are fragile organisms which require micro-aerophilic conditions for growth and do not survive or multiply very well on foods. However, the low infectious dose means that a small level of contamination may result in illness. Campylobacter may be transmitted by food, particularly poultry,[12] unpasteurised milk,[13] and contaminated water.[14] *Campylobacter* spp are especially common in birds but have also been isolated from a wide range of animals. Wild birds are considered to be an important reservoir of infection for domestic and food animals. Cases have also been associated with the consumption of pasteurised milk where the milk bottle tops had been pecked by birds, who presumably transferred the bacteria on their beaks.[15] Although many foods may be contaminated with campylobacter, it is considered by many authorities that poultry and poultry products are of particular importance as a source of human infection. *Campylobacter* spp do not multiply very effectively in most foods, however, *Campylobacter* spp may

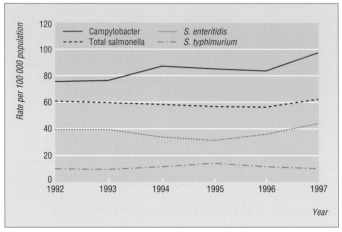

Principal faecal pathogens identified in humans: England and Wales 1992-97 (Source: PHLS CDSC)

---

**Recommendations to control transmission of *Campylobacter* spp in the food chain[16]**

Recommendations to control transmission of *Campylobacter* spp (and other foodborne pathogens) from farm to fork include:

- poultry industry complying with the highest possible degree of biosecurity measures
- industry development and implementation of evidence-based standard operating procedures, in order to prevent or minimise product contamination with *Campylobacter* spp
- food businesses should implement and document a food safety management system based on the principles of the Hazard Analysis Critical Control Point (HACCP)
- staff involved in food production should be appropriately trained in food safety to a level commensurate with their work activities
- the provision of a supply of potable water for food preparation
- consumers should practise basic good hygiene when handling food and should cook high-risk raw foods thoroughly[16]

survive through the food distribution system and because consumption of a small number of organisms (500 or less) may be associated with illness, proliferation in food is not a prerequisite for infection.[16]

In the United Kingdom there is a characteristic seasonal distribution of reports, with a peak in the early summer, in contrast to reports of salmonella which reach their maximum in the late summer and autumn. There are also regional variations in the reporting of campylobacter infections which may reflect a higher incidence in rural than urban populations.

### Salmonella (non-typhoid)

Salmonella is a genus made up of over 2200 serotypes. They are widely dispersed in nature, being found in the gastrointestinal tracts of domesticated and wild mammals, reptiles, birds, and insects (apart from *S. typhi* and *S. paratyphi* which only colonise humans). Although there is a vast range of serotypes, a small number predominate. Salmonella is the second most commonly reported bacterial cause of gastroenteritis after campylobacter. In England and Wales in 1997 there were 32 169 human cases of salmonellosis but four serotypes accounted for 90% of cases (*S. enteritidis* 22 806, *S. typhimurium* 4695, *S. hadar* 692, and *S. virchow* 650). Although the clinical management of most cases infected with the different serotypes is similar, for epidemiological purposes, it is important that isolates are sent to a reference laboratory for definitive typing. Salmonella can be phenotyped using serotyping, phage typing and antibiograms, and genotyped using molecular methods including plasmid profile analysis, pulsed field gel electrophoresis, and DNA sequencing. The National Reference Laboratory in England and Wales is the PHLS Laboratory of Enteric Pathogens. Most countries have such a facility and in the European Union all such labs are collaborating in the Enter-net Project to standardise methodology and share surveillance and outbreak data. Detailed typing can be used to link strains identified in humans, food samples, environment samples and livestock in the course of outbreak investigations. The standardisation of phage typing techniques, the electronic transfer of molecular typing patterns, formal and informal links established through international networks including Enter-net and the notification of national outbreaks to these networks are extremely important, particularly in the case of an international outbreak.

Incidence rates of infection are highest in children under 10. This may reflect increased susceptibility but is also likely to be due to these young children being brought to medical care and having faecal specimens submitted for examination. Most cases suffer from gastroenteritis with a subset (<1%) suffering from invasive disease.

Undercooked (or improperly heat treated) food from infected food animals is most commonly implicated. There has been a dramatic rise in human salmonellosis in the United Kingdom since the mid 1980s due to an unprecedented increase in one subtype, *S. enteritidis* phage type (PT) 4. The reservoir for this subtype is infected poultry. Humans become infected from consuming under-cooked poultry, raw eggs, dishes made from the same, or foods cross-contaminated from these.[17-19] Egg-associated salmonellosis is caused when *S. enteritidis* infects the ovaries of apparently healthy hens and these hens lay contaminated eggs. If the eggs are eaten raw or undercooked, salmonellosis may result. The increase in

**Traceability from plough to plate**

The plough to plate (or farm to fork) approach to food safety embraces all elements which have an impact on the safety of food, at every level of the food chain. The communication of information throughout the food chain is a critical element of this approach. This approach encompasses the production of all foods and can be applied not only to meat but also to milk, eggs, fish and other products from product from aquaculture, as well as fruit and vegetables.

**The Stages of Food Production in the traceability from farm to fork approach:**

Animal feed/fertiliser/chemical product manufacturers
↓↑
Primary production (**PLOUGH**) e.g. planting, breeding, rearing, growing, dairy production, fish production
↓↑
Transport of animals or of raw products
↓↑
Slaughtering and processing
↓↑
Transport of processed products
↓↑
Wholesale
↓↑
Transport of processed products
↓↑
Retailing e.g. restaurants, catering services, food stores
↓↑
Consumers (**PLATE**)

*S. enteritidis* PT4 in the United Kingdom has been seen in many countries and this pathogen is now a global problem.

Although *S. enteritidis* has declined by 50% since its peak year of 1997 and *S. typhimurium* by 40% in England and Wales since 1995, these serotypes continue to dominate. The decline in *S. enteritidis* phage type 4 (PT4) is the result of vaccination of poultry flocks but in its place new types are emerging.

In 2001 in England and Wales there was a significant increase in salmonellosis which is associated with a range of salmonellas that have links with foreign travel and the importation of food stuffs (for example, contaminated desiccated coconut).[20] Another emerging global problem is *S. typhimurium* definitive type 104 (DT 104). It is the second most prevalent salmonella found in humans in England and Wales, increasing from fewer than 250 in 1990 to 4006 cases in 1996. Over 90% of isolates are multi-antibiotic resistant to ampicillin, chloramphenicol, streptomycin, sulphonamides and tetracyclines, with a subset of the strains having reduced susceptibility to trimethoprim and ciprofloxacin.[21] This subtype is prevalent in cattle, sheep, pigs, and poultry, and therefore a wide array of foods can be contaminated. Reduced susceptibility to fluoroquinolone drugs has also emerged in the poultry-associated serotypes *S. hadar* and *S. virchow*. The development of these strains is a consequence of the use of antibiotics in animal husbandry.[22] This acquisition of resistance has resulted in a progressive reduction in options for the management of invasive salmonellosis in humans.

### Enterovirulent E. coli *including* E. coli *O157*

The enterovirulent *E. coli* include all those *E. coli* believed to be associated with diarrhoea. Enterotoxigenic *E. coli* are an important cause of travellers' diarrhoea, enteropathogenic *E. coli* are an important cause of childhood diarrhoea, enteroinvasive *E. coli* cause a disease that is similar to shigella-like dysentery, enteroaggregative *E. coli* have been associated with diarrhoeal disease in infants and travellers, and enterohaemorrhagic *E. coli* are associated with haemorrhagic colitis and haemolytic uraemic syndrome.

Of the latter, currently the most important is verocytoxin (VT) producing *E. coli* O157. It is now a major foodborne public health problem, with one outbreak in central Scotland in 1996 resulting in 500 cases and 20 deaths.[23] Diarrhoea caused by VTEC O157 is often accompanied by bleeding or haemorrhagic colitis and may be complicated by haemolytic uraemic syndrome (HUS) or thrombotic thrombocytopenic purpura.[25] HUS is most likely in children under 5 years and is a major cause of renal failure in children.

*E. coli* O157 is part of the normal gut flora of cattle primarily, and to a lesser extent sheep. Raw or undercooked minced beef or cooked meats cross-contaminated from raw meat are the high risk foods.[25–27] However, any food that could possibly be contaminated with ruminant faeces poses a risk and infections have been associated with vegetables, cheese, milk, fruit juice, and water. The organism is not particularly heat-resistant and is easily killed by cooking; however the low infective dose means that foods must be cooked thoroughly and be protected post-cooking from cross-contamination with raw foods. *E. coli* O157 first came to prominence as a human pathogen in 1982.[28] In addition to the foodborne route, infections are transmitted by the person to person route, particularly in nurseries and old people's homes, and by direct contact with farm animals.[26] Nobody knows where this strain of *E. coli* came from and, more worryingly, nobody knows where it is going to, as the incidence is increasing in many countries including the United Kingdom where rates of infection vary geographically. In 1996 the highest rate of infection was seen in

> **Low infectious dose of verocytotoxigenic *E. coli* (VTEC)**
>
> The number of VTEC required to cause illness is very low. The precise infectious dose is not known but it has been reported to be as low as 10 cells. VTEC can survive the high acidity of the stomach and with such small numbers, infection can occur without any growth of the bacteria in food.[24,25]

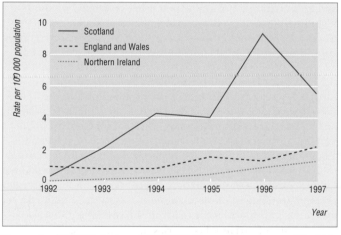

Human *E. coli* O157 infections: UK 1992-97 (Source: Department of Health)

Scotland with a rate of 9.25 per 100 000 population compared with 1.27 in England and Wales and 0.85 in Northern Ireland.

## Listeria monocytogenes

*L. monocytogenes* causes serious human illness such as perinatal infections, septicaemia, and meningitis. In pregnant women it can cause a flu-like illness, which can result in miscarriage, stillbirth or birth of a severely ill infant. More recently, it has been recognised that *L. monocytogenes* can cause mild gastrointestinal symptoms. Listeriosis is a comparatively rare but very serious human illness with a case fatality ratio of ~20%. Highly susceptible individuals include pregnant women, neonates, elderly people and immunocompromised individuals. *L. monocytogenes* is ubiquitous in the environment and so can be transferred to foods from a wide variety of sources. Foods associated with transmission are characteristically highly processed, have extended shelf lives at refrigeration temperatures, are capable of supporting the growth of *L. monocytogenes* and are consumed without further cooking. *L. monocytogenes* is psychrotrophic, —that is, potentially capable of growing, albeit slowly, at refrigeration temperatures as low as 0°C.[1]

## Clostridium botulinum

*C. botulinum* produces a neurotoxin which is one of the most poisonous substances known to man. Foodborne botulism occurs when food becomes contaminated with spores from the environment, which are not destroyed by initial cooking or processing. If the food provides a suitable environment for growth the spores will germinate leading to toxin production. The toxin itself is heat sensitive and so a further heat treatment of the food would prevent illness. Botulism can be prevented by using food preservation methods that are designed to inhibit the growth of *C. botulinum*. For example, low acid food, (pH > 4.4) canned foods are heat treated to 121°C for three minutes (known as the "botulism cook") or equivalent.[1]

## Parasites

Foodborne parasitic diseases are a major public health problem that affects millions of people, predominantly in non-industrialised countries. The incidence of parasitic disease associated with the consumption of foods of animal origin has declined in industrialised countries in recent years, where improvements in animal husbandry and meat inspection have led to considerable safety and quality gains. The situation in non-industrialised countries is very different in that these diseases are associated with poor standards of sanitation and hygiene, low educational standards, and extreme poverty.

Parasites are organisms that live on other living organisms known as hosts. They may be transmitted from animals to humans, from humans to humans, or from humans to animals. Foodborne parasitic disease occurs when the infective stages of parasites are eaten in raw or partially cooked protein foods, or in raw vegetables and fruits that are inadequately washed prior to consumption. These organisms then live and reproduce within the tissues and organs of infected human and animal hosts, and are often excreted in faeces. The parasites involved in foodborne disease usually have complex life cycles involving one or two intermediate hosts. The foodborne parasites known to cause disease in man are broadly classified as helminths (multicellular worms) and protozoa (single-celled microscopic organisms). These include the major helminthic groups of trematodes, nematodes, and cestodes and some of the emerging protozoan pathogens, such as cryptosporidia and cyclospora. The illnesses they can cause range from mild discomfort to debilitating illness and possibly death.[1,27,29]

---

**Individuals highly susceptible to listeriosis include**
- Pregnant women
- Neonates
- Elderly people
- Immunocompromised individuals

---

**Foodborne parasitic diseases**

Foodborne parasitic diseases are a major public health problem that affect millions of people, predominately in non-industrialised countries. The incidence of parasitic disease associated with the consumption of foods of animal origin has declined in industrialised countries in recent years, where improvements in animal husbandry and meat inspection have led to considerable safety and quality gains. The situation in non-industrialised countries is very different in that these diseases are associated with poor standards of sanitation and hygiene, low educational standards and extreme poverty.

## Principal foodborne parasites[1,27,29]

| Parasite | Food involved in transmission to man | Pathogenesis |
|---|---|---|
| **(a) Helminths** | | |
| (i) Trematodes | | |
| *Opisthorchis* (liver fluke) | Many species of freshwater fish including the family *Cyprinidae* (for example whitefish, carp, tench) Ingestion of infective larvae (metacercariae) in fish muscle and subcutaneous tissue | The liver flukes, *Opisthorchis viverrini*, *O. felineus* and *Clonorchis sinensis*, are biologically similar, foodborne trematodes which chronically infect the bile ducts and, more rarely, the pancreatic duct and gallbladder of human beings and other mammals |
| *Clonorchis* (liver fluke) | Many species (ca. 110) of freshwater fish, mainly *Cyprinidae* (carp, roach, dace). Ingestion of infective larvae (metacercariae) in fish muscle | |
| *Paragonimus* (lung fluke) | Raw, salted or partially cooked flesh of fresh and brackish-water crabs, crayfish and shrimps. (Wild boar meat suspected as a source of infection) | Paragonimiasis—symptoms include cough, hemoptysis and pleuritic chest pain |
| (ii) Cestodes (tape worm) | | Symptoms commonly are trivial or absent. Where worms attach to the jejunum patients develop B-12 deficiency anaemia. Massive infections may be associated with diarrhoea, obstruction of the bile duct or intestine and toxic symptoms |
| *Diphyllobothrium* | Humans acquire infection by eating raw or inadequately cooked fish | |
| (iii) Nematodes (round worm) | | |
| *Anisakis* | Humans acquire infection by eating raw or lightly cooked fish | Usually manifests as cramping, abdominal pain and vomiting |
| **(b) Protozoa** | | |
| *Giardia intestinalis* | Transmission is foodborne, waterborne (faecally contaminated food or water) or person to person spread | Chronic diarrhoea, malabsorption, weight loss |
| *Toxoplasma gondii* | Transmission is foodborne (from raw or inadequately cooked infected meat) waterborne or by faecal-oral route (infected cats) | Mostly asymptomatic. In severe cases: hepatitis, pneumonia, blindness, severe neurological disorders. Can also be transmitted transplacentally resulting in a spontaneous abortion, a stillborn, mental/physical retardation |
| *Cryptosporidium parvum* | Transmission is foodborne, waterborne, animal-person or by faecal-oral route | Often asymptomatic Abdominal cramps, vomiting, weight loss, diarrhoea |

*Cryptosporidium*

*Cryptosporidium parvum* is a coccidian protozoan parasite which was identified as an important human pathogen in 1976. Infection rates in the United Kingdom show variation in both age and seasonal distribution. The age distribution reflects endemicity; few infections occur under the age of 1 year, probably due to passive maternal immunity and protection from exposure to the environment. An almost logarithmic increase is observed in toddlers and young children, moderately high rates in young adults, and few cases after the age of 40 years. Seasonal peaks occur in the spring and late autumn. Cryptosporidiosis is a zoonoses with its primary reservoir in calves and lambs. The oocysts are resistant to chlorination and outbreaks associated with drinking water and swimming pools are common.[30,31] Cryptosporidium is highlighted here because it can contaminate the public water supply and extensive outbreaks of gastroenteritis can result.[30] Transmission can also occur by direct contact with animals and by the person to person route. Before the advent of effective antiretroviral therapy, cryptosporidiosis in patients infected with HIV was life threatening.

**Viral gastroenteritis (see box on page 96)**
Although primarily transmitted by the person to person route, transmission by the food or waterborne route has been documented for astrovirus and calicivirus (human calicivirus

and Norwalk-like virus).[32] Norwalk-like virus, also known as Small Round Structured Virus (SRSV), is the most commonly identified foodborne virus.[33] Humans are the reservoir for SRSV and shellfish, particularly oysters grown in sewage-contaminated water, are a source of infection. Infected foodhandlers are another source and can contaminate food during preparation. Aerosolisation of vomitus-containing virus particles has been proposed as a mode of transmission of the virus and may also be a source of food contamination. Clinical and epidemiological features, including stool culture negative for bacteria, duration of illness 12-60 hours, incubation period 24-48 hours and vomiting in >50% of cases, can assist in making the diagnosis when no laboratory results are available.[34] Sensitive detection assays have now revealed that shedding of the virus in faeces may continue for up to a week after the illness subsides.

# Principal chemicals affecting food safety

## Pesticide residues

Pesticides are chemicals or biological products used to control harmful or undesired organisms and plants, or to regulate the growth of plants as crop protection agents.

Pesticides can also be toxic to humans since certain biochemical pathways are relatively conserved across species as are some enzymes and hormones. In the context of food safety, exposure to pesticides is classified as acute or chronic. An acute intoxication usually has an immediate effect on the body whilst a chronic effect may reveal itself over the life span. The severity depends on the dose and the toxicity of the pesticide compound or breakdown product. Toxic effects that have been identified can include enzyme inhibition, endocrine disruption, and carcinogenic action, depending on the compound in question.

In Europe the control of pesticides is based on Council Directive No 91/414/EEC. Under this regulation, pesticides must be evaluated for safety based on dossiers prepared by their manufacturers. If a pesticide is accepted it is placed on a positive list with a maximum residue limit (MRL) assigned to it.

## Veterinary drug residues

Veterinary drugs include antibacterial compounds, hormones and non-steroidal anti-inflammatory preparations. As animal husbandry practices have intensified over the past few decades, antibacterial substances have been increasingly used as growth promoters to increase feed conversion efficiency and for prophylaxis and therapy to prevent outbreaks and treat disease. Similarly, hormones are administered to increase growth rate and meat yield.

The excessive use of antibacterial compounds in animal husbandry has raised concerns about the development of resistant bacteria and the effect that this may have on the usefulness of antibiotics in human medicine. There have also been concerns about the risk of allergic reactions in humans to antibacterial residues in food of animal origin.[1]

## Environmental/industrial contaminants

This group of contaminants are of environmental origin or are by-products of industrial processes. Polyhalogenated hydrocarbons (PHH) are a category of environmental contaminants that includes toxophene, dioxins, and polychlorinated biphenyls (PCBs). Certain PHH are manufactured for use in plastics, paints, transformers, and herbicides although their use is now either banned or severely

---

**Pesticide residues in food[1]**

- Insecticides
- Fungicides
- Herbicides
- Rodenticides
- Molluscicides
- Plant growth regulators

---

**Main types of veterinary drugs[1]**

| *Antibacterial compounds* | *Hormones* |
|---|---|
| • Aminoglycosides | • β-agonists |
| • β-lactams | • Resorcylic lactones |
| • Fluoroquinolones | • Steroids |
| • Macrolides | • Stilbenes |
| • Sulphonamides | • Thyrostat |
| • Tetracyclines | |
| • Quinolones | |

---

restricted. In most industrialised nations the compounds have become ubiquitous in the environment. Hence contamination of the food chain is inevitable and it has been estimated that in Western industrialised countries, 90% of human exposure is through ingestion of contaminated foods like fish and milk.

Foods that are rich sources of fats and oils tend to accumulate PHH because the compounds are lipophilic and bioaccumulate in lipid rich tissues and fluids. Oily fish from areas such as the Baltic Sea, where levels of PHH in the water are high, may contain elevated levels of these contaminants. Similarly, cows that graze on polluted pasture can accumulate unacceptable concentrations of PHH in their milk. A recent incident in Belgium introduced PCBs and dioxins into the food chain via contaminated animal feed resulting from the accidental incorporation of industrial oil into the feed ration.[1]

# Prevention and control of foodborne infectious disease

If the incidence of food poisoning is to be reduced, everyone from primary producers, workers throughout the industry to consumers has a role to play. Farms are the reservoir for many foodborne pathogens and these harmful microbes need to be controlled in livestock. Best husbandry practices will assist farmers to deliver livestock and produce free of pathogens and residues to the next link in the chain. Processors must have rigid process controls to ensure that the food is produced with safety paramount. The distribution, wholesale and retail networks must adhere to the best hygienic practices so that food is delivered to the point of sale in the best possible condition.

Modern food control programmes take consideration of the role of the food producers and food processors in managing the safety of their products. The various sectors of food production, processing and distribution possess knowledge about the safety and shelf-life of their products and have an important role in assisting regulators in achieving national food safety goals. One of the most effective ways for the food sector to protect the health of consumers is to base their food safety management programmes on the seven principles of the Hazard Analysis Critical Control Point (HACCP) system. European food hygiene law requires that food businesses identify the steps in their activities which are critical to ensuring food safety and make certain that adequate safety procedures are identified, implemented, maintained and reviewed.

Even with the best control measures in place a proportion of raw meat and poultry may contain harmful microbes. Food handlers, whether working in the commercial setting or in a domestic kitchen, must be aware of this and take appropriate hygienic precautions.

Raising awareness through continuous innovative education programmes for everyone from consumers including school children to workers throughout the food industry is the mainstay for reducing the incidence of foodborne infectious diseases. Foodhandlers must be aware of their responsibility to handle food hygienically. Infected humans are the reservoir for typhoidal salmonellas and SRSV but can potentially spread any infection by contaminating food during preparation if their personal hygiene is poor. Symptomatic individuals should be excluded from preparing food until they have been at least 48 hours symptom free for most microbes, and until microbiological clearance has been confirmed if infected with enteric salmonellas and VTEC.[35] Any individual incapable of

---

**The seven basic principles of a HACCP system***

1. Conduct a hazard analysis.
2. Determine the Critical Control Points (CCPs) in the process.
3. Establish critical limit(s) for each CCP.
4. Establish a monitoring programme to ensure control of the CCP.
5. Establish corrective action to be taken when monitoring indicates that a CCP is not under control.
6. Establish verification procedures to demonstrate the effectiveness of the HACCP system.
7. Establish documentation concerning all procedures and records appropriate to these principles and their application.

*HACCP means Hazard Analysis and Critical Control Points. It is a systematic approach to identifying and controlling hazards (microbiological, chemical, and physical) that could pose a threat to the production of safe food—in simple terms, it involves identifying what could go wrong and planning to prevent it.

---

**Prevention of food poisoning outbreaks[19]**

The same four readily preventable faults repeatedly contribute to outbreaks in food poisoning:

- grossly contaminated raw product
- inadequate refrigeration allowing harmful microbes to multiply at warm temperatures to dangerous levels
- cross contamination from raw to cooked food
- insufficient heat treatment when cooking[19]

practising basic personal hygiene should be excluded from working with food.

The table on page 106 provides a list of useful websites.

# New variant Creutzfeldt–Jakob disease (nvCJD): is it a foodborne disease?

The magnitude of the epidemic of bovine spongiform encephalopathy (BSE) in the United Kingdom is without precedent in the recorded history of the transmissible spongiform encephalopathies. The public health and the scientific issues have become entwined in the political and commercial response, to increasing national and international concern over the possibility of transmission of spongiform encephalopathy from cattle to man. Medical practitioners and other public health professionals are having to respond to the intense public anxiety regarding the risk of exposure to BSE contaminated material. Documented transmission of BSE to non-human primates indicates that such anxiety is not without some scientific foundation.[36] We are left facing possible present consequences of past events over which we now have no control.

In March 1996 the UK CJD Surveillance Unit described a distinct variant of CJD in 10 people aged under 42 (average age 27 years) with dates of illness since January 1995.[37] This variant had not been previously recognised and is characterised by behavioural change, ataxia, progressive cognitive impairment, and a prolonged duration of illness (up to 23 months) compared to classical CJD. In addition the EEG is not typical of classical CJD and the brain pathology, although showing marked spongiform change and extensive amyloid plaques, is also not typical. The most striking features of these cases are the extensive plaque formation and a pattern of prion protein immunostaining which is unique and remarkably consistent between cases. After reviewing the data on these variant CJD cases the UK Spongiform Encephalopathy Advisory Committee (SEAC) advised the British Government "that in the absence of any credible alternative, the most likely explanation at present is that these cases are linked to exposure to BSE material before the Specified Bovine Offal (SBO) ban was introduced in 1989".[38] The SBO ban prohibits the use of those tissues (brain, spinal cord, thymus, tonsils, spleen, and intestine) most likely to contain the infective agent of BSE in products for human consumption.

Ten nvCJD cases were announced in March 1996. By the end of June 2002, a total of 124 cases of nvCJD (number of deaths from definite or probable nvCJD: 115, number of probable nvCJD cases still alive: 9) had been reported in the United Kingdom. The overall median age at death was 28 (range 14-74 years). The median number of days from onset to diagnosis was 334 days and from onset to death 411 days. Of the 124 cases, 68 (55%) were male. The recent analyses showed that the underlying incidence is increasing by an estimated 18% per year based on date of symptom onset, or 20% per year based on date of death.[41] In relation to the number of nvCJD cases in countries other than the United Kingdom, as in March 2002 there were five definite and probable cases of nvCJD in France, one in Italy,[42] one in the Republic of Ireland and one in Hong Kong (reported to be associated with the United Kingdom).[43] With a possible incubation period of up to 25 years, nobody knows how many people in the United Kingdom and elsewhere worldwide may be currently incubating this new variant CJD. If further cases continue to appear, we could be witnessing the unfolding of one of the greatest man-made public health catastrophes ever.

## Possible vehicles associated with principal aetiological agents of food poisoning

| Aetiology | Principal possible vehicles |
| --- | --- |
| *Bacillus* species | Reheated rice |
| *Campylobacter* | Poultry, raw milk, water |
| *Clostridium perfringens* | Cooked red meat and poultry |
| *Clostridium botulinum* | Canned products, honey |
| *Cryptosporidium* | Water |
| *E. coli* (non-VTEC) | Salads, raw milk, vegetables, cheese, water |
| *E. coli* (VTEC) | Undercooked meat, unpasteurised milk and cheese, vegetables, water |
| Hepatitis A | Seafood, water, (any food contaminated by infected food handler) |
| *Listeria monocytogenes* | Cheese, paté |
| Salmonella (non-typhoid) | Poultry, eggs, red meat, dairy products |
| Salmonella (typhoid) | Water, (any food contaminated by sewage or infected food handler) |
| Scombrotoxin | Mackerel, tuna, and other scromboid fish |
| *Staph. aureus* | Food contaminated by infected food handler |
| SRSV | Oysters and other seafood (any food contaminated by infected food handler) |

Adapted from Department of Health (2000)[5]

## Factors reported to BSE agent support the responsibility for nvCJD in humans

There are several factors supporting the hypothesis that the BSE agent is responsible for the emergence of the new form of CJD in humans. These include:

- the temporal association—BSE came first followed by nvCJD
- the geographical association—the UK has had the bulk of the BSE cases and the majority of the nvCJD cases
- a report describing similar clinical, molecular, and neuropathological features in three BSE experimentally infected macaque monkeys[39]
- molecular typing of prion proteins from cases of BSE and nvCJD has revealed that they are indistinguishable from each other and different from sporadic CJD cases, supporting the hypothesis of a causal link[40]

## Useful web addresses

### Bulletins of foodborne diseases and communicable diseases

| | |
|---|---|
| Insititute de Veille Sanitaire | http://www.invs.sante.fr/ |
| EPI-Insight, National Disease Surveillance Centre, Ireland | http://www.ndsc.ie/Publications/EPI-Insight/ |
| Canada Communicable Disease Report | http://www.hc-sc.gc.ca/pphb-dgspsp/publicat/ccdr-rmtc/ |
| Communicable Disease Report, Public Health Laboratory Service, UK | http://www.phls.co.uk/publications/cdr/index.html |
| Communicable Diseases Intelligence, Australia | http://www.health.gov.au/pubs/cdi/cdihtml.htm |
| EuroSurveillance, European Union | http://www.eurosurveillance.org/eurosurv/index.htm |
| Infectious Agents Surveillance Report, NIH, Japan | http://www.nih.go.jp/ |
| Jaargang nummer Infectieziekten bulletin, the Netherlands | http://www.isis.rivm.nl/inf_bul/home_bul.html |
| Kansanterveyslaitos, Finland | http://www.ktl.fi/ |
| NSW Public Health Bulletin, NSW, Australia | http://www.health.nsw.gov.au/public-health/phb/phb.html |
| EPI-News, Statens Serum Institut, Denmark | http://www.ssi.dk/en/index.html |
| Weekly epidemiological report, WHO | http://www.who.int/wer |

### Food science, technology, food safety and public health

| | |
|---|---|
| Institute of Food Science and Technology | http://www.ifst.org/ |
| FoodNet, Canada | http://foodnet.fic.ca/ |
| International Food Information Council Foundation, USA | http://www.ific.org |
| National Food Safety Database, University of Florida, USA | http://www.foodsafety.org/ |
| Institute of Food Science and Technology | http://www.ifst.org.uk |
| Campden and Chorleywood Food Research Association | http://www.campden.co.uk |
| Leatherhead Food Research Association | http://www.lfra.co.uk |
| Food Communications Information Service, UCC | http://www.ucc.ie/fcis |
| Institute of Food Research | http://www.ifr.bbsrc.ac.uk |

### National and international food safety agencies

| | |
|---|---|
| Food and Agriculture Organization of United Nations (FAO) | http://www.fao.org/ |
| Organization for Economic Co-operation and Development (OECD) | http://www.oecd.org/EN/home/0,,EN-home-0-nodirectorate no-no-no-0,FF html |
| The Joint FAO/WHO Food Standards Program (Codex Alimentarius Commission) | http://www.codexalimentarius.net/ |
| World Health Organization, Food Safety Program | http://www.who.int/fsf/ |
| Food Standards Australia New Zealand (FSANZ) | http://www.foodstandards.gov.au |
| | http://www.foodstandards.govt.nz |
| The Danish Veterinary and Food Administration | http://www.lst.min.dk/java_enab/f_uk.html |
| Communicable Disease Surveillance Centre (CDSC) | http://www.phls.co.uk/ |
| Department of Health, UK | http://www.doh.gov.uk/ |
| Food Standards Agency, UK | http://www.foodstandards.gov.uk/ |
| INED "Mortalité, santé, épidémiologie", France | http://matisse.ined.fr/~mesle/ |
| Institut Pasteur, France | http://www.pasteur.fr/externe |
| Agence française de sécurité sanitaire des aliments (AFSSA), France | http://www.afssa.fr/ |
| Department for Environment, Food and Rural Affairs, UK | http://www.defra.gov.uk/ |
| Directorate-General, Health and Consumer Protection, European Union | http://europa.eu.int/comm/dgs/health_consumer/index_en.htm |
| Food Safety Authority of Ireland | http://www.fsai.ie |
| National Institute of Public Health and the Environment (RIVM), the Netherlands | http://www.rivm.nl/ |
| Canadian Food Inspection Agency (CFIA), Canada | http://www.inspection.gc.ca/english/toce.shtml |
| Center for Disease Control and Prevention (CDC), USA | http://www.cdc.gov/ |
| Food and Drug Administration (FDA), USA | http://vm.cfsan.fda.gov/ |
| Food Safety and Inspection Service (FSIS), USA | http://www.fsis.usda.gov/ |
| National Institutes of Health (NIH), USA | http://www.nih.gov/ |
| United States Department of Agriculture (USDA), USA | http://www.usda.gov/ |

# Conclusion

As society changes, so do the bacteria involved in foodborne disease and this trend is likely to continue. The globalisation of our food supply poses greater risks to consumer health from the mass production and distribution of foods and increased risk for food contamination. If the regulators and all stakeholders in the food production chain are to ensure that consumers' health is adequately protected and that they are provided with the reassurances that they are seeking, then issues such as BSE, dioxin contamination, antibiotic resistant bacteria, *Salmonella enteritidis* in poultry, *E. coli* O157, and the increasing incidence of campylobacter infection will have to be dealt with. The solution is sequential incremental risk reduction along the food chain with all stakeholders playing their part; also, the communication of any unavoidable residual risk to consumers with clear instructions on how to manage such risks. While there are specific control programmes required, and more research and surveillance needed to understand the epidemiology of different agents, increased hygiene standards across the food chain will have the effect of reducing foodborne disease.

The authors acknowledge the work of Dr David Thomkins, Consultant Microbiologist, Public Health Laboratory Leeds and his colleagues on the National Infectious Intestinal Diseases Study[5] team, in preparing the tables: Bacterial pathogens, protozoal pathogens, and viral pathogens.

## References

1 Reilly A, Tlustos C, Anderson W, O'Connor L, Foley B, Wall PG. Food safety: A public health issue of growing importance. In: Gibney MJ, Vorster HH, Kok FJ (eds). *Introduction to Human Nutrition, 2002*. USA: Blackwell Science Publishing Company, 2002.

2 Killalea D, Ward LR, Roberts D *et al*. International epidemiological and microbiological study of outbreak of *Salmonella agona* infection from ready to eat savoury snack. 1 England and Wales and United States. *BMJ* 1996; **313**: 1093-4.

3 US Bureau of the Census, International Population Reports, *An Aging World II*. US Government Printing Office, Washington DC, USA. 1992; **25**: 92-3.

4 Department of Health. *A report of the study of infectious intestinal disease in England*. London: Stationery Office, 2000.

5 Department of Health. *Management of outbreaks of foodborne illness*. London: Department of Health, 1994.

6 Wall PG, de Louvois J, Gilbert RJ, Rowe B. Food poisoning: notifications, laboratory reports and outbreaks: where do the statistics come from and what do they mean? CDR. *Communicable Dis Rep* **4**: R130-5.

7 Feldman RA, Banatvala N. The frequency of culturing stools from adults with diarrhoea in Great Britain. *Epidemiol Inf* 1994; **113**: 41-4.

8 Mead PS, Slutsker L, Dietz V *et al*. Food-related illness and death in the United States. *Emerg Infect Dis* 1999; **5**: 607-25.

9 Skirrow MB. Campylobacter enteritis: a new disease. *BMJ* 1997; **2**: 9-11.

10 Healing TD, Greenwood M, Pearson AD. Campylobacters and enteritis. *Rev Med Microbiol* 1992; **3**: 159-67.

11 Peabody RG, Ryan MJ, Wall PG. Outbreaks of campylobacter infection: rare events for a common pathogen. *Communicable Dis Rep* 1997; **7**: R33-7.

12 Humphrey TJ, Henley A, Lanning DG. The colonisation of broiler chickens with *Campylobacter jejuni*: some epidemiological investigations. *Epidemiol Infect* 1993; **110**: 601-7.

13 Djuretic T, Wall PG, Nichols G. General outbreaks of infectious intestinal disease associated with milk and dairy products in England and Wales: 1992-1996. *Communicable Dis Rep* 1997; **7**: R41-5.

14 Palmer SR, Gully PR, White JM *et al*. Water-borne outbreak of Campylobacter gastro-enteritis. *Lancet* 1983; **i**: 287-90.

15 Hudson SJ, Lightfoot NF, Coulson JC, Russell K, Sisson PR, Sobo AO. Jackdaws and magpies as vectors of milk borne human Campylobacter infection. *Epidemiol Infect* 1991; **107**: 363-72.

16 Food Safety Authority of Ireland. *Control of Campylobacter species in the food chain*. Report, Food Safety Authority of Ireland, Dublin, 2002.

17 Coyle E, Palmer S, Ribeiro C *et al*. *Salmonella enteritidis* phage type 4 infection: association with hens' eggs. *Lancet* 1988; **ii**: 1295-6.

18 Humphrey TJ. Contamination of egg shells and contents with *Salmonella enteritidis*: a review. *Int J Food Microbiol* 1994; **21**: 31-40.

19 Cowden JM, Wall PG, Adak G, Evans H, Le Baigue S, Ross D. Outbreak of foodborne infectious intestinal disease in England and Wales: 1992-1993. *Communicable Dis Rep* 1995; **5**: R109-17.

20 Ward LR, Threlfall EJ, O'Brien SJ. *The changing trends of salmonellosis in England and Wales*. Proceedings of the International Symposium on Salmonella and Salmonellosis, St. Brieuc, France, May 2002; pp. 393-6.

21 Threlfall EJ, Ward LR, Rowe B. Increasing incidence of resistance to trimethoprim and ciprofloxacin in epidemic *Salmonella typhimurium* DT104 in England and Wales. *Eurosurveillance* 1997; **2**: 81-4.

22 World Health Organization. *Medical impact of the use of antimicrobial drugs in food animals*. Report. Geneva: WHO, 1997.

23 The Pennington Group. *Report on the circumstances leading to the 1996 outbreak of infection with E. coli O157 in Central Scotland, the implications for food safety and the lessons to be learned*. Edinburgh: Stationery Office, 1997.

24 Doyle MP, Zhao T, Meng J, Zhao S. *Escherichia coli* O157:H7. In: Doyle MP, Beuchat LR, Montville TJ (eds). *Food Microbiology: Fundamentals and Frontiers*. Washington DC: ASM Press 1997, 171–91.

25 Food Safety Authority of Ireland. *The Prevention of E. coli O157:H7 Infection—A Shared Responsibility*. Report, Dublin: Food Safety Authority of Ireland, 1999.

26 Wall PG, Mcdonnell RJ, Adak GK, Cheasty T, Smith HR, Rowe B. General outbreaks of verocytotoxin producing *Escherichia coli* O157 in England and Wales from 1992-1994. *Communicable Dis Rep CDR Rev* 1996; **6**: R26-R33.

27 Reilly A, Käferstein F. Food safety and products from aquaculture. *J Appl Microbiol, Symposium Supplement* 1999; **85**: S249-57.

28 Riley LW, Remis RS, Helgerson SD *et al*. Haemorrhagic colitis associated with a rare *Escherichia coli* serotype. *N Engl J Med* 1983; **308**: 681-5.

29 Benenson AS. Control of communicable disease manual, *An Official Report of the American Public Health Association* 1995; American Public Health Association, Washington DC, USA.

30 Richardson AJ, Frankenburg RA, Buck AC *et al*. An outbreak of waterborne cryptosporidiosis in Swindon and Oxfordshire. *Epidemiol Infect* 1991; **107**: 485-95.

31 Smith HV. Environmental aspects of *Cryptosporidium* species: a review. *J R Soc Med* 1990; **83**: 629-31.

32 Hedberg CW, Osterholm MT. Outbreaks of foodborne and waterborne viral gastroenteritis. *Clin Microbiol Rev* 1993; **6**: 199-210.

33 Luthi TM, Wall PG, Evans HS, Caul EO. Outbreaks of foodborne and waterborne viral gastroenteritis in England and Wales: 1992-1994. *Communicable Dis Rep CDR Rev* 1996; **6**: R131-6.

34 Kaplan JE, Feldman R, Campbell DS, Lookabaugh C, William CG. The frequency of a Norwalk like pattern of illness in outbreaks of acute gastro-enteritis. *Am J Public Health* 1982; **72**: 1329-32.

35 Anon. The prevention of human transmission of gastrointestinal infections, infestations and bacterial intoxications. *Communicable Dis Rep* 1995; **5**: R158-72.

36 Baker HF, Ridley RM, Wells GAH. Experimental transmission of BSE and scrapie to the common marmoset. *Vet Rec* 1993; **132**: 406.

37 Will RG, Ironside JW, Zeidler M *et al*. A new variant of Creutzfeldt–Jakob disease in the UK. *Lancet* 1996; **347**: 921-5.

38 Calman K. New variant of Creutzfeldt–Jakob Disease (CJD). London: Department of Health 1996. PL/CMO (96)5.

39 Lasmezas CI, Deslys JP, Demaimay R *et al*. BSE transmission to macaques. *Nature* 1996; 381: 743-4.

40 Collinge J, Sidle KCL, Meads J, Ironside J, Hill AF. Molecular analysis of prion strain variation and the aetiology of new variant CJD. *Nature* 1996; **383**: 685-90.

41 Andrews N. Incidence trends and short term predictions for variant Creutzfeldt-Jakob disease in the United Kingdom—update. *Eurosurveillance Weekly* 2002; **6**: 020725.

42 Salmaso S. First case of vCJD reported in Italy. *Eurosurveillance Weekly* 2002; **6** (6), 020207.

43 Food Standards Agency. Minutes of the UK Food Standards Agency Board Meeting, 14th of March 2002, Exeter, UK. FSA paper number 02/05/01.

# 15   Food sensitivity

One man's meat is another's poison
                              Lucretius 96-55 BC

In affluent countries the idea is now widespread that a variety of symptoms (not just those of classical allergy) are caused by individual (hyper)sensitivity to certain foods or substances in them; that such sensitivity has become more common; and that food processing may have something to do with it. The media, various unorthodox practitioners, and some groups of lay people have spread the "news". Medical practitioners meanwhile are equipped with little information, most of it confusing, and no reliable diagnostic test to answer their patients' needs.

This is one of the most polarised topics in human nutrition. On one hand many lay people are concerned about sensitivity to food and believe that they suffer from it. On the other hand the medical and food science establishment has been fairly dismissive and declares that most food sensitivity (except adult lactase insufficiency) is uncommon.

The subject is at the interface between scientific immunology, food technology, and quackery. Good clinical research has been lacking, but recently a few academic departments have started to apply the methods of clinical science to unravel this confusing area. At present it is impossible to give estimates of the objectively confirmed prevalence of most types of sensitivity to food.

## A little epidemiology

Young et al.[1] sent questionnaires to 15 000 households, half across the UK, half in their local (High Wycombe) area. 20% of individuals who replied said they had some form of food intolerance. Those who did and were living locally were asked further standard questions. About half had relevant symptoms and some of them agreed to take eight, double-blind, placebo-controlled challenges with cows' milk, egg, wheat, soya, orange, prawns, nuts, and chocolate (disguised in cans of cornflour and suitable flavouring). Each challenge was taken for three days, followed by three days of placebo in random order. Nearly a quarter reacted. From this painstaking work the authors estimated that 2% of British adults have objectively verifiable sensitivity to the eight foods, and a few more may be sensitive to other foods less commonly reported in their questionnaire.

In children 5-7%[2] and 4-10%[3] are estimated to have allergy to one or more foods. This is most prevalent in the first three years of life and fades as children grow older for most foods but not usually for peanuts.

## Terminology

The words describing food sensitivity are imprecise and often used to mean different things.

- **Food allergy** is commonly used by lay people (and by doctors talking to patients) as the broad term, including non-immunological (and sometimes even psychosomatic) reactions. In technical communication the term 'allergy' should be confined to immunological reactions.[4-6]
- **Food sensitivity or hypersensitivity** is sometimes used in the narrow sense to mean only immunological reactions.
- **Adverse reaction to food** is not used in this chapter because it conveys no meaning of individual susceptibility and includes food poisoning (dealt with in chapter 14).
- **Pseudoallergic** and **anaphylactoid** reactions are used for, for example, asthma or angio-oedema after food with no immunological abnormalities detectable in the patient.
- **Food idiosyncrasy** is used in some classifications for non-allergic food intolerance.

The classification shown opposite is developed from and compatible with the definitions in the report of the Royal College of Physicians.[5]

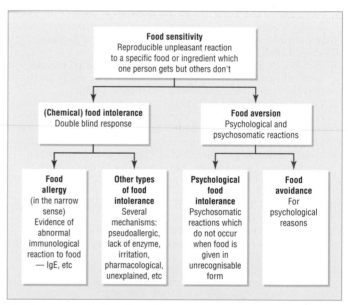

Classification of types of food sensitivity

## Diagnosis

Diagnosis of food sensitivity is easy when there is a characteristic early response to a food that is eaten at least occasionally. The patient often notices the association and its reproducibility and tells the doctor the diagnosis.

Diagnosis is more difficult, however, if the clinical reaction is delayed or varies or does not always happen, and if the food

## Four ways of presentation

- "Whenever I eat peanuts I get swollen lips, then itchy spots and I sometimes vomit"
- "I can't eat peanuts" (reason why, vague or based on a single episode long ago)
- "I wonder if this rash could be caused by something in my diet?"
- "I've given up eating peanuts because the lady in the health food shop (or the lady next door) says I must be allergic to them"

is eaten most days. Such reactions are also made more difficult to judge if someone else has already incriminated a food on circumstantial evidence or because of prejudice. There are no straightforward diagnostic tests for food sensitivity comparable with the electrocardiogram for coronary disease or the blood urea for renal failure.

**Skin tests**—Drops of extracts of one or more suspected food antigens are dropped on to the skin and the skin is then pricked or scratched through the drop. A positive response is a wheal and flare within 20 minutes. This indicates the ability of skin mast cells to degranulate in response to the antigen, because they have on their surface IgE specific to the food antigen. Reliability of the test result depends on the quality (specificity) and concentration of the antigen.

The **radioallergosorbent test** (RAST) is a radioimmunoassay performed on serum to show the presence of IgE specific for the food antigen. It is positive in association with IgE mediated food sensitivity.

The skin test and RAST are both sensitive and specific methods for detecting specific IgE, but they do need to be interpreted with care. The **presence** of IgE antibodies to a food does not mean that the patient is **clinically** allergic to it. Many atopic people have IgE antibodies but no symptoms, so positive results must be interpreted in conjunction with a careful history. Foods should not be restricted on the basis of a positive result if no clinical symptoms exist. On the other hand, a negative skin test (or RAST) result is good evidence that a reaction to food is **not** mediated by IgE. A negative skin test result does not exclude food sensitivity mediated by a mechanism other than the IgE immunological reaction.

### Dietary manipulation

The more general diagnostic procedure to indicate food sensitivity is dietary manipulation and recording of symptoms. Such procedures give diagnostic information in food sensitivity of all types. There are several strategies.

#### Diet diary

The patient or parent keeps a list of all foods eaten and notes any symptoms. This is simple and cheap and can be done at home for several weeks. It is liable to subjective bias, not suitable if the reaction was serious, and difficult to interpret if the responsible agent is present in several foods.

#### Temporary exclusion of one or a few suspected foods

Avoidance can be for about a week each time. This is an open trial, liable to subjective bias, but it causes little inconvenience. The method is not suitable if the reaction was serious. It is relatively easy to carry out for foods not eaten every day, such as strawberries and shellfish, but more difficult for wheat and milk, which are widely distributed in the diet.

#### Few foods (oligoantigenic) diet followed by reintroduction of foods one by one

All the foods that commonly provoke sensitivity reactions are eliminated from the diet for two or three weeks. One food is then added back every three to seven days. Elimination diets carry a risk of nutritional deficiency if taken for long or not properly managed.

#### Patient-blind or double-blind challenges

After the patient has been stabilised on a standard or elimination diet, foods or ingredients are given in capsules or incorporated into oligoantigenic masking foods. The patient is "blind" to what the foods are. Injection of adrenaline should be available if the reaction was of allergic type.

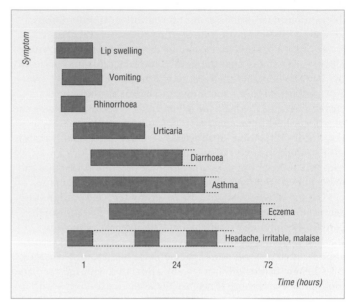

Time course of symptoms of intolerance[7]

### Responses expected with different types of food sensitivity

| Type of food sensitivity | Open trial | Blind trial | Immune response |
|---|---|---|---|
| Food allergy | + | + | + |
| Food intolerance | + | + | − |
| Psychosomatic | + | − | − |
| Food aversion | − | − | − |

### Few foods diets

- The meat least likely to cause reactions is *lamb*
- The least antigenic cereal is *rice*
- Vegetables: *peeled potatoes* and *lettuce*
- Fruits: *pears* (peeled)
- Fat: a refined vegetable *seed oil*, for example, (cold pressed) *sunflower* or *safflower*
- Drink: *water* and *sugar*
- If the diet continues for more than a week an uncoloured multivitamin supplement should be taken
- Other foods are included in some elimination diets, depending on the type of reaction and the suspected ingredients

# Clinical reactions

## Urticaria, angio-oedema and anaphylaxis

True food protein allergy, IgE mediated, is potentially the most serious sensitivity reaction to food, and the best understood. A small amount of ingested protein crosses the intestinal wall, and attaches to receptors on T lymphocytes. In an allergic response these secrete interleukin 4 which influences B lymphocytes to secrete IgE. Antibodies of this class bind to mast cells in the tissues and sensitise them. Then when the allergen contacts the sensitised mast cells they react by degranulation and liberation of histamine and other kinins. Reactions occur very quickly, starting with the oral allergy syndrome—lips, cheeks, tongue or throat swell and itch within minutes of contact with the food. Soon reactions may occur in the larynx (oedema, the most dangerous reaction), gastrointestinal tract (vomiting or diarrhoea), the skin (urticaria), and the bronchi (wheezing). Or several systems can be affected, with an acute drop of blood pressure and respiratory difficulty—**anaphylaxis**. Treatment of anaphylaxis is with prompt injection of adrenaline, followed by hydrocortisone.[8] For urticaria and other localised reaction the main line of treatment is with a non-sedative antihistamine.

Urticarial reactions can also be mediated without IgE, for example, be caused by eating large amounts of foods which contain histamine-releasing agents, such as, strawberries, shellfish, papaya, or those that contain histamine itself or other amines, such as some wines, fermented cheeses, and sausages.

**Chronic urticaria** is not usually associated with IgE-mediated food allergy and there is not usually a history linking it with a particular food. A minority of cases have been found sensitive to certain food additives—benzoic acid and compounds (E210, 211, 212, 213, 216, 218) or the azo dyes tartrazine (E102) or sunset yellow (E110).[10] This can be demonstrated by placebo-controlled challenge testing in a specialist clinic. Physical factors, for example, exercise and warmth, tend to cause urticaria on their own and may exacerbate a reaction to food.

## Asthma and rhinitis

Foods can precipitate some attacks of asthma in infancy but come well behind infections. The role of foods in asthma diminishes during childhood and it is an uncommon precipitant in adults. Inhalants, irritants, infections, pollens and moulds, changes in the weather, and exercise are then all more important. Food sensitivity asthma in adults is largely confined to those exposed to dusty grain, flour, coffee, etc, in their work.

Eggs, seafood, and nuts are among the foods most likely to provoke asthma in children. Skin tests are usually positive, indicating that IgE is implicated, but if the skin test is positive for a food in an asthmatic child, asthma may not follow a double blind challenge. In addition, the response to foods is sometimes psychosomatic.

The food preservatives sulphur dioxide ($SO_2$) and sodium metabisulphite can aggravate bronchospasm in established asthmatics. These patients are very sensitive to the irritant effect of $SO_2$ gas, which is liberated from sodium metabisulphite in acid foods and inhaled in low concentration as the food is swallowed.

## Eczema

Infantile eczema and flexural eczema in adults are associated with high serum titres of IgE and often with multiple positive skin tests. In infantile eczema the response to food taking or elimination is slower and less clear cut than in urticaria.

---

**Foods that can cause allergic reactions including anaphylaxis**

- Cows' milk (esp. young children)
- Hens' eggs (esp. young children)
- Peanuts
- Tree nuts: brazil, almond, hazel
- Fish
- Shellfish
- *Also* wheat, legumes (peas, soya), fruits (citrus, strawberries, apples), vegetables (tomato, celery), sesame, etc

**Peanuts** top the list of foods responsible for anaphylaxis. Most fatal reactions have occurred from foods eaten outside the sufferer's home. Waiters, hosts, and food-pack labels cannot always be relied on. People with peanut allergy must be constantly vigilant with any unfamiliar food and consider carrying self-injectable adrenaline. In atopic families the lactating mother should not eat peanuts (or products containing peanuts) herself or give any to the child for at least three years.[9]

---

**Foods likely to contain tartrazine (food colour E102) include:**

| | |
|---|---|
| • fruit squash and cordial | • instant puddings |
| • coloured fizzy drinks | • coloured sweets |
| • pickles | • filled chocolates |
| • bottled sauces | • jelly |
| • salad cream | • ice cream and lollies |
| • cakes (shop bought) | • jam |
| • cake mix | • marmalade |
| • soups (packets and tins) | • curry powder |
| • custard | • mustard |
| | • yoghurt |

Tartrazine is water soluble and gives a pleasant lemon yellow colour to foods. It is also used in some medicine capsules. Incidence of sensitivity appears to be between 1 in 10 000 and 1 in 1000.

Tartrazine is one of several permitted azo colours. It has been the most tested and incriminated in reactions, but some of the other colours (if eaten in comparable "dosage") might possibly cause reactions in the rare people who are sensitive to tartrazine.

---

**Foods likely to contain sulphur dioxide**

- Wines, chilled fruit juices
- Pickled onions, dried fruits
- Commercial precut chips
- Salads in salad bars*
- Fresh fruit salad in hotels*

*From "stay fresh" spray

---

Statistically significant responses to skin tests have been reported in infants apparently sensitive to a food—for example, exacerbation after milk or improvement after withdrawing egg. A controlled trial showed improvement in 14 out of 20 children with infantile eczema when egg and milk were removed. Elemental diets (glucose, oil, amino acid mixture, vitamins, and minerals), though expensive, have been helpful in severe infantile eczema. Breast feeding reduces the chance of eczema but only partly in babies with a strong atopic family history. In such cases the mother should avoid eating common allergenic foods.

In adults with eczema a response to few foods diets is less likely.

## Migraine

Tension, relaxation, menstruation, bright lights, and hypoglycaemia are among the major precipitants of migraine. Foods can also precipitate attacks. The different factors can be cumulative; several may be needed before an attack occurs. Attacks may come on many hours after eating a provoking food. Suggestibility and placebo effect have been well established in the responses of migraine sufferers.

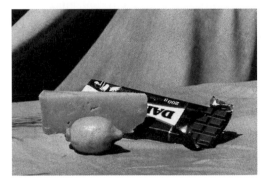
Foods reported to precipitate migraine

Chocolate, cheese, and citrus fruits are reported to precipitate migraine. They contain pressor amines—tyramine, phenylethylamine, and synephrine, respectively. Alcoholic drinks are another precipitant, notably related to cluster headaches: red wines and some other drinks contain histamine. Other attacks may come about from foods that produce nausea, such as fatty foods. Nitrates, found in some sausages, occasionally cause headaches ("hot dog headache").

True food allergy via IgE is not the usual mechanism in migraine. In a trial at Great Ormond Street, in children with severe recurrent migraine most recovered on an exclusion diet. Reintroduction of foods, first "open", later disguised, showed that cows' milk, eggs, chocolate, orange, and wheat were most likely to provoke an attack and tartrazine less commonly.

## Gastrointestinal reactions

Many different gastrointestinal sensitivity reactions to food are known and they can act through several different mechanisms. Early symptoms are lip swelling, tingling in the mouth or throat, and vomiting. Later symptoms include diarrhoea, bloating, or even steatorrhoea. Remote symptoms—urticaria, asthma, headache, joint pains—can be associated.

In young children immediate intolerance is not uncommon to cows' milk or egg white, nuts, seafood, and some fruits. Tolerance increases with age. Cows' milk allergy can produce a variety of effects, including gastrointestinal bleeding or protein losing enteropathy; eosinophilia may be present.

### Coeliac disease

Sensitivity to wheat gluten is the cause of coeliac disease with jejunal atrophy. It took from 1888, when coeliac disease was classically described, to 1953 before it was found that a fraction of wheat was responsible. A few other foods have been linked with occasional mucosal damage in children, such as cows' milk and soya. (See diets for gluten-sensitive enteropathy in chapter 13.)

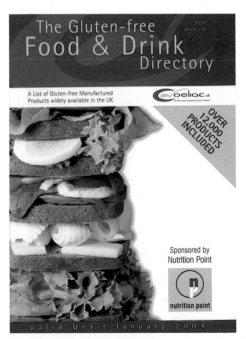
The Gluten-free Food & Drink directory (reproduced with permission from Coeliac UK)

### Infantile colic

When it occurs, this lasts for about the first three months. It occurs at least as often in breast fed as in bottle fed infants. In the former there is no consistent evidence that the colic is related to anything the mother eats.

### Irritable bowel syndrome

Evidence for food sensitivity in the irritable bowel syndrome is conflicting. One study, which performed exclusion and double-blind challenge, indicated that food sensitivity was common: wheat, dairy foods, maize, some fruits, tea, and coffee were mostly implicated. Another study could not show food sensitivity in most patients.

*Intestinal lactase insufficiency*
This is the rule in most adults of Asian and African origin and seen in a minority of white people. There is diarrhoea, abdominal distension, discomfort, and flatus after milk, but this usually has to be a cupful or more.

## Attention-deficit/hyperactivity disorder
Feingold in the USA suggested that children (usually boys) with overactivity, short attention span, and impulsive behaviour might improve on a diet which omitted foods containing artificial colours or natural salicylates, or both. Although organisations of parents of difficult children have had faith in this hypothesis, objective confirmation is sparse. Most double-blind tests with food colours reported significant effects in either none or only one or two of the hyperactive children tested, and much of the information Feingold used on the salicylate content of foods was wrong. The salicylate content of most diets, by modern specific analysis, is only 1-2 mg/day.[11] Nevertheless, there are some children with a combination of overactivity and physical symptoms (rashes, rhinitis, headaches) suggestive of food sensitivity that have improved on an elimination diet, at Great Ormond Street. They appeared on challenge to be sensitive to different foods, but tartrazine and benzoic acid were top of the list.[12]

## Arthritis
Gouty arthritis is aggravated by alcohol and by high purine and high protein diets. Although most patients with rheumatoid arthritis do not respond to food exclusions or challenges, a patient whose arthritis was clearly shown to be aggravated by milk and cheese was reported from the Hammersmith Hospital. A small minority of similarly reacting rheumatoid patients was found in a subsequent study in Florida.[13]

## Pseudo food allergy[14]
Apparent reactions to food are quite often psychological rather than organic in origin. Patients may be convinced, but on circumstantial or no real evidence, that they are sensitive to certain foods. These beliefs are encouraged by some popular books and unorthodox practitioners, and are not easy for the busy general practitioner to change. Avoiding a broad range of foods carries a risk of malnutrition. Parents have also been reported as having inflicted supposed allergies on their children—a variant of Meadow's syndrome.

**Specialist food "allergy" (sensitivity) clinics** are available at some of the teaching hospitals, such as Addenbrooks, Cambridge; Great Ormond Street, London; Guy's, London, etc.

**Food intolerance databanks** have been set up in several European countries. In the United Kingdom the Leatherhead Food Research Association manages the databank.

## Some less common food sensitivities
- *Favism*—haemolytic anaemia after eating broad beans. The basic defect is red blood cell glucose-6-phosphate dehydrogenase deficiency.
- *Bitter lemon purpura*—"bitter lemon" contains quinine, which may rarely precipitate thrombocytopenic purpura.
- *Chinese restaurant syndrome*—as first described, the symptoms were facial pressure, burning sensation in upper trunk and shoulders, and chest pain soon after eating foods rich in monosodium glutamate, particularly Chinese wonton soup. But delayed headache and nausea have subsequently been found to be more common, and asthma has sometimes been precipitated.
- *Sensitivity to tea or coffee*, or both—these common social beverages can cause a variety of pharmacological effects, for example, vomiting, headaches, tachycardia, which have sometimes been proved by objective tests.[6]

## References
1 Young E, Stoneham MD, Petruckevitch A, Barton J, Rona R. A population study of food intolerance. *Lancet* 1994; **343:** 1127-30.
2 Moneret-Vautrin DA. Food allergy and intolerance in infancy. In: Walker AF, Rolls BA (eds). *Infant Nutrition*. London: Chapman & Hall, 1994.
3 Bindslev-Jensen C. ABC of allergies: food allergy. *BMJ* 1998; **316:** 1299-302.
4 Lessof MH. *Food allergy and other adverse reactions to food*. Brussels: ILSI Europe, 1994.
5 Royal College of Physicians and the British Nutrition Foundation. Food intolerance and food aversion. *J R Coll Phys Lond* 1984; **18:** 2-41.
6 American Academy of Allergy and Immunology Committee on Adverse Reactions to Foods. National Institute of Allergy and Infectious Diseases. *Adverse reactions to foods*. (NIH Publication No 84-2442.) Bethesda, MD: National Institutes of Health, 1984.
7 Lessof MH. Reactions to food in adults. In: Lessof MH (ed). *Clinical reactions to food*. Chichester: John Wiley, 1983.
8 Ewan PW. ABC of allergies: anaphylaxis. *BMJ* 1998; **316:** 1442-5.
9 Sampson HA. Managing peanut allergy. *BMJ* 1996; **312:** 1050-1.
10 Greaves MW. Current concepts: chronic urticaria. *New Engl J Med* 1995; **332:** 1767-72.
11 Janssen PLTMK, Hollman PCH, Reichman E, Venema DP, van Staveren WA, Katan MB. Urinary salicylate excretion in subjects eating a variety of diets shows that amounts of bioavailable salicylates in foods are low. *Am J Clin Nutr* 1996; **64:** 743-7.
12 Egger J. Food allergy and the central nervous system. In: Reinhardt D, Schmidt E (eds). *Food Allergy, Nestle Nutrition Workshop Series*, vol 17. New York: Raven Press, 1988.
13 Panush RS. Nutritional therapy for rheumatic diseases. *Ann Intern Med* 1987; **106:** 619-21.
14 Pearson DJ. Pseudo food allergy. *BMJ* 1986; **292:** 221-2.

## Further reading
Buttriss J. (ed) *Adverse Reactions to Food. The report of a British Nutrition foundation Task Force*. Oxford: Blackwell Science, 2002.

# 16    Processing food

In the guessing game, "Animal, vegetable, or mineral?" nearly all foods are animal or vegetable or the two combined. What we eat is other organisms, some of them—fruits and cereals—still viable. The basic material of our foods has an anatomy and a histology. It is made of cells which contain numerous enzymes and biochemical compounds that are the same as or similar to those in the human body. Foods are also inhabited by micro-organisms. These multiply after slaughter or harvesting and nearly all our basic foodstuffs deteriorate rapidly because of autolytic decay and microbial activity. Foods can become dangerous because of these unless we treat them in some way. Cereal grains are the major exception. They have a lower water content and normally keep for years when dry at ambient temperatures. The major early civilisations were built on this property, and even today the only staple foods that are kept in savings banks are the cereals. Insect activity also leads to appreciable losses of food.

## Why foods have to be processed or prepared

(1) Foods are preserved so that they can be kept edible for longer. Preservation reduces wastage and hence cost. It enables people in affluent communities to eat their favourite foods all the year round and also enables us to benefit from economies of scale by growing large quantities of a food on large areas of suitable land. Preservation helps to feed the growing world population.

(2) Processing or preparation makes foods safe to eat by destroying or retarding the growth of pathogenic micro-organisms (such as salmonella, clostridia, or fungi) or inactivating natural toxins (such as trypsin inhibitors and goitrogens).

(3) Processing or preparation improves the attractiveness of food, its flavour, and its appearance. This is not a frivolous function. Poorly prepared food is often the chief complaint of patients in hospitals and nursing homes.

(4) Processing also provides convenience. In Mrs Beaton's time most women spent their lives working for hours each day in the kitchen. Modern convenience foods have liberated women in countries like Britain. Much of the work that used to be done by hand in the Victorian kitchen is now done by machines, some controlled by computer, in the food processing plant or factory.

## Methods of food preservation and processing

### Drying
Traditionally this was sun drying or smoking, but nowadays tunnel drying, spray drying, and freeze drying produce concentrated forms of the foods—for example, milk powder or instant coffee powder. Bacteria, which require water, cannot grow and autolytic enzymes are inhibited.

### Freezing
This prevents bacterial growth because bacterial enzyme activity slows then stops as temperature is lowered. In addition, water in the food is not in an available form.

---

**Doctors need to know about food**

- "Doctors need to know as much about foods as they do about drugs."
- "Each medical school should have an expert on the biochemistry of foods among their preclinical lecturers."

*Two recommendations from the International Union of Nutritional Sciences Workshop on Nutrition Education for Medical Practitioners*, held at the Royal College of Physicians, London, March 1984.[1]

---

**Food technology**

- **Handling after harvest**—Foods must be kept at the best temperature, atmosphere, etc, between the farm and market or factory.
- **Food processing** is treatment of food in a plant or factory before it is sold in the shop.
- **Food preparation** is treatment of food in the kitchen, at home, in a catering establishment or take-away shop. It is a wider term than "cooking", which implies the use of heat.
- Between each treatment stage food has to be **stored**; the conditions affect how long it keeps and its quality.

---

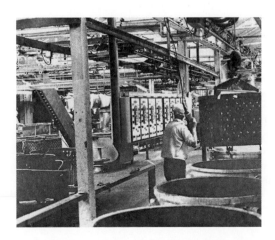

*Refrigeration*
Does not destroy micro-organisms but ensures that those present cannot multiply or do so only slowly; it also slows autolysis by enzymes in the food.

*Addition of salt or sugar*
This is a third way of lowering the "water activity" by increasing osmotic pressure and preventing bacterial growth, just as sugar has been shown to reduce infection in wounds.

*Acidification*
Acids also prevents microbial growth, for example, foods pickled in vinegar.

*Heat*
This is used in several ways. Blanching (1-8 min at 100°C depending on the food) before freezing and canning inactivates enzymes, that would otherwise continue autolysis of the food. Pasteurisation of milk (72°C for 15 seconds) destroys pathogenic organisms but not others. Cooking destroys all or nearly all organisms (except spore formers, depending on conditions). Sterilisation of canned and other sealed foods is performed by subjecting the food to a high temperature with or without pressure.

*Food irradiation*
A new technique, food irradiation, is useful for replacing ethylene oxide in sterilising spices (whose flavour would change on heating). It can also extend the shelf life of strawberries and mushrooms, inhibit sprouting of potatoes and onions, and destroy pathogens on poultry.[2]

*Fermentation*
This produces acid or ethanol, or both, which inhibit pathogenic and spoilage organisms.

*Chemical preservatives*
Benzoic acid, propionic acid, and sorbic acid, naturally present in cranberries, Gruyère cheese, and rowanberries, respectively, are added to certain specified foods in controlled amounts to prevent microbial growth. Sodium metabisulphite, which liberates sulphur dioxide in the food, is used for the same purpose.

*Packaging*
Once a food has been heat sterilised reinfection is prevented by sealing it in a can or airtight plastic bag or multilayer paper or plastic carton. Packaging of unsterilised food, though not preventing bacterial growth, reduces contamination and prevents loss of water through evaporation, etc.

*Separation methods*
Unlike the methods above these are not used to preserve foods. Milling produces different fractions of cereal flours. Pressing produces oils from oil seeds and juice from fruit.

**Fresh or processed?**
Most "fresh" fruit in the greengrocers comes from overseas or has been stored for weeks or months. "Fresh" vegetables too, though mostly home grown, are often stored. Bananas are picked in the tropics before they are ripe, shipped and stored at a controlled even temperature (>13°C), and ripened by exposure to ethylene gas (which is given off naturally by ripening fruit). Oranges are picked ripe, shipped, and stored at a lower temperature (3°C) in dry air with a raised carbon dioxide level. The skins have to be protected from mould

---

**From the earliest civilisations**
Some of the most important processes used for our foods go back to the earliest civilisations

- The Sumerians had a simple dairy industry. Butter is mentioned several times in the Bible (for example, Isaiah vii, 15).
- The ancient Egyptians brewed beer and discovered how to make raised bread. Beer has been called "liquid bread".

---

**Many processes are very old**

- Wine was part of the way of life of the ancient Greeks. Wine and raisins (another very old food) are two different ways of preserving the energy of grapes in palatable forms.
- Salted pork—forerunner of our ham and bacon—was a common meat for the ancient Greeks.
- Cheese is mentioned in the Bible (for example, II Samuel xvii, 29). It is a remarkable method for preserving the energy, calcium, and other nutrients of milk.
- Jam, another way of preserving fruit, was being made long before the Industrial Revolution.

---

**Nutrients per 100 g in wholemeal (100%) and white [breadmaking] (72%) wheat flour[3]**

| Nutrients | Wholemeal | White |
|---|---|---|
| Energy kJ (kcal) | 1318 (314) | 1451 (346) |
| Protein (g) | 12.7 | 11.5 |
| Fat (g) | 2.2 | 1.4 |
| Starch (g) | 62 | 74 |
| Sugars (g) | 2.1 | 1.4 |
| Dietary fibre (g) | 8.6 | 3.7 |
| Thiamin (mg) | 0.47 | 0.32* |
| Riboflavin (mg) | 0.09 | 0.03 |
| Niacin (mg) | 5.7 | 2.0* |
| Vitamin B-6 (mg) | 0.5 | 0.15 |
| Total folate (µg) | 57 | 31 |
| Vitamin E (mg) | 1.4 | 0.3 |
| Iron (mg) | 3.9 | 2.1* |
| Zinc (mg) | 2.9 | 0.9 |
| Calcium (mg) | 38 | 140* |
| Total phosphorus (mg) | 320 | 120 |
| Phytate phosphorus (mg) | 240 | 30 |

*As fortified in the UK. *Note:* These are wheat **flours**. In bread nutrient contents are lower because over a third of the fresh weight is water

infection, for example, by treating with fungicides mixed with waxes after they have been washed. Although these fruits have been in artificial environments, they are intact and alive and their cells are absorbing oxygen and producing carbon dioxide.

Likewise, it is worth money to understand what factors determine tenderness and flavour in meat. There is a speciality of meat science, which shares some of the histological and biochemical knowledge used by clinicians who specialise in muscular diseases.[4] Before slaughter, animals should have adequate muscle glycogen. This is converted to lactic acid, which acts as a weak preservative. Fresh meat is tough because of rigor mortis. This disperses during hanging in a controlled chilled temperature of $-1.4\,°C$ and the meat is tenderised.

## Food additives

Salt, vinegar, nitrates, and sugar have been used for centuries and are still among the most used food preservatives today. Hops are a traditional preservative for beer. Many of history's great voyages of exploration were made in search of food additives. Marco Polo journeyed to the East to obtain exotic spices. Cortez brought back vanilla from the Aztecs.

Food additive controls in Europe are now harmonised throughout the EU. The use of food additives is subject to strict legislative controls and they are only permitted if considered safe following scrutiny by independent experts, particularly the EC Scientific Committee for Food. To ensure that safe intake levels are not exceeded, many of the additives are only permitted in certain foods and up to specified maximum levels.

- **Preservatives** such as nitrates in bacon and ham and sulphur dioxide in dried fruit prolong the shelf life of foods by protecting them against deterioration caused by micro-organisms.
- **Antioxidants** are used to prevent the slow oxidation of oils and fats by atmospheric oxygen and development of rancidity.
- **Emulsifiers** keep oil and aqueous phase together in sauces. Lecithin is an example.
- **Humectants** prevent foods from drying out. Glycerol is an example.
- **Food acids** are acids that occur naturally. They are used for flavour or for technical reasons—for example, to adjust the pH in certain jams so that the pectin sets—and can also act as preservatives.
- **Anti-caking agents** stop lumps forming in powdery foods.
- **Thickeners** may be vegetable gums, cellulose derivatives, or starch derivatives.
- **Added nutrients** are now given by name on the label. A number of foods are fortified or enriched with nutrients— for example, margarine includes vitamins A and D, flour and bread and some breakfast cereals contain some B vitamins, and iron, and textured vegetable proteins contain vitamin B-12.
- **Miscellaneous**—Other additives include: flour treatment agents, firming agents, stabilisers, flavour enhancers, propellants, and glazing agents.
- **Colours**—Forty-three colours are permitted in the European community. More than half of them are natural, for example, beetroot red, chlorophyll and various carotenoids. Twenty of the permitted colours, such as some azo dyes and erythrosine (an iodine compound), are synthetic.
- **Flavourings**—Flavourings are added to foods in minute quantities and without hazard to public health. They are either natural flavour preparations (for example, essential oils) or chemically defined flavouring substances. These may be natural (isolated from products of plant or animal origin,

**EC code number for food additives on labels (some examples)**

| | |
|---|---|
| *Preservatives* | |
| Benzoic acid | E210 |
| Propionic acid | E280 |
| Sorbic acid | E200 |
| Sodium metabisulphite | E223 |
| *Antioxidants* | |
| Butylated hydroxyanisole (BHA) | E320 |
| Butylated hydroxytoluene (BHT) | E321 |
| Propyl gallate | E310 |
| Tocopherols | E306-309 |
| *Emulsifiers* | |
| Monoglycerides and diglycerides of fatty acids | E471 |
| Lecithins | E322 |
| *Humectants* | |
| Glycerol | E422 |
| Sorbitol | E420 |
| *Acids* | |
| Acetic acid | E260 |
| Citric acid | E330 |
| Malic acid | E296 |
| *Anti-caking agents* | |
| Calcium phosphate | E341 |
| Magnesium carbonate | E504 |
| *Thickeners* | |
| Guar gum | E412 |
| Locust bean gum | E410 |
| Pectin | E440 |
| Carboxymethylcellulose | E466 |
| *Colours—natural* | |
| Beetroot red | E162 |
| Chlorophyll | E140 |
| β-carotene | E160(a) |
| *Colours—synthetic* | |
| Tartrazine | E102 |
| Brown FK | E154 |
| Erythrosine | E127 |
| *Flavour enhancers* | |
| Monosodium glutamate | E621 |
| Sodium inosinate | E631 |

for example, menthol from peppermint oil) or nature-identical (made synthetically but chemically identical to a substance that occurs naturally, for example, citral) or artificial (not yet found in nature, for example, ethyl vanillin). There is no EU-wide flavouring legislation at present, but the EU is working towards creation of a list of permitted flavouring substances. The names of individual flavours are not declared on labels and they are not in the E code, but if flavourings are used this is mentioned (non-specifically) in the ingredients list. Flavour recipes in food are regarded as trade secrets.

- **Artificial sweeteners** permitted under EU law include saccharin, aspartame, and acesulfame K.

## Contaminants

Unintentional additives can get into foods somewhere along the chain from farm to plate. Examples are pesticides, other farm chemicals, veterinary residues, drugs, heavy metals (lead, cadmium, mercury, and arsenic), industrial chemicals—for example, polycyclic aromatic hydrocarbons and polychlorinated biphenyls (PCBs), atmospheric and water pollutants, radionuclides, and phthalate plasticisers. Foods should be monitored for most of these by government agencies, such as, in Britain, the Food Standards Agency.

## Foods and ingredients derived from gene technology[5-8]

Direct genetic manipulation of our food production is new and controversial. For centuries desirable genetic evolution was achieved by selective breeding of plants and animals used for food, mainly for external characters, recently for chemical composition. Rape plants were selectively bred in Canada '*to not*' express the characteristic (but potentially toxic) erucic acid in their seed oil—hence canola oil. With the traditional selective breeding many genes change one way or the other, along with the desired modification. With the new GM (genetically modified) technology a single gene from another species or an extra copy of an indigenous gene is inserted into the plant or animal, on a virus or bacterium, or is shot in on gold particles. The source of the new gene may be from a very different species; genes isolated from fish have been inserted into strawberries to give resistance to cold.

Gene technology is being developed—or already used—for several purposes:

- to make it easier to grow the food, for example, to introduce resistance to an endemic plant virus or to a particular herbicide that keeps the weeds down ("Roundup Ready" soyabeans)
- to make processing easier, for example, to reduce a spoilage enzyme and so prolong shelf life
- to make a food more palatable, for example, "Flavr Savr" tomatoes
- to produce a desired change in nutritional composition, for example, rice which contains (pro-vitamin A) $\beta$-carotene in the grain.

A primary aim of regulatory authorities is to determine if there can be any difference between, say, GM maize and conventional maize as food that could affect health—loss of nutrient(s) or appearance of a potential toxin or allergen. This is the concept of **substantial equivalence** and is the responsibility of food standards agencies. But the question of approving GM crops also has environmental and legal aspects. Not all GM crops are used for food (for example cotton, carnations).

---

**Foods can be altered with gene technology in five ways:**

- a chemically defined substance, obtained by gene technology, is used in production of the foods, for example, porcine somatotrophin (to improve the growth of pigs) or chymosin (replacing rennet in cheese making)
- less well defined ingredients in the food, for example, starch from insect-resistant maize, mycoprotein from genetically modified yeast
- foods/drinks produced using genetically modified organisms (GMOs), for example, wine or beer from yeast modified to result in an altered flavour profile
- transgenic plants or animals—that is, containing new or altered DNA, for example, soyabeans containing a gene that makes them resistant to a particular herbicide ("Roundup Ready" soyabeans)
- foods in which the genetically modified micro-organism is still present, for example, a "live" yoghurt with new properties.

---

**Why all the fuss about GM foods?**

- The process of GM technology is not natural. People object on religious grounds.
- Multinationals are controlling agribusiness vertically and globally. Though the inserted genes are natural, GM seeds are patented. Farmers have to contract with the seed company not to re-plant the seeds they harvest.
- GM crops will not help peasant farmers in developing countries who cannot afford to pay the premium and then not re-use seeds after harvest. Yields may not necessarily be better. The market price may be lower if the demand is for non-GM.
- The first generation of foods from GM crops has no advantage for consumers. Maize that is resistant to a herbicide does not taste any better, is not more nutritious and could possibly have some deleterious effect long term.
- Antibiotic resistant genes have often been used as markers for successful implantation of the new gene in seedling plants.
- There may be environmental damage, for example spread by pollen to weeds of the same botanical family, resulting in "superweeds", or "superbugs".
- GM food crops are based on a concept of fighting, rather than adapting to the ecology. We would be placing living things in an environment where there is no evolutionary history of how to accommodate them.

The growing of GM crops has to be considered and approved by a country's Department of the Environment. Here the **precautionary principle** should be used, and approval to grow a GM crop should start with experimental plots, well separated from conventional crops of the same botanical family.

The United States has been more permissive and the European Union has been and still is very cautious about approving GM foods. In the United States about 30% of the soyabeans now grown, and a lot of the maize, is from plants genetically modified to be resistant to the herbicide glyphosate ("Roundup"). These foods are not segregated or labelled in the wholesale markets; there is no way they can be identified by simple chemical analysis and they are likely to be present of course in soya and maize products being exported from north America. But these soyabeans and maize plants are not permitted to be grown in the European Union at present.

In the European Union multiple authorities, both national and in Brussels, both environmental and food authorities, have to scrutinise applications to grow GM plants. Consumers want any GM foods eventually approved, to be clearly labelled. Major supermarkets have a policy of not stocking GM foods and are giving increased shelf space to "organic" foods, a term which now covers non-GM.

In mid 2002 food aid maize shipped from the America to Zambia was impounded and not distributed to hungry people. The government feared that some might be be sown with the result that next year's maize could not be exported to Europe.

Scientific developments in plant breeding have made a huge leap. Regulators, politicians and consumers are in disarray. Meanwhile there is no present likelihood that doctors will be able to diagnose any disease caused by eating a GM food.

## Are our foods safe?

Britain had the first food safety legislation in the world, the Sale of Food and Drugs Act 1875; this and subsequent acts have been replaced by the Food Act 1984. Food safety became the responsibility of the Food Standards Agency in 2000. Its expert committees are in regular informal communication with the EC Scientific Committee for food, the Joint FAO/WHO Expert Committee on Food Additives, the US Food and Drug Administration, and food toxicologists round the world.

Deliberate food additives are not intrinsically toxic substances. They have been tested in several animal species and are kept under review continuously by food toxicologists. Amounts permitted in foods are such that the maximum intake does not exceed the acceptable daily intake (usually 1/100 the highest level that has no effect in animal tests). Toxicological tests have not so far systematically examined the chances of hypersensitivity reactions in man, and such occasional reactions to tartrazine, sulphur dioxide, and monosodium glutamate are described in chapter 15.

Whereas some natural components in the diet are risk factors for certain types of cancer (chapter 3), the World Cancer Research Fund's expert panel[9] agrees with previous reviewers that intentional food additives do not cause cancer (when used in quantities prescribed by the regulations).

## Losses of nutrients

Some losses of nutrients occur during food processing but they are qualitatively and quantitatively similar to the losses that happen in domestic cooking. Most processes in the food factory are scaled up versions of one or another home recipe. Factory processes are standardised and controlled, but home

---

**Potentially toxic substances in foods**

**Natural**

| | |
|---|---|
| Inherent, naturally occurring | Usually present in the food and affect everyone if they eat enough, for example, solanine in potatoes |
| Toxin resulting from abnormal conditions of animal or plant used for food | For example, neurotoxic mussel poisoning; honey from bees feeding on rhododendron nectar |
| Consumer abnormally sensitive | For example, coeliac disease from wheat gluten; allergy to particular food; or drug induced, for example, cheese reaction |
| Contamination by pathogenic bacteria | Acute illness, usually gastrointestinal, for example, infection with *Salmonella* spp, or campylobacters or toxins produced by *Staphylococcus aureus* or *Clostridium botulinum* (food may not appear spoiled) |
| Mycotoxins | Food mouldy or spoiled, for example, aflatoxin $B_1$, from *Aspergillus flavus*, is a liver carcinogen |

**Manmade**

| | |
|---|---|
| Unintentional additives: manmade chemicals used in agriculture and animal husbandry | For example, fungicides on grain, insecticides on fruit, antibiotics or hormones given to animals |
| Environmental pollution | For example, organic mercury, cadmium, polychlorinated biphenyls, and radioactive fallout can affect any stage of food chain |
| Intentional food additives: preservatives, emulsifiers, flavours, colours, etc | The most thoroughly tested and monitored of all chemicals in food |

---

**Testing food additives**

- Acute toxicity is tested in male and female animals of at least three species.
- Distribution of the compound in the body and its metabolism are studied.
- Short-term feeding trials are done on at least two species of animal (one non-rodent).
- Long-term toxicity is assessed in at least one metabolically appropriate animal species.
- Reproduction studies involve giving the compound to experimental animals over at least two generations.
- Testing for mutagenicity (in bacteria) and carcinogenicity (in tissue culture) is undertaken.
- Observations in man are reviewed.

cooking varies from excellent to bad. Nutrient losses are roughly predictable and can easily be measured by analysis at different stages.

Two vitamins are more unstable than the others when heated, vitamin C and folate, but whereas vitamin C lasts better in acid medium, folate does not. Thiamin (vitamin $B_1$) is moderately unstable when heated. Riboflavin decomposes in ultraviolet light. Water soluble vitamins dissolve into the cooking water and the more water used the more vitamins are likely to be wasted. Mineral nutrients are stable but can also be washed out if large amounts of cooking water are used. Lysine, the limiting amino acid in cereals, is the most unstable of the essential amino acids. The golden crust of bread is coloured by a complex of sugars and lysine which becomes biologically unavailable. There is some loss of linoleic acid in oils when they are reused for frying, especially at high temperatures.

Losses of **vitamin C** are worth considering in detail. The factors that cause the oxidative breakdown of vitamin C are tissue damage (which liberates ascorbic acid oxidase) by bruising or freezing of leafy vegetables, heating in alkaline water—for example, with sodium bicarbonate added—contact with copper, and leaching into the processing or cooking water. Moderate losses occur between harvesting and cooking fresh vegetables and when a bottle of fruit juice is opened and kept at room temperature. There is little difference in losses of vitamin C between these three methods of cooking: boiling, microwave, and pressure cooking, but the less water used the less vitamin is thrown away in the water. There are substantial losses of vitamin C when cooked vegetables are kept warm before they are served, or refrigerated until the next day.

**Percentage retention of vitamin C in peas after different stages of preparation (after Mapson)[10]**

| Fresh | Frozen | Canned | Air dried |
|---|---|---|---|
| — | Blanching 75 | Blanching 70 | Blanching 75 |
| — | Freezing 75 | Canning 63 | Drying 45 |
| — | Thawing 71 | Diffusion 40 | — |
| Cooking 44 | Cooking 39 | Heating 36 | Cooking 25 |

**Effect of different conditions on stability of nutrients in foods (based on Harris and Karmas[11])**

| Nutrients | Effect of solutions | | | Effect of exposure to | | | Cooking losses (% range) |
|---|---|---|---|---|---|---|---|
| | Acid | Neutral | Alkaline | Oxygen | Light | Heat | |
| **Vitamins** | | | | | | | |
| Vitamin A | U | S | S | U | U | U | 0-40 |
| Vitamin D | | S | U | U | U | U | 0-40 |
| Vitamin E | S | S | S | U | U | U | 0-55 |
| Thiamin | S | U | U | U | S | U | 0-80 |
| Riboflavin | S | S | U | S | U | U | 0-60 |
| Niacin | S | S | S | S | S | S | 0-50 |
| Folate | U | U | S | U | U | U | 0-80 |
| Vitamin C | S | U | U | U | U | U | 0-100 |
| **Amino acids** | | | | | | | |
| Leucine, isoleucine, methionine, valine and phenylalanine | S | S | S | S | S | S | 0-10 |
| Lysine | S | S | S | S | S | U | 0-40 |
| Tryptophan | U | S | S | S | U | S | 0-15 |
| Threonine | U | S | U | S | S | U | 0-20 |
| **Mineral salts** | S | S | S | S | S | S | 0-3 |

U = unstable, S = stable

On average, losses of vitamin C in cooking may be taken as 70%—that is, 30% retention—in leafy vegetables and 40% in root vegetables. Food tables usually give values for cooked vegetables, as well as for the raw food (see table opposite).

# Perspective

- Some loss of nutrients is inevitable in food processing, but for most nutrients losses are small.
- Manufacturing losses, when they occur, are often in place of similar losses through cooking at home.

**Vitamin C content in raw and cooked peas and mangetout[3]**

| | mg/100 g |
|---|---|
| Peas | |
| raw | 24 |
| boiled | 16 |
| frozen, boiled | 12 |
| canned, reheated | 1 |
| Mangetout peas | |
| raw | 54 |
| boiled | 28 |
| stir fried in oil | 51 |

- The importance of the losses in a particular food has to be considered in relation to the whole diet. If a food makes only a small contribution to the intake of nutrients, processing losses are not of practical importance. On the other hand, changes in any food that makes a major contribution to nutrient supply—for example, milk for babies and cereals in some adults—need continued vigilance.

- There are some beneficial effects of processing or preparation: destruction of trypsin inhibitor in legumes and liberation of bound niacin in cereals. Nutrient enrichment is possible.

- Other advantages of food processing are protection from pathogenic organisms, better flavour, and cheaper price. Often the ultimate choice is between dried, canned, or frozen peas (say) in late winter or no peas at all.

## Geography of food processing

Last century cows were kept in towns because there was no way of preventing milk from souring.

To provide the milk, cheese, yoghurt, and cream for the people of London today about 0.5 million cows are needed. They in turn each need about 7 acres of farm land to feed them through the year. From these 3.5 million acres scattered across the south of England fresh milk is pooled, transported, pasteurised, bottled, and distributed or processed in other ways. Other foods—fruits, meat, fish in Britain—may come from half way around the world. This complex movement and distribution of foods would be impossible without food processing.

## References

1 Truswell AS (rapporteur). Nutrition education for medical students and practitioners: report of a workshop. *UN University Food Nutr Bull* 1984; **6**: 75-81.

2 *Food irradiation. A technique for preserving and improving the safety of food.* Published by WHO in collaboration with FAO. Geneva: WHO, 1988.

3 Holland B, Welch AA, Unwin ID, Buss DH, Paul AA, Southgate DAT. *McCance & Widdowson's the composition of foods,* 5th edn. Cambridge: Royal Society of Chemistry, 1991.

4 Lawrie RA. *Meat science,* 6th edn. Cambridge: Woodhead, 1998.

5 Dixon B. The paradoxes of genetically modified foods. *BMJ* 1999; **318**: 547-8.

6 Horton R. Genetically modified foods: "absurd" concern or welcome dialogue? *Lancet* 1999; **354**: 1314-15.

7 Gaskell G, Bauer MW, Durant J, Allum NC. Worlds apart? The reception of genetically modified foods in Europe and the US. *Science* 1999; **285**: 384-7.

8 The grim reaper. *The Economist* 2002; Aug 24: 42-43.

9 World Cancer Research Fund in association with American Institute for Cancer Research. *Food, nutrition and the prevention of cancer: a global perspective.* Washington DC: American Institute for Cancer Research, 1997.

10 Mapson LW. Effect of processing on the vitamin content of foods. *Br Med Bull* 1956; **12**: 73-7.

11 Harris RS, Karmas E. *Nutritional evaluation of food processing,* 2nd edn. Westport, CT: Avi, 1975.

# 17   Nutritional support

Nigel Reynolds, Christopher R Pennington

Nutritional support is required for the prevention of starvation and the treatment of malnutrition in patients who are unable to ingest or absorb sufficient nutrients. There is controversial evidence that the provision of specific nutrient substrates may modify the response to disease. This chapter will review current concepts with respect to the need for nutritional support, the route of nutrient delivery, the prescription of nutrient substances, and the quality of nutritional management.

## The problem of malnutrition

Studies have demonstrated that malnutrition is common in hospital patients although often it goes unrecognised. Unless nutritional management is initiated nutritional status declines in most patients during hospital stay, particularly in those who are malnourished on admission. Furthermore, nutritional depletion has been shown to continue for two months after discharge in malnourished postoperative patients.

Malnutrition is defined in terms of tissue wasting which may arise through starvation and the metabolic action of cytokines generated in response to tissue injury. There is evidence that nutrient deprivation is of major importance in most patients through a reluctance or inability to eat, the lack of available food for prolonged periods in hospital, and impaired intestinal function. Common causes of malnutrition are given alongside.

**Malnutrition in hospital patients**

| Study* | Patients (no) | Type of patients | % Mal- nourished |
|---|---|---|---|
| **Prevalence of malnutrition in hospital patients** | | | |
| Bistrian et al. 1974 | 131 | General surgical | 50.0 |
| Bistrian et al. 1976 | 251 | General medical | 44.0 |
| Hill et al. 1977 | 105 | General surgical | 50.0 |
| **Incidence of malnutrition on admission to hospital** | | | |
| Willard et al. 1980 | 200 | General medical General surgical | 31.5 |
| Bastow et al. 1983 | 744 | Orthopaedic surgical | 52.8 |
| Zador and Truswell 1989 | 84 | General surgical | 14.0 |
| Larsson et al. 1990 | 501 | Care of elderly | 28.5 |
| Cederholm et al. 1993 | 200 | General medical | 20.0 |
| McWhirter and Pennington 1994 | 500 | General medical General surgical Orthopaedic surgical Respiratory medicine Care of elderly | 40.0 |
| Giner et al. 1996 | 129 | Intensive care | 43 |

* (For details of the studies see Pennington 1998)[1]

**Some causes of malnutrition in hospital patients**

**Anorexia**
- Depression
- Chronic disease

**Inability to eat**
- Neurological disorders
- Swallowing disorders

**Intestinal disease**
- Inflammatory bowel disease
- Radiation enteritis
- Gluten enteropathy
- Short bowel syndrome
- Hollow visceral myopathy

**Inflammatory response to infection**

Studies of starvation in normal healthy subjects reveal that death is likely from 60 days when weight loss in excess of 30% has been sustained. The time before tissue loss becomes irreversible is significantly reduced in hospital patients who have already lost weight before admission and in whom the process is accelerated in the presence of inflammatory mediators. Cytokines lead to proteolysis and lipolysis combined with the suppression of appetite.

There are other reasons for the early recognition of malnutrition and where appropriate the provision of nutritional support. When patients are metabolically stressed through infection or trauma, tissue wasting can only be retarded not reversed. Data from the Minnesota experiment and from re-feeding patients with anorexia nervosa have demonstrated that a very long time is required for tissue

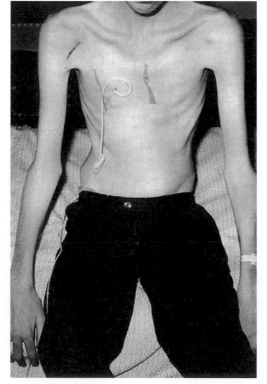

A malnourished patient

repletion. Of more importance is the fact that organ function is impaired by starvation, long before current indices of nutritional status become abnormal. Thus obese subjects who starved for two weeks demonstrated loss of muscle power and increased muscle fatiguability of comparable magnitude to malnourished hospital patients. This has implications for the mobilisation of patients after surgery and illness. Furthermore respiratory muscles are also affected, adding to the risk of clinical complications of malnutrition. Other clinically important consequences of nutritional depletion include impairment of wound healing, and of immune response and digestive function.

## The recognition of malnutrition

There is no single clinical method that will reliably diagnose malnutrition. The measurement of weight and height is used to calculate the Body Mass Index (BMI) by the formula: weight (kg) divided by the height$^2$ (m). The normal range is 20-25. Adult patients with values of 19 or below are malnourished. Information from the BMI may be supplemented by measuring the mid-arm muscle circumference and triceps skinfold thickness which respectively correlate with protein and fat stores. Values are compared with standard reference ranges for the patient population (see page 72).

There are significant limitations in the interpretation of these measurements. They are affected by changes in the hydration status and inter-observer error, and the patient may suffer from the effects of starvation due to impaired organ function long before such measurements become abnormal. Some clinicians employ hand grip dynamometry as a method of detecting nutritional influences on muscle power. All these measurements are time consuming. Nutritional screening of all patients admitted to hospital has been recommended as a simple method of detecting patients at nutritional risk who may merit further investigation. Such a scheme is summarised in the box opposite.

## The role of nutritional support

Nutritional support is clearly indicated in patients who are unable to eat or who have prolonged intestinal failure. Under these circumstances it is required to prevent death from starvation. When used to treat malnutrition, nutritional support will reduce morbidity in many patient groups and some of the studies which demonstrated benefit are summarised in the table opposite. There are other studies in which no benefit or increased morbidity has been observed with nutritional treatment. Many of these studies were characterised by the inappropriate use of nutritional support and in particular parenteral nutrition with excessive substrate administration.

Nutritional support may be administered in the form of oral supplements, enteral tube feeding or parenteral (intravenous) nutrition. Estimates suggest that 3-4% of hospital beds are occupied by patients who are receiving nutritional support by parenteral or enteral tube feeding. Approximately four times the number of patients are tube fed compared to those who receive parenteral nutrition.

## Enteral nutrition

### Oral supplements
Oral supplements containing the recommended provision of micronutrients (vitamins and trace elements) should be used when it is anticipated that they will provide a large part of the diet. These preparations include a range of flavours and when

### Some of the effects of malnutrition
**Impaired mental function**
- Apathy, fatigue, poor cognition

**Impaired muscle function**
- Respiratory failure
- Delayed mobilisation

**Impaired immune function**
- Increased incidence of infection

**Miscellaneous**
- Impaired thermogenic response
- Impaired wound healing

### Nutritional screening*
**Questions**
- Reduced food consumption
- Unintentional weight loss

**Measurements**
- Weight
- Height

*Reproduced from Lennard-Jones et al. 1995[2]

### Randomised controlled studies which examine the influence of nutritional support on the length of hospital stay (LOS) (Adapted from Booth and Morgan 1995[3])

| Study* | Patient group | Nutritional management | Reduction of LOS days |
|---|---|---|---|
| Bastow et al. 1983 | 122 elderly females with fracture of neck of femur | Nocturnal nasogastric supplementary EN | 9 (in very thin group) |
| Askanazi et al. 1986 | 35 radical cystectomy | Postoperative PN | 7 |
| Delmi et al. 1990 | 59 elderly patients with fracture of neck of femur | Oral supplements postoperatively | 16 |
| Rana et al. 1992 | 40 patients undergoing moderate or major abdominal surgery | Oral supplements postoperatively | 3.3 |
| Eisenberg et al. 1993 | 459, 86% general surgical, 14% general medical | Preoperative PN | 0 |
| Mac Burney et al. 1994 | 43 bone-marrow transplant patients | Glutamine-supplemented PN | 7 |
| Bower et al. 1995 | 368 intensive care patients | Early EN with formula supplemented with argenine, nucleosides, and fish oil | 8 (in patients who tolerated at least 821 ml per day) |
| Keele et al. 1997 | 100 patients following moderate or major abdominal surgery | Postoperative supplements | 0 |

*For details of the studies see Booth and Morgan 1995[3] and Pennington[1]
EN enteral nutrition; PN parenteral nutrition

121

used between meals they do not significantly reduce the consumption of food. Oral supplements augment dietary intake in patients who experience difficulty in taking an adequate diet. They are unsuitable when patients are profoundly anorexic or suffer from swallowing disorders.

## Enteral tube feeding

Enteral nutrition delivered by tube is cheaper, safer, and more physiological than parenteral nutrition. In particular, in common with oral nutrition, it stimulates intestinal and biliary motility and provides a greater range of nutrients. These include glutamine and short chain fatty acids, important substrates for the enterocyte and colonocyte respectively, yet which are not part of routine parenteral nutrition prescriptions because of potential problems with the stability of the solution. Enteral nutrition may have a role in the protection of the mucosal barrier function in the ill patient, although studies on the prevention of intestinal translocation of micro-organisms by enteral nutrition in the animal model have not been replicated in the human. Some of the indications for enteral tube feeding are summarised in the box opposite. The ability to infuse nutrients over prolonged periods can fully exploit residual intestinal function in patients with intestinal impairment.

The methods of delivering enteral tube feeding are given in table opposite. Post-pyloric placement is required for patients with gastric stasis, notably in the postoperative period in the critically ill patient. Percutaneous tubes are needed when prolonged treatment is envisaged, notably in patients with swallowing disorders due to chronic neurological disease. This approach is also useful in the younger patient with cystic fibrosis. These younger patients may prefer to have a conventional gastrostomy replaced with a button gastrostomy giving a more acceptable cosmetic appearance.

Enteral feeding solutions most commonly used are based on whole protein substrates and are termed polymeric. Occasionally feeds with a low sodium content are useful in patients with liver cirrhosis and some patients with intestinal failure may benefit from a peptide feed in which much of the lipid is in the form of medium chain triglycerides. Feeds supplemented with glutamine, arginine, nucleotides, and fish oils have been formulated for nutritional support in the critically ill patient. So far there is no convincing clinical evidence to support the use of these more expensive products. However, polymeric feeds containing fibre are useful for the regulation of bowel function in patients who are dependent on artificial nutritional support, particularly elderly patients with chronic neurological disease.

The complications of enteral feeding may be considered in three groups:

(1) Metabolic complications include disorders of glucose and electrolyte balance. Very malnourished patients are prone to a condition termed the **re-feeding syndrome**. During starvation the body adapts to use less carbohydrate and more fat metabolism such that metabolic tolerance of carbohydrates can be impaired. With the introduction of artificial nutritional support there is rapid intracellular passage of phosphate, magnesium, and potassium resulting in low serum concentrations. Thiamin depletion can be dangerous in this situation, so the vitamin should be routinely provided. There are potentially serious life-threatening effects on cardiac, bone marrow, brain, and respiratory function. Intravenous replacement of electrolytes may be required.

(2) Gastrointestinal symptoms are common. Diarrhoea is often associated with the use of antibiotics which suppress the

### Some indications for enteral tube feeding

| Problem | Examples |
| --- | --- |
| Anorexia | Cirrhosis, Crohn's disease, some forms of malignancy |
| Swallowing disorders | Cerebrovascular disease, motor neurone disease, oesophageal stricture |
| Gastric stasis | Postoperative patient, intensive care patient |
| Intestinal malfunction | Crohn's disease, cystic fibrosis |

### Examples of common methods of enteral tube feeding

| Route | Placement | Comment |
| --- | --- | --- |
| Nasogastric | Nurse or patient | Easy access<br>Commonly displaced<br>Suitable for short-term or intermittent feeding |
| Nasojejunal | Surgeon at operation<br>Endoscopist | Useful in patients with gastric stasis, postoperative or ITU<br>Readily displaced |
| Percutaneous gastrostomy | Endoscopist<br>Radiologist using fluoroscopy<br>Surgeon laparoscopically | More suitable for prolonged feeding<br>Relatively safe<br>Can be converted to a button gastrostomy |
| Percutaneous jejunostomy | Surgeon at operation<br>Endoscopist | Alternative to parenteral nutrition for some postoperative patients<br>Significant short- and long-term morbidity |

(Reproduced from Lennard-Jones et al. 1995[2])

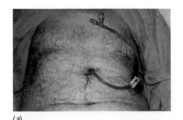 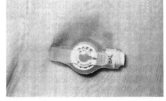

(a)     (b)

(a) A gastrostomy tube, (b) a button gastrostomy. (Reproduced from Pennington CR, 1998[4] by kind permission of The Medicine Publishing Company)

activity of colonic bacteria, thus reducing the availability of short-chain fatty acids from fibre. Short-chain fatty acids are an important fuel for the colonocyte; they stimulate sodium and water transport across the colon. The problem of diarrhoea can be reduced with fibre-containing feeds and possibly by post-pyloric feeding.

(3) Complications of nutrient delivery include pneumonia as a result of aspiration or displacement of the gastric tube. Stomal infection is common in patients with percutaneous feeding tubes; peritonitis can occur when the stomach or jejunum are not opposed to the abdominal wall at the time of percutaneous tube insertion.

# Parenteral nutrition

Parenteral nutrition is needed when the intestinal tract is unavailable or intestinal function is inadequate. Examples of some potential indications for short-term and prolonged parenteral nutrition are given in the box opposite.

The nutrient solution is compounded in a large multilayer bag under sterile conditions in the pharmacy, or provided as a standard solution available commercially. The solution contains glucose, lipid, amino acids, electrolytes, minerals, vitamins, and trace elements. Typically the volume ranges from 2 to 3 litres, the non-protein energy provision is 20-40 kcal per kg and the nitrogen provision 0.2-0.3 g per kg. These solutions contain all the essential amino acids, but not all the non-essential amino acids are included because of potential problems with the stability of the lipid solution. There is evidence that under some circumstances some of these "non-essential" amino acids are required. Thus in the stressed patient glutamine is considered to be conditionally essential. There is debate about the potential benefit of adding glutamine, in the form of dipeptides, to the parenteral nutrition prescription in critically ill patients to improve immune and gut barrier function. Furthermore as conventional fat solutions contain n−6 fatty acids that promote the formation of pro-inflammatory cytokines, there may be theoretical merit in deploying structured lipids which contain n−3 fatty acids. More clinical evidence is needed to support the use of these newer substrates.

In hospital parenteral nutrition is commonly needed for only two weeks, when it is conveniently administered by finebore peripheral cannulae. Peripheral cannulae have the advantage of avoiding the risks of central vein cannulation but have the drawback that it may be difficult to meet predicted energy and protein needs using tolerable volumes of fluid and lipid. The hypertonic nature of nutrient solutions can lead to phlebitis and loss of venous access. Critically ill patients and patients who need prolonged parenteral nutrition require central venous access. Venous access for parenteral nutrition is summarised in the box opposite.

Parenteral nutrition is infused continuously in the stressed unstable patient. Cyclical feeding, with overnight infusion and a heparin lock during the day, has metabolic advantages in the majority of patients as mobilisation can be facilitated. The complications of parenteral nutrition are summarised in the box on page 124. Catheter-related infection can be prevented with appropriate protocols dictating catheter care and guiding the training of staff and patients. The hepatobiliary complications which accompany prolonged treatment in some patients may reflect the lack of enteral nutrition, with the formation of biliary sludge or the excess administration of glucose or other nutrients. There is good evidence that nutritional care of a high standard can be most cost-effectively established by using multidisciplinary nutritional support teams.

## Some indications for parenteral nutrition

**Short-term**
- Severe inflammatory bowel disease
- Mucositis following chemotherapy
- Patients with multiorgan failure
- Major surgery
- Severe acute pancreatitis

**Long-term**
- Inflammatory disease
  Crohn's disease, radiation enteritis
- Motility disorders
  Hollow visceral myopathy, scleroderma
- Short bowel syndrome
  Mesenteric infarction, Crohn's disease

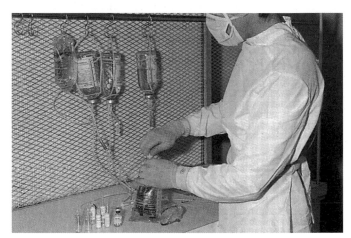

Parenteral nutrition solution compounded in the pharmacy

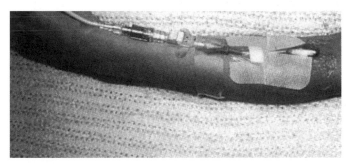

Peripheral parenteral nutrition catheter

## Venous access for parenteral nutrition

| | |
|---|---|
| Peripheral parenteral nutrition | Venflon<br>Ultrafine 15 cm cannula |
| Peripherally inserted central catheter | PICC Line |
| Central parenteral nutrition | Non-cuffed catheter with detachable hub<br>Cuffed Broviac type of catheter<br>Subcutaneous vascular port |

## Some complications of parenteral nutrition

**Nutritional and metabolic**
- Problems of glucose homoeostasis
- Electrolyte imbalance
- Micronutrient deficiencies
- Micronutrient excess, for example manganese

**Catheter-related**
- Infection: exit site, tunnel, lumen
- Occlusion: lipid, fibrin
- Central vein thrombosis
- Fracture of catheter

**Effect on other organ systems**
- Liver disease
- Biliary disease
- Osteoporosis

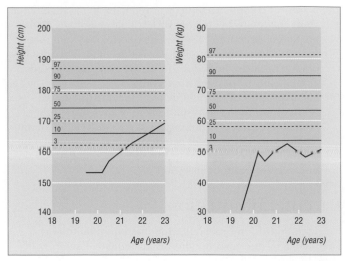

Growth charts demonstrating belated growth between the ages of 20 and 23 years. (Reproduced from Pennington CR, 1998[4] by kind permission of The Medicine Publishing Company)

## References

1 Pennington CR. Disease associated with malnutrition in the year 2000. *Postgrad Med J* 1998; **74**: 65-71.
2 Lennard-Jones JE, Arrowsmith H, Davison C, Denham AF, Micklewright A. Screening by nurses and junior doctors to detect malnutrition when patients are first assessed in hospital. *Clin Nutr* 1995; **14**: 336-40.
3 Booth K, Morgan S. *Financial issues for clinical nutrition in NHS hospitals.* Lancaster: Nutricia Clinical Care, Lancaster University 1995, pp 9-10.
4 Pennington CR. Artificial nutrition. *Medicine* 1998: **26**; 22–6.

The author, Christopher Pennington, sadly passed away in 2002.

## Further reading

Elia M. Changing concepts of nutrient requirements in disease: implications for artificial nutritional support. *Lancet* 1995; **345**: 1279-84.
McWhirter JP, Pennington CR. The incidence and recognition of malnutrition in hospital. *BMJ* 1994; **308**: 945-8.

# 18   Some principles

There are two questions affecting health about any food.

(1) Is it safe, or will it harm me (*a*) immediately or (*b*) later if I
eat it repeatedly?
(2) Is it good for me?

## Is it "food"?

For a food one has not eaten before question 1(*a*) predominates.
If it has not been contaminated or infected the answer depends
ultimately on folklore. In every culture there are parts of
plants and animals that the group recognises as food but other
cultures do not. Only a minority of plants can be expected
to be freely edible. For most plants it would be an evolutionary
advantage to possess a toxin that discourages animals from
eating it. Our folklore about which plants are edible comes
down from unknown ancestors who took the risk of eating an
unfamiliar plant, sometimes with unfortunate results.

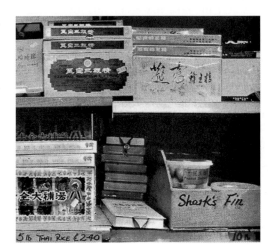

## Is this food good for me?

Simple trial and error by people with primitive technology
cannot answer questions 1(*b*) or 2. One of the difficulties for
professionals who give advice about healthy diets is that there is
no immediate symptom of well-being corresponding to the
surge of amino acids or vitamins that blood samples can show.
The feelings of satiety and of inner warmth after a meal are
much the same after a good nutritious one as after a meal that
contains only "empty calories". One rare exception is the
gratifying faecal results that occur within hours of eating wheat
bran in people inclined to constipation. This is probably why
the fibre hypothesis was accepted by lay people years before it
was well supported by scientific human experiments. The only
reliable way to answer questions 1(*b*) and 2 is by the methods
of nutritional science.

## Origins of our scientific knowledge about human nutrition

### Comparative and evolutionary
Homo sapiens and their predecessors have been on the earth
one million years or more. Ninety-nine per cent of this time
our ancestors lived as hunter-gatherers. Agriculture started only
10 000 years ago. There has not been enough time for our
species to evolve new metabolic mechanisms required by the
recent food supply. Natural selection, which must work chiefly
via reproductive success, has been distorted by inequality of
wealth and lately by technology. It is difficult to see how it
could modify diseases that start in middle age. But presumably
our bodies have evolved well-adapted for doing what hunter-
gatherers did and eating what they ate. We have information
from archaeological records and from studies of the few, fast
disappearing groups of contemporary hunter-gatherers.[1,2]

### Experiments of nature and travellers' tales
From people who eat different foods from us, under stable
conditions or during a disaster, we can form hypotheses about
the physiological effects of different food patterns that we
could not easily persuade our fellow countrymen to adopt.

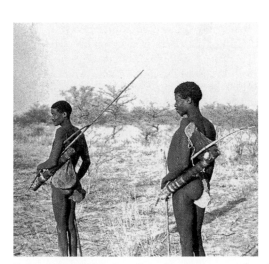

Hunter-gatherers were lean. Some groups ate more plant than animal foods;
others (especially in the cold northern winters) ate mostly meat (not only
the muscle) or seafoods. They ate a large variety of foods, depending on the
season but had no salt or alcohol and concentrated sugar only rarely (as
wild honey) and only occasionally cereal. The photograph shows hunters
about to set out, !Kung bushmen in the northern Kalahari, Botswana (taken
by the author in 1968[1])

We have, for example, learnt about the physiological role of
ω-3 polyunsaturated fatty acids from the Eskimos,[3] and
about deficiency diseases from nutritional experiences of
prisoners of war.[4]

### Epidemiological studies

These studies range in the power of their design. Associations
and correlations of disease characteristics and dietary variables
do not prove cause and effect, but prospective studies, especially
if repeated in different groups, give valuable information on the
relation between usual diets and chronic diseases.[5]

### Animal experiments

Animal experiments were the principal technique for working
out the vitamins.[6] The right animal model has to be used.
Understanding of scurvy was static and controversial until
Norwegian workers found (in 1910) that guinea pigs are
susceptible like man because, unlike most animals, they cannot
synthesise ascorbic acid from glucose.

### Clinical records

Clinical records have been informative about the role of diet in
disease, including inborn errors of metabolism. Information
about requirements for trace elements has come from
experiences with total parenteral nutrition.[7]

### Food analysis

The independent variables in nutritional epidemiology and in
dietetic treatment of disease are food constituents. Food
analysis is work that is never finished; foods keep changing and
demand develops for constituents not measured before, such as
different types of fatty acids and potentially protective
phytochemicals. To facilitate international sharing of what food
composition data there is INFOODS (the International
Network of Food Data Systems) set up in 1983.

### Human experiments and trials

These last from hours to years and many different variables can
be measured.

### Evidence-based nutrition advice[8]

Official dietary guidelines and (if permitted) health claims on
foods should be judged on the best available evidence. For
judging the efficacy of drugs the best evidence is
a meta-analysis or systematic review of all randomised
controlled trials (RCTs) of the effect of drug versus placebo on
disease outcome. These are paid for by pharmaceutical
companies as part of the cost of developing new drugs. For
nutrition RCTs with disease outcome are scarce. Available
evidence may be epidemiological—cohort/prospective studies
are more reliable than case-control or ecological studies. Or
they may be short-term controlled trials with a physiological
variable as outcome, for example plasma lipids or blood
pressure. The evidence, say about vegetables and health, will
never consist mostly of RCTs. Emphasis instead has to be on **all**
the evidence, including animal studies and molecular biology
and critical interpretation of the observational epidemiology.

# The three groups of substances in foods

### Energy and nutrients

Man needs oxygen, water and enough food energy (calories),
9 or more indispensable amino acids in proteins, essential fatty
acids (ω-6 and ω-3 polyunsaturated) a small amount of

---

**Some examples of human experiments and trials**

- Intervention trial of low saturated fat diet in half of 850
  middle-aged male veterans in Los Angeles over five years
- Trials of vitamin C against placebo for preventing colds during
  winter
- Experimental depletion of a single nutrient in human volunteers
- Long-term testing of the value of novel protein foods
- Experiments measuring energy expenditure
- Metabolic studies—for example, to assess the effect of diet on
  plasma cholesterol
- Absorption and uptake studies—for example, glycaemic index
  after different foods containing carbohydrates

---

**The three groups of substances in the edible portion of
foods**

**Energy and nutrients**
**Water and packing**
**Other substances**
Colour, flavouring, etc.
Natural non-nutritive substances, some of which appear to be
protective, some of which are potentially toxic

carbohydrate, 13 vitamins, and 17 elements scattered across the upper half of the periodic table (in addition to hydrogen, carbon, nitrogen, and oxygen: see figure on page 126).

Together they add up to over 40 nutrients, many of which are normally taken for granted; the minor nutrients are present in sufficient amounts in a diet of mixed foods. But for long-term total parenteral nutrition all the minor vitamins and trace elements must be included in the required postabsorptive amounts.

For some of the nutrients **you can have too much of a good thing**. Generous intakes of saturated fat raise the plasma cholesterol concentration and contribute to coronary heart disease. People with high salt intakes have more hypertension. Too much food energy leads to obesity.

## Water and packing

All foods contain water. In many it is more than half the weight. The percentage of water is higher in some fruits and vegetables than in milk. The more water a food contains, the fewer calories. But this water has to be counted in the diet of patients with anuria. The "packing" of plant foods—that is, dietary fibre—is not all inert. Some fractions have physiological effects: arabinoxylans (hemicelluloses) of wheat increase faecal bulk and speed colonic transit; pectins slow absorption of lipids and glucose.

## All the rest

There are many other substances in most foods. They include flavours and colours.

### Potentially beneficial substances

It has long been noticed that higher intakes of vegetables and fruits are associated with lower rates of chronic degenerative diseases.[10] In the 1970s this was attributed to fibre or β-carotene or vitamin C. But in the 1990s it looked as if other bioactive substances that are not among the classical nutrients might also be protective. Some of these have antioxidant activity, and antioxidants in food and drink have attracted research interest since publication of the oxidised LDL hypothesis of atherogenesis. But phytochemicals may act by other mechanisms; one group are weak oestrogens, phytoestrogens. Evidence about these substances is indirect, mostly epidemiological association[11] or effects *in vitro* or in animals. Some promising possibilities are shown in the box opposite.

### Potentially toxic substances

In most natural foods there are inherent substances that are potentially toxic but usually present in small amounts—for example, solanine in potatoes, nitrates and oxalates in spinach, thyroid antagonists in brassica vegetables, cyanogenetic glycosides in cassava and apricot stones, etc. Then there are substances that only some people are sensitive to—for example, in some people wheat causes gluten enteropathy, broad beans favism, and cheese a tyramine effect in patients taking monoamine oxidase inhibitors.

Other toxins get into foods when their environment is unusual—for example, toxic shellfish after a "red tide"—or if polluted with industrial contaminants, such as methyl mercury, polychlorinated biphenyls, etc. Microbiological infection can produce very potent toxins, such as botulism and aflatoxin. Deliberate food additives are not known to be toxic—if they were they would not be permitted by international or national food administrations. A few can cause sensitivity reactions in a minority of people (see chapter 15 on food sensitivity).

## Amount of adult requirements for different nutrients

| Adult daily requirements in foods | Essential nutrients for man |
| --- | --- |
| 2-10 µg | Vitamin D, Vitamin B-12 |
| c 50 µg | Vitamin K, Se, biotin, Cr |
| c 100 µg | Biotin, I, Mo |
| 200-400 µg | Folate |
| 1-2 mg | Vitamin A, thiamin, riboflavin, vitamin B-6, F, Cu |
| c 5 mg | Mn, pantothenate |
| c 15 mg | Niacin, vitamin E, Zn, Fe |
| c 50 mg | Vitamin C |
| 300 mg | Mg |
| c 1 g | Ca, P |
| 1-5 g | Na, Cl, K, essential fatty acids |
| c 50 g | Protein (10 or more essential amino acids) |
| 50-100 g | Available carbohydrate |
| 1 kg (litre) | Water |

Figures are approximate and in places rounded. The range of requirements for different nutrients is about $10^9$

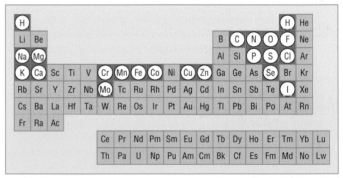

Periodic table of the elements. Those essential for man are blocked in. In addition, boron, silicon, nickel, arsenic, and vanadium are still under consideration as ultra-trace nutrients[9]

## Non-nutrient bioactive substances in food and drink that might help protect against chronic diseases

- **Carotenoids** other than β-carotene: *lycopene* (red pigment of tomatoes) and *lutein* (xanthophyll, in leafy vegetables). Though not pro-vitamin A they are antioxidants, are absorbed and seen in the plasma, and lutein is one of the pigments of the retinal macula lutea.
- **Polyphenols (flavonoids)**, antioxidants that occur in tea (especially green tea), wine (especially red)[12]: *catechins*; and in apples and onions: for example, *quercetin*.
- **Phytoestrogens**, especially isoflavones in soya: *genistein* and *daidzein*. Higher consumption of soya and soya products in East Asia might contribute to the lower incidences of breast and prostate cancers in that region.[13]

# Patterns of nutrients in different foods

If animals are fed only one food sooner or later they will become ill and die. No single food contains all the essential nutrients. Wheat (wholemeal flour) lacks vitamins A, B-12, C, and D and is very low in iron and calcium (if unfortified); beef (muscle) contains little or no calcium, vitamins A, C, or dietary fibre. On the other hand, wheat is a good source of dietary fibre and beef of iron and vitamin B-12. The two together provide more nutrients than either alone but between them have no vitamin C or D and hardly any calcium. Addition of citrus fruit or salad brings vitamin C into the mixture, and milk or cheese adds the missing calcium and a little vitamin D.

This is the theory behind the "basic four" food groups for educating the public about nutrition. Each group has some deficiencies which the other three make up between them. You should aim to eat each day from each of: the bread and cereals group; the meat, poultry, and fish group; the vegetable and fruit group; and the milk group.

### Variety

It is not enough to have daily servings of the same food from each group. One should also choose variety within food groups for two reasons. First, the characteristic nutrients in each group vary greatly for individual foods. Among fruits the vitamin C ranges from negligible (for dried fruits, grapes, and figs) up to 115-180 mg/100 g for stewed blackcurrants and canned guavas (this is in the British food tables; the international range goes up to about 3000 mg/100 g).[14]

Second, natural toxins do not follow any of our arbitrary groupings of foods. The wider the variety of individual foods that people eat, the less their chance of acquiring harmful amounts of the toxins that are inevitable in foods but usually in small and subclinical amounts.

### Blending dietary guidelines with food groups

The four groups are intended to minimise deficiency of traditional nutrients—protein, calcium, vitamin C, etc. In affluent countries, however, more disease is probably caused by too much fat, salt, and alcohol and not enough fibre. So we have to modify the older message. In the United States the Departments of Agriculture and of Health use a pyramid for nutrition education.[15] In the base (largest) layer ("eat most") is the cereal food group. The middle layer ("eat moderately") is for the vegetable group and the fruit group. The upper (smallest) layer ("eat least") is for the dairy group and the meat, etc, group. The areas allocated to each group convey broad quantitative recommendations and are accompanied by recommendations for numbers of servings. The divided plate on page 37 is based on the same principle.

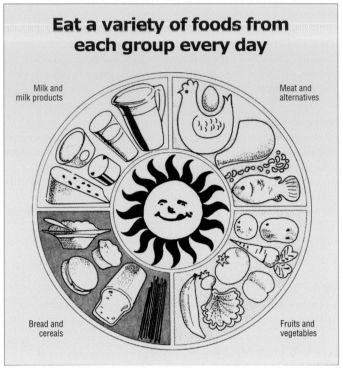

A Canadian food guide

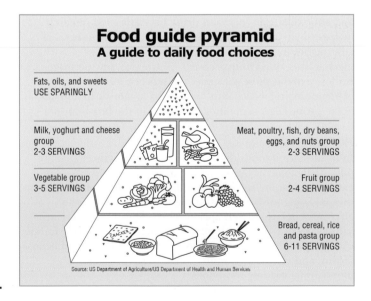

---

### Possible modifications of four food groups to incorporate dietary guidelines

- **Bread**—Yes, but wholegrain and with lower salt. Prefer lower fat, low salt *cakes* and *biscuits*
- **Meat**—Lean cuts with the fat removed and not fried. Alternate with *fish* (grilled) and *legumes*
- **Vegetables** slightly cooked, not with salt
- **Fruit** fresh, not canned in syrup or dried
- **Milk** with half or all the cream removed

### Junk foods and nutritious foods

Whether a food is nutritionally bad or good depends on the rest of the diet. As Hippocrates taught, "All things in nutriment are good or bad relatively". An extra portion of saturated fat is bad in Britain but would be good for starving children in north east Africa. An orange does nothing for someone who takes vitamin C tablets but is important for an elderly person who eats no vegetables. Value judgements about foods are being made all the time; they are nearly always subjective and often wrong.

A good objective method is to work out for a typical serving of the food its provisions of important nutrients, as a percentage of their recommended dietary intakes, compared with its content of energy (calories), also as a percentage of a standard daily intake. For each nutrient:

$$\text{the index of nutritional quantity} = \frac{\text{nutrient as \% standard}}{\text{energy as \% standard}}$$

"Nutrient dense" foods have high ratios of important nutrients to energy (calories).

The profile of indices for major nutrients can be put in an array. Other components in the food, like cholesterol, saturated fatty acids, and dietary fibre can be treated in a similar way by using a dietary goal as the standard.

The table below, modified from an American book,[17] shows that egg contains a smaller proportion of fat per energy (calories) than butter; the fat is less saturated and egg is also a good source of protein and some other nutrients. Egg and butter both contain some vitamin A but egg contains thiamin, riboflavin, iron, calcium, protein—not found in butter. However, an egg contains much more cholesterol than $\frac{1}{2}$ oz (14g) butter.

Calculations of this type should be made before authorities advise communities to eat more or less of a food. Applying them to the 1995 Department of Health recommendations[18] about diet to prevent cardiovascular disease means that the amount of butter eaten should be reduced more than the amount of egg, because reduced saturated fat is recommended but current cholesterol intake is not considered excessive. In the United States, however, a dietary guideline[15] advises against high levels of dietary cholesterol and so recommends the general public to moderate its consumption of egg yolks.

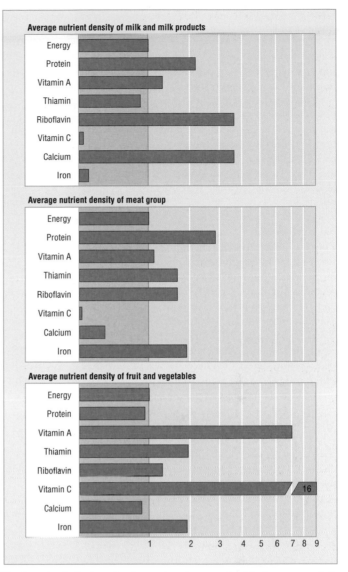

Nutrient density is the ratio of a nutrient (expressed as % of recommended daily intake) to energy (expressed as % of a standard energy intake). In the total diet of mixed foods the density for each nutrient should exceed 1.0. (From Hansen[16])

### Indices of nutritional quality (INQ) for butter and egg

| | Butter ($\frac{1}{2}$ oz; 14 g) | | | Egg (50 g), hard boiled | | |
|---|---|---|---|---|---|---|
| | Amount | % of standard | INQ | Amount | % of standard | INQ |
| Energy (kcal) | 100 | 5 | 1.0 | 80 | 4 | 1.0 |
| Vitamin A (mg) | 0.129 | 11 | 2.2 | 0.078 | 7 | 1.6 |
| Thiamin (mg) | 0 | 0 | 0 | 0.04 | 4 | 1.0 |
| Riboflavin (mg) | 0 | 0 | 0 | 0.14 | 12 | 2.9 |
| Niacin (mg) | 0 | 0 | 0 | 0.03 | 0 | 0 |
| Vitamin C (mg) | 0 | 0 | 0 | 0 | 0 | 0 |
| Iron (mg) | 0 | 0 | 0 | 1.0 | 6 | 1.5 |
| Calcium (mg) | 3 | 0 | 0.07 | 28.0 | 3 | 0.8 |
| Potassium (mg) | 4 | 0 | 0.02 | 65 | 1 | 0.3 |
| Protein (g) | 0 | 0 | 0 | 6 | 12 | 3.0 |
| Carbohydrate (g) | 0 | 0 | 0 | 1 | 0 | 0.1 |
| Fat (g) | 12 | 15 | 3.1 | 6 | 8 | 1.9 |
| Oleic acid (g)* | 2.9 | 12 | 2.4 | 2 | 8 | 2.0 |
| Linoleic acid (g) | 0.3 | 2 | 0.3 | 0.6 | 3 | 0.8 |
| Saturated fatty acids (g)* | 7.2 | 25 | 5.1 | 1.7 | 6 | 1.5 |
| Cholesterol (mg)* | 32 | 11 | 2.2 | 225 | 75 | 19 |

Based on Hansen RG *et al.*[17] [The standards they used are energy 2000 kcal (8.4 MJ), vitamin A 1.2 mg, thiamin 1 mg, vitamin C 60 mg, riboflavin 1.2 mg, niacin 14 mg, iron 16 mg, calcium 900 mg, potassium 5000 mg, protein 50 g, carbohydrate 275 g, fat 78 g, oleic acid 24.5 g, linoleic acid 20 g, saturated fatty acids 28.5 g.] I have taken 300 mg as standard for cholesterol. These are all intakes per day
*Not essential nutrients

## Calories do count

The law of conservation of energy applies to human nutrition as in the rest of nature. Atwater established this around 1900. A little more heat may be produced after some foods or in some people but the more calories (or kilojoules) you eat the more you can expect to store as adipose tissue.

Foods differ in their calorie content from 32 kJ/100 g (7 kcal/100 g) for celery, up to 3.7 MJ/100 g (899 kcal/100 g) for vegetable oils—a 128-fold range. This great range depends on the different energy values of fat, alcohol, protein, and carbohydrate and how much these are diluted by water. It is useful for doctors to know the energy values of average servings of common foods (there is a short list in chapter 11 on obesity).

## No perfect diet

There are several diets that appear (in our present state of knowledge) to be good. We can advise on a better diet for Mr Smith or, as in a United States report, make recommendations "towards healthful diets", but there is no best diet. The reason is that man is an omnivore with enzyme systems that can adapt to ranges of intakes of many food components. There is, for example, an inducible enzyme, sucrase, in the small intestinal epithelium; if people eat sucrose this enzyme appears and digests it. There are several enzymes in the liver which oxidise amino acids; their activity increases when protein intake is high and falls in people on low protein diets.

## The dose determines the effect

When the intake of one essential nutrient is varied, with the rest of the diet adequate in other nutrients and energy, the individual's state of health is likely to be very poor if intakes of the essential nutrient are inadequate and sustained. Health improves as the intake is increased, up to the nutritional requirement level. Above this, it has been thought that the state of health remains on a plateau up until the nutrient intake becomes undesirably high, beyond which toxicity may be seen. Recent experience with some nutrients suggests, however, that above the requirement level, which cures deficiency disease, there can be an optimal range of intake. The individual may not feel or function differently but has a reduced risk of degenerative disease or more favourable biochemical profile. Folate is a good example. Above the level that cures or prevents megaloblastic anaemia women have a reduced risk of a malformed baby, and older adults are less likely to have a raised plasma homocysteine.

## Replacement

For every food you remove from the diet another has to take its place. This principle is prominent in the design and interpretation of nutritional experiments. Does consumption of milk raise or lower the plasma cholesterol concentration? To test this an adequate but physiological amount of milk is to be given in a middle two or three week period. The plasma cholesterol value is measured at the end of this period and at the end of equal length control periods before and after.[19] But what should be given to replace the calories of the milk in the control periods? If nothing is given the periods will not be isocaloric.

To some extent the effect of milk on plasma cholesterol could be manipulated by the choice of the control food. We do not want to influence the experiment so might ask, "If people here stop drinking milk what would they drink (or eat) in its place: beer, water, fruit juice, fizzy drink, etc?" A similar situation applies in outpatients when the doctor or dietitian instructs a patient to cut out one food from his/her diet.

**Energy values as metabolised in the body of the main energy-yielding groups of food components (Atwater factors)**

|  | kcal/g | kJ/g |
| --- | --- | --- |
| Fat | 9 | 37 |
| Alcohol | 7 | 29 |
| Protein | 4 | 17 |
| Carbohydrate* | 3.75 | 16 |

*This is for available carbohydrate. The energy provided by dietary fibre from its fermentation to volatile fatty acids in the large intestine is less than half this amount

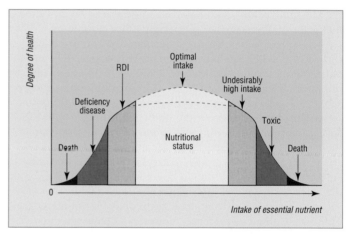

Ingestion of the RDI should guarantee no deficiency disease but beyond the RDI there may still be additional health benefits (for example, partial protection from a degenerative disease). The top of the dome beyond the RDI is then the optimal intake range. RDI corresponds to Reference Nutrient Intake. (Adapted from Truswell[20])

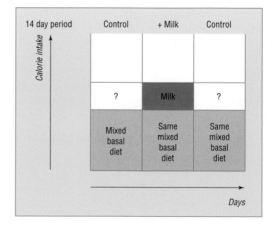

Unless he/she is to lose weight he/she will sooner or later choose other food(s) as replacement, which may affect the outcome.

## Some concluding proverbs

People have been thinking about the safety and goodness of food, as well as its social roles and tastiness, ever since the Garden of Eden or its evolutionary counterpart. So it is perhaps not surprising that a number of proverbs about food and eating are being confirmed by nutritional science.

*Moderation in all things*
The recommendation of many expert committees on nutrition. Do not eat too much or too little of anything, and do not follow one of the extreme unorthodox regimens.

*Man cannot live by bread alone*
Though the original was about spiritual nourishment, it is also true that people have to eat more than one (type of) food.

*Variety is the spice of life*
You should eat a mixed and varied choice of foods.

*Enough is as good as a feast*
More leads to obesity. People's energy requirements differ. "Enough" is an individual amount.

*You can have too much of a good thing*
For example, saturated fat, salt, dietary cholesterol, vitamins A, D, and B-6, and alcohol.

*One man's meat is another man's poison*
The subject of chapter 15 on food sensitivity. For each of us there are foods we dislike and may well be foods that can make us ill.

*There's no accounting for taste*
Taste has to be considered in planning therapeutic diets.

*A little of what you fancy does you good*
Dietary prescriptions are sometimes more rigid than they need be. This proverb also speaks of the placebo effect; if someone believes a food is doing him good he may feel better for a time after eating it.

*Old habits die hard*
Food habits must be respected. Prescribed dietary changes are likely to be followed better if they are fitted into the least strongly held of an individual's food habits.

*There's many a slip twixt cup and lip*
People do not necessarily eat what they intend or say they eat. That patient you just put on a diabetic diet may not have understood you.

## References

1 Truswell AS, Hansen JDL. Medical research among the !Kung. In: Lee RB, De Vore I (eds) *Kalahari hunter-gatherers*. Cambridge, MA: Harvard University Press, 1976.

2 Eaton SB, Eaton SB III, Konner MJ. Paleolithic nutrition revised: a twelve-year retrospective on its nature and implications. *Eur J Clin Nutr* 1997; **51**: 207-16.

3 Leaf A, Weber PC. Cardiovascular effects of n-3 fatty acids. *N Engl J Med* 1988; **318**: 549-57.

4 de Wardener HE, Lennox B. Cerebral beriberi (Wernicke's encephalopathy). *Lancet* 1947; **1**: 11-17.

5 Hu FB, Stampfer MJ, Manson JE *et al.* Dietary fat intake and the risk of coronary heart disease in women. *N Engl J Med* 1997; **337**: 1491-9.

6 Widdowson EM. Animals in the service of human nutrition. In: Taylor TG, Jenkins NG (eds) *Proceedings of the XVIII International Congress of Nutrition (Brighton, 1985)*. London: John Libbey, 1986:52–7.

7 Freund H, Atamian S, Fischer JE. Chromium deficiency during total parenteral nutrition. *JAMA* 1979; **241**: 496-8.

8 Truswell AS. Levels and kinds of evidence for public health nutrition. *Lancet* 2001; **357**: 1061-2.

9 Nielsen FH. Other trace elements. In: Ziegler EE, Filer LJ (eds) *Present knowledge in nutrition*, 7th edn, Washington DC: ILSI Press, 1996.

10 Steinmetz KA, Potter JD. Vegetables, fruit and cancer prevention: a review. *J Am Diet Assoc* 1996; **96**: 1027-39.

11 Hertog MGL, Feskens EJM, Hollman PCH, Katan MB, Kromhout D. Dietary antioxidant flavonoids and risk of coronary heart disease: the Zutphen Elderly Study. *Lancet* 1993; **342**: 1007-11.

12 Frankel EN, Waterhouse AL, Teissedre PL. Principal phenolic phytochemicals in selected Californian wines and their antioxidant activity in inhibiting oxidation of human low-density lipoproteins. *J Agric Food Chem* 1995; **43**: 890-4.

13 Adlerkreutz H, Markkanen H, Watanabe S. Plasma concentrations of phytoestrogens in Japanese men. *Lancet* 1993; **342**: 1209-10.

14 Brand JC, Cherikoff V, Lee A, Truswell AS. An outstanding food source of vitamin C. *Lancet* 1982; **ii**: 873.

15 US Department of Agriculture; US Department of Health & Human Services. *Dietary guidelines for Americans*, 5th edn. *Home and Garden Bulletin no 232*. Beltsville, MD: Food and Nutrition Information Center, USDA, 2000.

16 Hansen RG. An index of food quality. *Nutr Rev* 1973; **51**: 1-7.

17 Hansen RG, Wyse BW, Sorenson AW. *Nutritional quality index of foods*. Westport, CT: Avi Press, 1979.

18 Department of Health. *Nutritional aspects of cardiovascular disease. Report of the Cardiovascular Review Group, Committee on Medical Aspects of Food Policy*. London: HMSO, 1995.

19 Roberts DCK, Truswell AS, Sullivan DR. Milk, plasma cholesterol and controls in nutritional experiments. *Atherosclerosis* 1982; **42**: 323-5.

20 Truswell AS. New vitamin research: antioxidants and folate. Introduction. *Asia Pacific J Clin Nutr* 1993; **2** (Suppl 1): 1-3.

# Index

Page numbers in bold refer to figures, those in italics refer to tables or boxed material

# Index

# Index

# Index

# The complete ABC series

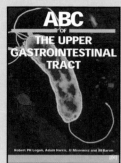

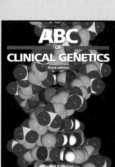

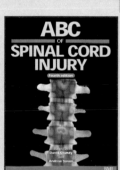

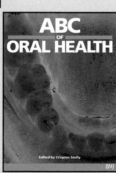

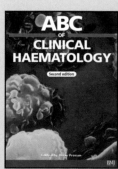

ABC of AIDS
**ABC of Alcohol**
ABC of Allergies
**ABC of Antenatal Care**
ABC of Antithrombotic Therapy
**ABC of Asthma**
ABC of Arterial and Venous Disease
**ABC of Arterial and Venous Disease, CD ROM**
ABC of Brain Stem Death
**ABC of Breast Diseases**
ABC of Child Abuse
**ABC of Clinical Electrocardiography**
ABC of Clinical Genetics
**ABC of Clinical Haematology**
ABC of Colorectal Cancer
**ABC of Colorectal Diseases**
ABC of Complementary Medicine
**ABC of Dermatology (includes CD ROM)**
ABC of Diabetes
**ABC of Emergency Radiology**
ABC of Eyes (includes CD ROM)
**ABC of the First Year**
ABC of Heart Failure
**ABC of Hypertension**
ABC of Intensive Care
**ABC of Labour Care**
ABC of Learning and Teaching in Medicine
**ABC of Liver, Pancreas and Gall Bladder**
ABC of Major Trauma
**ABC of Mental Health**
ABC of Nutrition
**ABC of Occupational and Environmental Medicine**
ABC of One to Seven
**ABC of Oral Health**
ABC of Otolaryngology
**ABC of Palliative Care**
ABC of Psychological Medicine
**ABC of Resuscitation**
ABC of Rheumatology
**ABC of Sexual Health**
ABC of Sexually Transmitted Diseases
**ABC of Spinal Cord Injury**
ABC of Sports Medicine
**ABC of Transfusion**
ABC of the Upper Gastrointestinal Tract
**ABC of Urology**

## Titles are available from all good medical bookshops or visit:

# www.abc.bmjbooks.com